HIPPOCRATES' HANDMAIDENS:
WOMEN MARRIED TO PHYSICIANS
Esther M. Nitzberg

SOME ADVANCE REVIEWS

Ms. Nitzberg's incisive, intuitive, and provocative treatise is a sensitive and compelling depiction not only of medical marriages but all traditional professional marriages. The text is beautifully written and is laced with rich imagery and anecdotes which have a ring of familiarity that captures the reader. The author's candid autobiographical style is refreshing and provides the passion which makes this book a winner.

Steven E. Katz, MD
Professor and Executive Vice-Chairman
Department of Psychiatry, New York University Medical Center;
Director of Psychiatry, Bellevue Hospital Center, New York

This book is based on the author's personal experience of being a physician's wife, extensive interviewing of other physician's wives, and findings of empirical research. The author provides a penetrating excursion into the world of the physician's wife, her helpmate role, and the entanglement of the medical marriage and the medical profession. The many personal and family problems that result from medical marriages and suggestions for constructive change are insightfully discussed.

Barbara R. Lorch, PhD
Professor of Sociology
University of Colorado

D1509584

Hippocrates' Handmaidens
Women Married to Physicians

HAWORTH Women's Studies
Ellen Cole and Esther Rothblum
Senior Co-Editors

New, Recent, and Forthcoming Titles

When Husbands Come Out of the Closet by Jean Schaar Gochros

Prisoners of Ritual: An Odyssey into Female Circumcision in Africa by Hanny Lightfoot-Klein

Foundations for a Feminist Restructuring of the Academic Disciplines edited by Michele A. Paludi and Gertrude A. Steuernagel

Hippocrates' Handmaidens: Women Married to Physicians by Esther M. Nitzberg

Waiting: A Diary of Loss and Hope in Pregnancy by Ellen Judith Reich

God's Country: A Case Against Theocracy by Sandy Rapp

Women and Aging: Celebrating Ourselves by Ruth Raymond Thone

A Woman's Odyssey into Africa: Tracks Across a Life by Hanny Lightfoot-Klein

Women's Conflicts About Eating and Sexuality: The Relationship Between Food and Sex by Rosalyn M. Meadow and Lillie Weiss

Hippocrates' Handmaidens
Women Married to Physicians

Esther M. Nitzberg

Harrington Park Press
New York • London • Sydney

ISBN 0-918393-81-7

Published by

Harrington Park Press, 10 Alice Street, Binghamton, NY 13904-1580.
EUROSPAN/Harrington, 3 Henrietta Street, London WC2E 8LU England
ASTAM/Haworth, 162-168 Parramatta Road, Stanmore (Sydney), N.S.W. 2048 Australia

Harrington Park Press is a subsidiary of The Haworth Press, Inc., 10 Alice Street, Binghamton, NY 13904-1580.

Cover design by Marshall Andrews.

Library of Congress Cataloging-in-Publication Data

Nitzberg, Esther M.
    Hippocrates' handmaidens : women married to physicians / Esther M. Nitzberg.
       p. cm.
    Includes bibliographical references and index.
    ISBN 0-918393-81-7
    1. Physicians' wives—Psychology. 2. Physicians' wives—Mental health. I. Title.
R707.2.N57   1990b
306.872′08861—dc20
                                                    90-41946
                                                    CIP

This book is dedicated to the women who graciously and generously allowed me into their confidence — and to our silent sisters everywhere.

My thanks also to Jerry, Jim, Mark, Bill, and Eric Nitzberg and to Vicki Chirco, Terri Appling, Miljana Bovan, Pat Florin, Jean McLaughlin, Anna Trelstad, Dori Appel, and Colleen Pyke for their help, support, and love.

ABOUT THE AUTHOR

Esther M. Nitzberg, MA, NCC, has been a clinical counselor and stress reduction therapist for 15 years. In addition to counseling, she writes, works in radio and television, and lectures on stress, marriage, and current issues of particular interest to women. She is affiliated with the National Board of Clinical Counselors, the American Association of Counseling and Development, and The Association of Applied Psychophysiology and Biofeedback. Ms. Nitzberg currently lives in Ashland, Oregon with her husband of 31 years — a doctor.

CONTENTS

The Sign on the Doctors' Lounge

On the door of the staff physicians' lounge in a mid-sized local hospital in a mid-sized town is a small but significant sign saying,

"When I come back, I want to be a doctor's wife!"

This is a very private joke among the "docs." It is their way of perpetuating the myth that a doctor's wife has the best of all possible lives, a charmed and enviable existence. There is a distinct note of hostility and aggression in the meaning of the sign. That he begrudges her financial dependence on him, that he stereotypes her and is somehow oppressed by her underlies the words. Also hidden in that statement is an arrogance and vanity, his presumption of her total satisfaction and gratification for her sought-after position.

When a physician explained the sign on the door to me, with the blessing and brotherhood of his fellow doctors who must all believe that what they offer as husbands is beyond comprehension, I was horrified. The very men who make trite jests and backstabbing comments about their wives are the same men who quietly depend on and owe their very comfort and existence to these women. I am offended and frightened by the attitudes that at once laugh at her while maintaining an aggressively condescending stance. I am not convinced that a doctor's wife would feel complimented or supported by the implication of that motto.

Prologue:
A Talk on the Medical Marriage —
No Questions, Please!

Last spring I attended a county Medical Society meeting. This one was unusual — spouses were invited. The program topic was "Medical Marriage: Special Problems and Solutions." There were almost 200 people in attendance, the largest group ever for this county.

Why was it so well attended? The speaker was a locally respected counselor known to work with couples and to whom the doctors refer their patients whose marriages are in trouble. The surprisingly large attendance reflected the curiosity about the medical marriage. Is it special? Is it unusual? Each attendee listened and wondered how he or she measured up to the speaker's descriptions of the doctor-spouse combination.

This meeting was of particular interest to me for my research. The speaker consulted me, in fact, for input on the subject, because although she dealt with numerous marital problems and had given workshops on communication, assertiveness, and other interpersonal issues, the idea of addressing a group of physicians and their wives terrified her.

Should she confront, be logical and orderly, fill the room with facts and statistics, deal with feminist issues? Which approach would work? She wanted to be heard, respected, and appreciated (to keep the referrals coming?) but felt insecure, intimidated, and inadequate to address the specialness of a doctor's marriage. She never married a doctor nor was she a doctor's child — growing up in a doctor's family gives one a closer perspective.

She asked me for input about medical couples. What is the mystery? What are the closely guarded secrets? I shared what I'd gleaned from marriage to a doctor and disclosed discoveries from my last two years of broader inquiry. I gave her a brief job description of the doctor's wife: the loyalty and reserve required to defend, protect, and support her husband while attending to all the private and personal items in his life. I shared the following from my interview with a 34-year-old married eight years:

> Do you know what it's like being married to God? I sometimes have to pick out his clothes for the next day! He's supposed to know everything, but I keep the records, do all the parenting, make all the appointments; anything to do with our home and social life is my job.

And the young newlywed who said:

> It isn't at all what I thought. Allen never tells me how he feels and expects me to field his calls and protect him from the outside world. I married him because I love him, but I got a representation of an institution rather than a man.

I illuminated more details of the marriage our mothers hold so dear. Sharon, mother of three, described how after 18 years of marriage:

> It still baffles me. Bruce is never around when I need him. But when the phone rings and the hospital calls, he's so willing and ready to go. I can't tell him how I feel; he gets so uptight, defensive, and then I feel guilty. After all, he does save lives and heal the sick.

I continued:

> Both the doctor's wife and her husband may be depressed, isolated, confused, overworked, and overly responsible. Neither can seek help for themselves or their children because he's supposed to know all, and both are to be strong and guarded—whatever the price. Though he deals with life and death every day, he may ignore what's happening under his own roof.

The speaker revealed this information to the group. The people were silent, mildly alert, respectful, but somehow different than at other meetings. The talk was general and overly simplistic, as is the case when there are only 35 minutes to discuss what should fill many books. A cultural endowment that begins long before medical school and marriage and permeates our entire society is hard to address briefly.

The audience was squirmy and uncomfortable when "denial" was mentioned over and over. The worlds "feelings" and "sharing" touched a sensitive chord. I imagined that everyone was trying to determine if they were being talked about when the speaker said, "Don't have an affair under any circumstances if you are feeling hurt, frustrated, in transition, and unloved in your marriage." She told the doctors to cut down on their meetings, the wives to get babysitters in order to spend more regular time with their husbands, and both to "take showers together regularly, encourage intimacy and closeness." She even handed out communication tips on how to express love and affection and settle conflicts—all the right pieces of information for a group interested in improving the health of their marriages.

Why was the group quiet, sullen, uncomfortable? She preambled her presentation with a request for a 15-minute concluding question period. When that time came, no one asked a single question. Not one! This silence demonstrated the ultimate example of how competition and loyalty keep the doctor quiet, and his wife, his shadow, quiet. In front of peers, he supports the institution of medicine and she supports him.

This was a talk about communication by a professional to a group of professionals, and no one interacted. They feared exposure. Even the speaker intimated:

> I don't really want to tangle with you—a group of doctors, unapproachable, critical, analytical. I'll read my talk verbatim from my notes, make no eye contact, stay behind the podium, and give conflicting messages about how to share and communicate.

She maintained distance and diplomacy. Dealing with enraged doctors and spouses was too scary. (There were some female doctors in attendance, but they were a small minority.)

An outsider was among us, pretending to know our lives inside and out, privy to special information – thanks to me – but still she was an outsider. The group implied:

> Go ahead, we dare you to touch us, criticize us, find faults. We are the healers, the caretakers of society. Our wives are the bearers of our heavy burdens and we will walk through life together: solemnly, stoically and with dignity. Don't treat us as if we suffer the same flaws as others.

The speaker mentioned denial and the audience denied her mention of the word. Oh, some people tried to relax even as their peers scrutinized them from all sides. How should they respond to: "Take time to smell the roses, be with your children more, support your wife's career, listen, affairs, second marriages, your wife's crying for more niceties, affection . . ." and on and on? How after a lifetime of strength and reserve can emotions be expressed?

The women's silence surprised me more than the men's. Here was a chance to relate, to empathize with those who live the identical experience. Their unique view was being exposed as human, and hope was offered for solving problems. No confrontation, no cross-examination. Am I to assume there was no insight, no curiosity or real interest, only annoyance?

Women are often portrayed as more verbal, more articulate, as wearing their feelings on their sleeves. Why did they roll up their sleeves in the face of this chance to share and encourage others? "Express now or forever hold your peace," I thought. But I was guilty too; I kept quiet. "Don't speak now, don't tread on the speaker's toes, it's her podium tonight!" I too feared the risk of being singled out. Perhaps my thoughts would be twisted or manipulated. I might unwittingly divulge a family secret. What could that be? I too hurt sometimes. I too find joy and pleasure in my specialness, though infrequently. *What cost silence?* We learn nothing but further isolation and separation.

I attended this meeting as a doctor's wife, a counselor, an observer, and a researcher. I wanted information for my book. I needed feedback and affirmation for myself and my marriage. So did the others. Why was this group so untouchable? Or was it arrogance that made them close down when facing perceived criticism?

The wives sharing their responses the next day indicated the talk was too general, too simple, unrealistic. "She wasn't talking about us." Some wives felt they, too, were type A obsessive personalities, working compulsively at everything they did, whether paid or unpaid. "She didn't really address things that related to me," was the overtone. The undertone was awareness, fear, uneasiness, squeamishness, and a great defensiveness that comes when the heart of a value system is questioned and confronted.

Where are the facts? What about other couples? Who says we're different from politicians' wives, executives' wives, officers' wives, anyone married to a person in the public sphere? Some of us are quite happy — we love our work, we love our life, our meetings, our recognition, our supportiveness. There is quiet protest, especially when facts and figures are not presented. In truth, figures are kept secret, especially from researchers looking at the doctor's wife.

How can this cycle of impermeability be broken? The wall around the medical profession that the wives unknowingly help support with both hands is uncertain. Their hands are chapped, strong, delicate, or manicured. Their hands write checks, wash the dishes, diaper babies, run a business, attend school, nurse patients at the hospital, wring in frustration at times, applaud with joy at others. Yet these same hands couldn't be raised to ask a question of an expert on problems and solutions of the medical marriage. The wall may come tumbling down.

Preface

To review the literature and separate the perspective of women married to physicians from their husbands and from the institution of medicine itself was impossible. In fact, the medical profession has been distinctly intertwined with the female gender since its inception as a profession.

Before medical care and healing became a male domain, it was the job of women as healers of physical illness, as emotional support givers for those who suffered mental anguish and crisis, as midwives to educate and help birth babies and to care completely for the new mother and child. Women in prehistory are thought to have been responsible for health care as well as influential in decisions in all areas of living, creating, and social organization.

Recently discovered evidence and methods of data and time analysis of prehistorical information have shed new light on this time, earlier than 5,000 years ago. It appears that the people living then were part of cooperative groups that strongly encouraged female nurturing, a life-enhancing value commonly attributed to women. At this time women were goddesses not only deified, but responsible for the caretaking and inner workings of the societies. Valuing birth, living, and death in ways more integrated with the natural environment, it appears that these people were living in great harmony with each other and nature.

Formerly, healing and preserving life were natural to the more humane and gentle societies, and were the domain of women. Throughout history women have been healers, but as men became aggressors rather than peace-lovers, women as leaders were no longer revered. Men took over property, commerce, spirituality, and healing. Though even today a few women are healers in some societies, cultures, and communities, history has been filled with the mass extinction of women known as witches. Later all people performing healing arts were overpowered and cast aside by "professional, scientific" men. "Doctors" would be in charge. These new doctors would be healing mostly women, and in so doing would soon dictate how to give birth, rear children, live our lives, and even how to die.

This book is about what it's like to be a woman married to a doctor in a time when our population hardly remembers midwives or lay healers as women who were trusted, loved, respected, and depended upon by families and larger social groups.

The kinder, more caring world view in which people cooperated and valued both sexes equally for their contribution and potential and when life-giving and the mutual benefit of all people and nature were prized, has been long overshadowed by a more rough and tough, "macho" view of capture and control. It is in this more authoritarian, more violent, less nurturing modern world that technological medicine and doctors have emerged. Remarkable technological and scientific wonders and miracles also have emerged.

The doctor's wife is a woman, a patient, a wife, and the invisible partner of these men of medicine. She lives in this paradox of control by men who are captains of this caregiving ship of today's health.

What is it like for her to be caught between the traditionally feminine world view of partnership, helping, sharing, connecting, nurturing, creating, and caring, and her husband's training and practice views, which embraces machismo, hierarchy, strength, power, domination, authoritarianism, patriarchal view of medicine and the world?

Once men won the struggle for world view, the gentleness, softness, and humanitarianism was left behind. The capital which could have been used for healing was earmarked for weapons and violence instead of life giving and the prevention of suffering.

The doctor's wife is like other women in the struggle. She is no longer part of the creative, collective effort but has been powerfully pushed aside, and like women all over the world, she has been made into the proverbial handmaiden. Unlike her historical counterpart, she is not in charge of herself, her body, or her destiny, or that of her children. She spends her life doing the bidding of a gender which is dedicated to healing while simultaneously embracing force, sterility, and technology. She provides the soft, female perspective to the men heading a profession that ironically values healing and life while perpetuating authority, fear, and control.

Here is her story.

Introduction

The doctor's wife is the last great stronghold of the feminine mystique in America today. She is an educated, articulate, socially correct woman who stopped in the middle of her own career training or surrendered a career to become Mrs. Doctor So and So.

Why is the hold of traditionalism so strong? Many young doctors' wives still live the ideals of the 1950s. How do the medical system and our society collude to maintain this world view? What is the relationship between the experience of doctors' wives and the women's movement? Where does dependency become interdependency?

Mothers still view the doctor as the choice catch for their daughters. Society preserves the notion that "My son-in-law the doctor provides the status, security, and influence that enables his wife to live happily ever after."

I was a '50s woman, a feminine mystique woman. Marriage — to a doctor — and bearing children was the American dream. Being a doctor myself wasn't an option. When dating, I was not aware that I was subconsciously choosing a medical student. My mother thought a doctor would be the most charming prince of all, the knight on the whitest horse. She could not imagine life with a doctor as anything less than perfect.

Throughout my 32 years of marriage, I have been intrigued by the notion that there is a special mystique to being a doctor's wife. Since medicine itself is so mysterious, the unique privileges afforded the medical family, the separateness, and the demands and responsibilities upon the doctors have all provoked my curiosity further. Our society is absolutely preoccupied with medicine and "The Doctor." Books, television, and movies abound with the life of the proverbial Dr. Kildare and General Hospital, but little or no information is shared about the woman he marries.

Why all the secrecy? Auxiliary groups that have done research on doctors' wives were reluctant and uncooperative about sharing their findings with me, another doctor's wife! I was informed that the states of Oregon, Florida, New Jersey, and Ohio, among others, have published extensive research and compiled statistics regarding physician impairment and medical family impairment, and the numbers are increasing yearly. Over the five years of my research for this book, after numerous phone calls and written requests to these states, the National Auxiliary, and numerous county auxiliary offices, I have not yet received any materials of this nature. The American Medical Association — the association of physicians themselves — has repeatedly referred me back to these groups. To call these incidents coincidental would be kind. Rather, I am inclined to say that information gleaned by these associations is deliberately kept from the public and designed to remain within the medical community.* Why so secretive and protective? Is there something to hide?

How do other doctors' wives feel about their lives? How do they deal with their daily existence? Are they secure in the knowledge that they are well-respected members of society? For the past 12 years I have been a counselor doing stress management and chronic pain control through biofeedback therapy with individuals, couples, and families — many medical families. In addition to my clinical observations, over the past two years I have extensively interviewed 125 doctors' wives and facilitated groups of other professionals' wives. (To protect their privacy, real names were not used.) Included were first, second, or third marriages. Each was married to a doctor at the time of the interview. Three had married a doctor a second time.

Clearly the experience of the doctor's wife reflects problems that are universal. Included is the complex relationship between our dependency on the medical profession and the influence of the women's movement on how we view dependency. The role of the doctor's wife is a metaphor for women's struggle to become more independent, responsible, and fully equal human beings.

---

*I am still awaiting the names and numbers of physicians' wives currently in political office in the United States, information I requested several times from the American Medical Association Political Action Committee.

She feels great responsibility, requires strength, needs protectiveness, and often uses blind faith to follow and steadfastly adhere to the rules and aura of the medical life. Her self is submerged, questioned, or denied. I am calling this conflict "dependency-related identity anxiety," akin to our society's dependency-related health anxiety.

Her life of affluence, or "privilege by proxy," is a catch-22. She appears to have it all, on the surface she is materially secure, but that very security isolates her from other women and from society. She is discriminated against by feminists and nonfeminists alike. Finally, she is overlooked or ignored by social reformers who are embarrassed by her wealth and cannot imagine the reality of her human needs. The women's movement loses, and so perhaps do all women.

I have divided the book into four sections. To introduce this material, I have included a look at women and their doctor-husbands, as well as a historical perspective. Part I is the personal view and experience of the doctor's wife, Part II includes her experiences with her "husband the doctor," and Part III offers her experiences that uniquely interact with society. Part IV concludes with the doctor-wife doctor-patient metaphor, and offers suggestions for change.

As part of the process of researching and writing this book, poetry emerged as an alternative means to present this material. I've included those of my poems which I felt complemented or clarified a point.

My goal was understanding and discovery both for me and for the reader. The experience of doing research, giving talks, having group discussions, and then putting them together here has been therapeutic and required honesty to the core of my being. I am deeply grateful to have had the opportunity to share with others and unravel some of the misunderstandings and myths that surround the life of the doctor's wife.

THE WOMAN WHO MARRIES A DOCTOR:
PERSONALITY TYPE OR CLUSTER
OF CHARACTERISTICS

> I'm glad I have Carolyn; nobody else could put up with me or
> this kind of life. — Raymond

The doctor's wife has been called a narcissist; an overly dependent personality type; a weak, helpless woman who exaggerates or overdramatizes her difficulties (histrionic); one who exhibits or experiences an overabundance of physical complaints rather than express them psychologically (somatizes). She's been described as selfish, self-centered, overly compliant, submissive, passive, unable to deal with conflict, repressive of her real feelings, living vicariously through her husband and children, prone to use alcohol and/or other drugs, prone to suicide to resolve her problems, and usually experiencing poor sexual functioning as well as a dissatisfactory sexual and emotional relationship in her marriage. There are probably some negative and recriminating characteristics that can be found elsewhere in the literature.

She has also been described as educated, articulate, overly competent, overly responsible, perfectionistic, mildly compulsive, over-achieving, demanding, extravagant, narrow-minded, empty-headed, gracious, a wonderful hostess, organized, business-minded, creative, empathic, sympathetic, a superior caretaker, reserved, flamboyant, quiet, controlled, controlling, helpless, helpful, overly independent, unable to be intimate, codependent, enabling, possessive, intelligent, thoughtful, not very intelligent, too thoughtful, practical, pragmatic, and the list goes on.

What is the point? These adjectives could describe all women, and specifically those married to doctors, but do not take into account the influence and effects of the doctor-husband and the demands of his profession upon the life of the doctor's wife. The average person sees her as a privileged and special woman, if she is seen at all. For women married to doctors, that stereotyping reinforces her retreat into the shadows and into the hands of the traditional medical marriage, in which the husband-doctor is viewed as "God" and she as his handmaiden or guardian angel, invisible and uniquely interdependent. Every day, in small and subtle as well as large and obvious ways, her husband's work, responsibilities, and very presence infringe upon her life, backed by the entire institution of medicine and our society.

It would be a presumptuous oversimplification to conclude that a woman married to a physician has a special cluster of personality characteristics which makes her either especially suited to the job or not well matched to the task. In addition, such presumption feeds right into the hands of a system that views life in a hierarchical, ranking order system of either/or, black/white, better/worse—the same view which values domination and power over others rather than personal power as responsibility for oneself and for and to others.

What I will say is that these women encompass a great breadth and depth of traits and characteristics. We have no idea of their potential because the lifestyle in the traditional male-ordered and conceived world disregards the potential and value of the female except to procreate, produce, and support according to the whims of their doctor-husbands.

Is she different? Yes, because she will lose sleep for one-third to one-half of her married nights, disturbed by her husband's patient-related calls; because her social existence will revolve around his hospital, university, or private practice; because she will spend much of her time waiting, accommodating, adjusting, and handling alone the responsibilities of the home and children; because in her world she will always be second, and perhaps lesser than second; because the doctor's wife, unlike the wives of men in most walks of life, is asked to be a wife to a profession and way of life, quietly, unobtrusively, without complaint. Unlike the professor, the diplomat, the executive, the plumber, or the movie maker, the doctor is a doctor 24 hours a day. His public and colleagues expect and encourage that view. His wife, if she was never married to a nonphysician, grows to believe in her subservience, and like the public, she will forever take a back seat to his reputation and influence.

In her role as doctor's wife, she demonstrates initiative and is flexible, creative, organized, spontaneous, resilient, determined, and compassionate. The traits of dependence, supportiveness, and interactiveness are those which demonstrate concern for others before herself. Those qualities which make her a great teacher and good wife, such as listening, preparedness, open-mindedness, and holistic thinking—especially when linked with intuitiveness, generosity, selfless regard for others, altruism, connection to others (plus multitudes which I have not stated here)—are generally said to be negative traits or are somehow used against her by the male world. Her caring concern, charity, and willingness to look beyond herself to assist others in efforts affecting the world at large, i.e., environmental pollution, nuclear disarmament, and assistance to the homeless and hungry worldwide, are undeniably admirable, if not essential, qualities to our future existence. Yet she is seen as weak, dependent, inferior and, after all, "only a woman."

How can I describe a cluster of traits when doctors' wives embody all that is wonderful and complicated in womanhood? My saddest realization from developing this book was the knowledge that no matter which traits or behaviors she chooses to develop or deny, the doctor's wife is caught in a world view obliterating feminine values, and even females themselves. She lives in a traditional world, in the most traditional marriage, wife to the epitome of traditional professionals. Her female qualities—her sensitivity, her nurturing, her awareness of natural life-giving systems in nature and her connection to it, her ability and need to be connected to others in a loving way—are tolerated at best and insulted or considered part of the "illness" of womanhood at worst.

Does the doctor's wife differ from other women? Yes, in that she will give up more of herself in her lifetime than many other women. She will be asked to sacrifice more and receive less emotional support. She will have money and its advantages, but less power over its disposition. She will be overly involved in her husband's profession, but wield less influence on the direction it takes. She foregoes her own development for the support and development of her husband and children. If satisfied in the traditional role, she foregoes personal achievement for vicarious respect and applause, all the while inconspicuous, ignored, an ornament or fixture to be engaged and exhibited when necessary. She may avoid conflict because as a woman the welfare of those close to her and her harmonious interaction with them are essential to her. She sees herself in connection or in relation to others. Stifled by her husband's need to see himself as an independent, separate, strong, closed-mouthed professional, she may at times find her life as his wife frustrating, unrewarding, empty, and confusing.

But how much is she like other women?

A great deal, and I hope that the sisterhood available to her will maintain her feminine perspective and enable her to hope and work for a changing world of partnership, united against oppression.

As women, as doctors' wives, we can look around and see the values that are contrary to a lasting, harmonious environment and world. To say that a doctor's wife is a certain type misses the point. She is a human, a female, with both unique and shared qualities of other humans. It is her situation and our long-held belief system in her inherent inferiority, I am convinced, that either develop and encourage, or retard and discourage, certain strengths and certain less useful characteristics. To be in a subordinate role, to live with fear of domination and its reprisals, to live with punishment either direct or indirect for certain thoughts or behaviors, in other words to be dominated, is not going to enable her to develop to her full potential, to "actualize," as Maslow has said. Maslow defines self-actualization

> as ongoing actualization of potentials, capacities, talents, as fulfillment of mission (or call, fate, destiny or vocation), as a fuller knowledge of, and acceptance of, the person's own intrinsic nature, as an unceasing trend toward unity, integration or synergy within the person. (1968, p. 25)

At best, she will be a product and a pawn of her restricted environment. Over time, the traditional medical marriage obliterates her selfhood.

The doctor's wife is in a unique position. Unlike others, her lifestyle remains reminiscent of the women of the '50s, often both privileged and powerless. However, if she is able to look at herself and the system in which she is co-partner, she may be better able to influence change than her husband. Knowledge of her domination and willingness to share her experience can be the beginning of a new lifestyle for the medical marriage. I believe that as she insists upon greater equality in her marriage, challenges the system which supports her inequality, and increases her self-esteem, the benefits will extend far into our health care system and society.

A BRIEF LOOK AT PERSONALITY CHARACTERISTICS COMMONLY SHARED BY MALE PHYSICIANS IN THE U.S.

> Phillip has always been an old-fashioned doctor, totally dedicated to his work and to his profession, even if it sometimes means sacrificing me and the kids. — Theresa

In this writing I was committed to the least possible reference to the physician himself. It was an impossible task. I have tried not to draw attention to the specialty, age, or other characteristics of the physician unless directly quoting his wife. Television, movies, newspaper stories, and book and magazine articles have filled us with wonderful images of doctors and their private and professional existence over the last 20 to 30 years. The public has an insatiable appetite for familiarizing ourselves with who these people are and what makes them tick. Often, however, the public view thrives on the popular image, causing even less awareness of the reality.

There has been a great deal written and postulated about becoming a physician: the personality profile, their selection process for medical education, the training. More to the point the making of a physician and his life thereafter have been analyzed and judged. At the risk of oversimplification, I will briefly sketch an overview of characteristics of the husbands of the women in this book, realizing the potential for stereotyping the physician.

Although much that has been written about him is gleaned from work with those in distress, there does seem to be a cluster of traits found to a greater or lesser degree in males who enter medical school and then go on to practice medicine. The forthcoming description gathered from a review of the literature, comments from wives, and my impressions from social and clinical contacts over the years as a doctor's wife and therapist is presented in broad contrast to the more extensive personal interviews of the women reported in this book, and is meant to be understood as a backdrop against which her life and experiences evolve. Naturally, an individual male physician is unlikely to bear all these traits. Rather, he may recognize some or many in himself or his colleagues at any given time.

Suffice it to say that a young man entering medical school is apt to be awkward socially, overly bookish in the areas of hard science, not strongly interested in social sciences or humanities, and uninterested in reading nonscientific material. His need for adulation, admiration, public respect, and appreciation is higher than that of the average person. He is generally intelligent if not above average, and dedicated to hard, long hours of study in his field. There is a compulsive and controlled aspect to his demeanor and personality. A moderate percentage grew up in households in which at least one parent was alcoholic. He is, therefore, likely to have a "hero" or "rescue" complex. He may have a great need to control his health and body. Perhaps he lived with illness in childhood, either in his family or himself. Or he learned of medicine through another physician in his family. Orderliness, organization, high achievement, and perfectionism are all essential to his gaining acceptance into medical school. Throughout his schooling, denial of personal pleasures and fun have become a habit, and earning top grades at all costs, the norm. Dating, partying, learning about communication with others, especially the opposite sex, is deferred for book work. To be admitted to medical school, competition is the watchword, even if that means occasionally stepping on others' toes to get a better grade or project an advantageous image.

Medical students have come from all sorts of families, but more often from middle-class, professional parents. They may or may not have always wanted to be a doctor, but likely have been extremely aware of the advantages in our society accorded to the profession. Their father may have been a physician, and their mother may have admired and doted on her would-be-doctor son and her husband.

Entering medical school, many are idealistic and really want to help others. They will give up much personal freedom and pleasure to this end. Some want only the prestige, money, and power that attends the field. Most are drawn by their great need to help others and to have others dependent upon them, and then by their desire for gratitude and respect. Most are unable to look inward or to develop introspection. Clearly, facts and scientific findings soon overwhelm any of their former abilities to touch human feelings or to delve into human motivation and behavior, with the exception of those becoming psychiatrists.

Much is written on medical training itself. Briefly, the early idealism is generally obliterated by excrutiating training hours and humiliation from teachers, residents, and other MDs. Whatever altruism existed upon entering medical school is systematically ground down by training, like the army drill sergeant who gradually and deliberately breaks the humanity and vulnerability of the new recruit. An arrogance and unrealistic sense of self and power is infused over the years of medical school into the soon-to-be MD. He practices delayed gratification throughout his training, and ultimately continues to deny himself personal rewards. Gruelling lack of sleep along with inhuman intellectual, physical, and emotional demands break him in to the life he will lead when he practices medicine. Eventually self-absorption and self-preoccupation will accompany self-sacrifice and humanitarianism.

Anger is repressed along with other feelings such as compassion, fear, doubt, and humility. However, of the range of emotions, anger comes to be the most comfortable and socially acceptable to express. Quick decision making, ability to give orders, certainty of thought, increased ability to absorb enormous amounts of new scientific information are honed to perfection. Sense of humor is sometimes distorted, sharp, biting, and hostile to protect against the denied pain and agony of dealing daily with life and death. Medical students are taught to be logical, hard-driving, and ambitious to succeed. They learn to solve problems by prescribing pills and ordering tests or x-rays, rather than listening or sharing feelings.

Following graduation, he is likely to become a clinical, reserved, quick tempered, overly stressed, compulsive, perfectionistic, narrowly focused man with unrealistic expectations of himself and others, covering insecurity and doubts at the enormity of his task with outward assuredness, distance, and perhaps an overly inflated view of himself and his place in the world. "Being rigid, emotionally inhibited, over dutiful, and unable to relax easily does not make one a tremendously exciting husband. . . . Their talk has a superior, self-righteous and arrogant quality which . . . is terribly off-putting and alienating in marriage" (Myers, 1988, p. 58).

Soon-to-be wives are usually met in college or medical school — often accidentally because social life takes a back seat to academic preparation. High school sweethearts, nurses, and medical receptionists make up some of those who will marry young doctors. Older doctors married to wife number two or three will also marry helping professionals, especially in the medical field, because they are most accessible. Others are met in ways all people meet, fall in love, and marry. However, there is much less attention paid to long courtships since a doctor has little time, interest, or ability to interact in an equal give-and-take manner. Articulation is often limited to science or medicine; he is so involved in his work that his conversation becomes one-tracked.

Please refer to bibliography for references and further explanation of this extremely bare bones overview of a physician (Myers, 1988; Smith, 1987; Gerber, 1983; Pearson, 1982; Derdeyn, 1979; Vaillant, 1972, 1970). I am well aware of the dedication and value of these men and the honor of the medical profession. However, his personality and style do influence and often determine the direction of his wife's world.

The Doctor's Wife —
A Historical Perspective

My mother bids me bind my hair
with bands of rosy hue.
Tie up my braids with ribbon rare
and lace my bodice blue.

by Anne (Howe) Hunter
music by Josef Hayden, late 1700s

I reviewed related historical literature in the hope of tracing changes in the role of doctor's wife. Medicine has certainly changed: the technology; the group practice; specialization; life-saving drugs; the threat of malpractice; and finally, an increase in the number of female physicians, perhaps foreshadowing a return to women as the primary healers in society. In this chapter I present a brief look at the role of the doctor's wife in modern history. In my review I was and am constantly amazed at the tenacity of her position and how slowly, if at all, changes occur. We will see striking similarities between the view of the doctor's wife in the 1700s, for example, and that of the late twentieth century. Her experience, her presence, her influence, and her reticence to think of herself as an individual are astonishingly consistent throughout this period.

Researchers credit Hippocrates, the noted Greek physician recognized as the father of medicine, for his contributions that separated medicine from mere superstition and philosophic speculation. In reference to his personal life, historians note that Hippocrates was the child of a physician father. But nowhere in my historical search have I found reference to a Mrs. Hippocrates; neither wife nor mother surfaces as having any role in his successes, writings, and breakthroughs. Today, as her husband or future husband swears to the Hippocratic oath, the little woman on the sidelines accepts the role of handmaiden to the male doctor, a role consistent in history, rich in monetary return, but impoverished in emotional growth.

Women married to physicians have kept quiet. Very little is available regarding their experience. But then, as we will see, the paragon of the doctor's wife is to be a self-effacing, staunch supporter of her husband and his work. So it is not surprising that women, who regard their role as secondary and supportive and are required to remain in the background in order to be successful in their role, stay in the shadows without leaving records of their deeds behind. Remarkably, what little comments I have found from women married to physicians were written by physicians or were on occasion reported in medical periodicals such as *Medical Economics*.

In a lovely compilation entitled "Wives of Some Famous Doctors," the President's Address presented by Sir Weldon Dalrymple-Champneys to the Royal Medical Society of London in 1959, the author refers to women from as early as the 1500s. In this talk Dalrymple-Champneys chose six women to highlight, either for their own "personal claims to distinction or who seem to have played an important, though unobtrusive, part in the blossoming of their husband's genius" (1959, p. 937). I will note here that "unobtrusive" is a recurring word in any description of a doctor's wife. Also, the fact that these women were married to famous men of their time is probably what brought them recognition at all.

Margaret (Giggs) Clement, married in 1530 to Dr. John Clement, had a "devotion, aided no doubt by her wisdom and unwavering faith both in her religion and in her husband's virtues and attainments, which must have been of inestimable succor to him" (Dalrymple-Champneys, 1959, p. 938).

Margaret Giggs was raised in the household of Sir Thomas More along with his daughters. More describes her as "very wise and well learned, and very virtuous too." Algebra was her favorite subject. In choosing to study this, she was "unique among her sex" (Dalrymple-Champneys, 1959). More says in his second book, *A Dialogue of Comfort Against Tribulation*, that Margaret studied "physicke" and helped him when he had tertian fever that baffled two physicians during his tower imprisonment. So it is thought that she was a help to her husband in his medical studies. She was nurse to the boy who later became King Edward VI, who it is believed called her "Mother Jak," which is inscribed on a wonderful drawing of her head done by Keolbein and preserved in the Royal collection (Dalrymple-Champneys, 1959).

Elizabeth (Browne) Harvey was the daughter of Dr. Lancelot Browne, physician to Queen Elizabeth I and King James I. She married Dr. William Harvey in 1604 at 24 years of age. Elizabeth has been immortalized in a book written by Dr. Harvey (famous for his discovery that blood circulates rather than stands still). In his 283-page book he recounts a brief story of their parrot, to which Elizabeth was extremely devoted. He goes into an extensive description of the parrot, and finally reports that while his wife stroked its back as usual, the bird died in her lap. They always assumed the parrot to be male. Upon postmortem examination, to his great astonishment he found Elizabeth's parrot was a female (Dalrymple-Champneys, 1959; McClinton 1942). This tale was recounted in a rather flippant manner, making Elizabeth seem an eccentric from Dr. Harvey's perspective.

Anne (Howe) Hunter, also the daughter of a famous surgeon, married John Hunter in 1771 after a prolonged engagement, as they were "without funds." She was 29 to his 43 years. She evidently loved entertaining and being surrounded by people in the arts and music. Her husband was uncouth, antisocial, and eccentric in his work habits, but she tolerated his work on original research projects. He was known for his variety; at any one time, he might be found dissecting his array of animals — a whale, leopards, lions, and a famous bull — conducting experiments, and involving himself as his own research subject. The noises and smells throughout the home were outrageous. In the only reference Dr. Hunter made of his wife, it is reported that upon returning home to his work one evening, he complained about a strange collection of Anne's musical friends. Horrified and impatient, he evidently made an unpleasant scene. She was a poet and musician in her own right, one of her poems being set to her friend Haydn's music. Mrs. Hunter's poem:

My mother bids me bind my hair
with bands of rosy hue.
Tie up my braids with ribbons rare
and lace my bodice blue. (McClinton, 1942, p. 475)

This song was sung at young girls' recitals for long years thereafter (McClinton, 1942, p. 475).

Agnes (Syne) Lister married Joseph Lister in 1856. He was said to have given up his Quaker religion for her. She did much to aid his career. There are references to her writing his speeches at the last minute, and of her husband, Joseph, kindly remarking in letters to his father of "Aggie's" suggestions as to words and arrangements or sentences. She allegedly wrote for seven hours one day and eight the next, and was considered invaluable. They were together for 37 years, with no children. Dalrymple-Champney suggests:

> She was not only a wife, but a mother to him; she had entered into all his scientific work with humility but rare understanding, and had helped him clerically and with wise advice, tirelessly, patiently, proudly and lovingly. (1959, p. 942)

Grace Revere Osler, or Lady Osler, the great granddaughter of Paul Revere, married Dr. Samuel Gross in 1876 and was called an inspiration to her husband, whose best work was done after his marriage. "Not only was his wife a most successful hostess, but she was tireless in her charitable work in public and private" (Dalrymple-Champneys, 1959, p. 943). Dr. Gross died in 1889, and in 1892 Grace married Dr. William Osler, a man she knew as a colleague of her first husband. She refused to marry Osler, though, until he completed the textbook he was working on. Dr. Osler, having written his much applauded textbook of medicine, became one of the darlings of the soon-to-be-new "scientific" medicine. He became the first full-time professor at the Johns Hopkins School of Medicine, the first accredited medical school and model for all those to come in the United States. It included laboratories; courses in biology, anatomy, and physiology; and staffed full-time professors in related fields. Dr. Osler was indeed an elite in the class of physicians. He would be the model of what is now the traditional physician: respectable, upper-class, pedigreed, educated, and revered.

Yet we hear little if nothing of his wife. From writings about him, they must have traveled in high society and royal circles, both in this country and abroad. He was quite influential in the thought and training of new physicians of his time. I expect that the next quotes from him establish his beliefs about the role of his wife, and influenced the role expectations of doctors' wives for a long time to come. Their marriage was described as:

> an ideal marriage in which as in other cases the wife, realizing her husband's greatness and the inestimable benefits he was conferring on mankind, was *content that he should put his work first and was glad and proud to be the creator of the happy home* from which he constantly drew strength and to which he never returned without finding inspiration, understanding and consolation. [Emphasis added]. (Darlymple-Champneys, 1959, p. 943-4)

Dr. Osler wrote in a letter to a doctor about to marry, saying:

> There must be trust, gentleness and consideration. A doctor needs a woman who will look after his house and rear his children; a woman whose first care will be for the home. Make her feel she's your partner arranging a side of the business in which she should have her say, and her way — console her and take notice about the house and the children, and keep to yourself as far as possible the outside affairs relating to the practice. (Darlymple-Champneys, 1959, p. 944)

Osler continued in an address entitled "The Student Life":

> What about the wife and babies, if you have them? Leave them! Heavy are your responsibilities to those nearest and dearest, they are outweighed by the responsibilities to yourself, to the profession and to the public. *Your wife will be glad to bear her share in the sacrifice you make. Lady Grace was*

glad to do so . . . [Emphasis added]. (Darlymple-Champneys, 1959, p. 944)

Evidently she was, or she didn't say otherwise for posterity. She did go on to be quite the hostess. Even the birth of a baby was not to deter her from her duties to her husband and his profession, including working to train nurses. She took on the total responsibility of the planning and preparation necessary when the family relocated from Philadelphia to Oxford, England in 1905. Before her death she was responsible for helping to biographize her husband and catalogue his books for a collection at McGill University in Canada.

Mary Elizabeth Steel married David Bruce in 1849. Mary has the distinction of being one of the few wives whose husband wanted her to be openly recognized for her contributions to his career success, although apparently waiting until he was on his deathbed to acknowledge Mary's efforts. He said:

If any notice is taken of my scientific work when I am gone, I should like it to be known that Mary is entitled to as much credit as I am. (Scarlett, 1965, p. 354)

It is suspected that Mary fueled his fire in the investigation and eventual discovery of the etiology of Malta fever and the influence of the tsetse fly which was until then the bane of the tropics. "Mrs. Bruce was able to rejoice in his triumph, in which she has played an important but, as usual, unobtrusive part" (Darlymple-Champneys, 1959, p. 945). Eventually she studied in the laboratory along with her husband. She perfected the art of microscopy and was elected Honorary Fellow of the Royal Microscopical Society. She and her husband worked together in the South African bush for two years, then did their final discovery work on the tsetse fly and trypanosomiasis in animals. During the South African war she worked alongside him in a military hospital and received the Royal Red Cross for her nursing work. Later, working together, they both provided the facts connecting the tsetse fly and and the transmission of sleeping sickness.

They were together for 50 years, and she was so modest that even her intimate friends never heard her allude to her own share in the research accomplishments (Darlymple-Champneys, 1959, p. 946).

Another doctor to speak of the influence of his wife was Dr. Robert Koch. Without Frau Koch, his discovery of the tubercle bacillus "would have been delayed at least" (Scarlett, 1965, p. 354). She is also credited with solving other research puzzles for him. In her frugal way, Frau Koch saved from household monies to purchase Dr. Koch a microscope on his 28th birthday.

In 1870 another selfless and frugal wife, Mrs. Mayo, having saved and sacrificed by mortgaging their house in Rochester, Minnesota, purchased a microscope for her husband's work. She reportedly said, "Well if you can do better by the people with this new microscope, we should buy it." Perhaps the origin of the famed Mayo Clinic can be traced to Mrs. Mayo's foresight and sacrificial purchase of the microscope for her husband's work (McClinton, 1942, p. 476).

Reluctant and stingy reference to these women is the watchword. When she has been referred to, it has been much more common to advise her on how to be a good doctor's wife. In 1893, Mrs. Ellen Firebaugh published *The Physician's Wife and All Things That Pertain to Her Life*. She opened with the fact that Aesculapius, the god of medicine, had a wife but she remained anonymous. Her daughter, Hygeia, did become more visible.

Mrs. Firebaugh listed the attributes necessary to be a doctor's wife: tact, discretion, and reduced curiosity about her husband's work. She essentially encouraged her readers to stay out of the doctoring business and to avoid pushing the doctor to betray professional confidences.

She goes on to say that physicians' wives are forever "debarred" from occasional hysterical fits. He "knows the symptoms," so the fit will get you nowhere. "It would be much better for the doctor's wife if she never got sick, if she could so arrange matters." Any other woman in the world has the privilege or right of choosing her own physician, but she must choose her husband for her physician, "whether she wants him or not." And when money is scarce, "The doctor's toilet must not suffer greatly. When it becomes necessary for one of the two to dress shabbily for a time, by all means let it be the wife! . . . Humility, true and unaffected, is one of the loveliest virtues, and let us hope every physician's wife knows something of its meaning" (Rome, 1976, p. 19).

More advice is readily found. In *Medical Economics*, a highly regarded journal for physicians, suggestions were written in the 1920s by anonymous physicians' wives. There is little mention of how it feels to be in her shoes, but extensive helpful hints for her survival are supplied. Some titles include, "Just What Can *WE* Do About the Future?" by a physician's wife, and "Why Not Consider the Doctor's Wife?" She may be very important to the success of the physician as the money manager and saver. She may actually collect the moneys from patients. In this article the author describes the great handicap unmarried physicians are under. A wife can save his money, help him in business, protect him from nervous female patients, decorate the office. "Cleanliness combined with artistic arrangement is the goal toward which we strive. Check on the other offices, make sure yours have all the up-to-date lighting, ventilation, magazines, comfortable furniture . . ." (*Medical Economics*, October 1928, p. 61). Perhaps if all this were publicly acknowledged the doctor would be greatly indebted to his wife. Quietly and without complaint, these women viewed their role as essential, proper, rewarding and satisfying.

Some 1920s advice written by a doctor's wife in the article, "Some Fibs I Tell for My Husband's Sake," continues, "I have learned to lie boldly, freely, glibly, joyously . . . but I never had to lie to cover a mistake on my husband's part." In a follow-up article a few months later entitled, "That Isn't the Half of Being a Doctor's Wife," one woman replied, "Worse than personal lying, however, is the fact that we have to teach our children to lie, our maids to lie, and if dogs could talk, we would have to make liars of them too" (*Medical Economics*, July 1928, p. 29). In addition to covering and intercepting calls for the doctor, including fabrications based on her concern that her husband had worked hard enough and needed time to rest, another reader replies, "I am on twenty-four-hour duty and I can lie and lie when lying is necessary to save my husband an unnecessary call" (*Medical Economics*, July 1928, p. 32).

Another article in *Medical Economics*, "Daddy Has a Patient," gives hints as to management of the children while Dad is working in an office in the home. There is also reference to teaching the kids to lie to protect Dad.

Remember these are from the 1920s. Again I am struck by the similar issues and injunctions given to the doctor's wife throughout modern history: secrecy, protectiveness, sacrifice, support, reverence for her husband, continued self-effacing attitudes. Overwhelmingly, the unobtrusive shadow figure.

It is interesting to note that the bylines in these early ('20s and '30s) articles in *Medical Economics* first identified the author as "a doctor's wife," then "Mrs. J. Jones, a doctor's wife," then Jane Jones at the bottom of the page, described as the wife of Dr. So and So Jones, physician from _____. Perhaps this was a sign of her increasing visibility and individuality at the time of the early '30s. In the '20s, '30s, and early '40s the voice of women grew stronger, peaking during the war when doctors' wives helped with the war effort and volunteered time whenever they were able. After the war, women, especially middle- and upper-middle-class women, were driven into the home again, not to be heard from much until the late '60s and early '70s. Even then, while pockets of women were becoming more educated, increasingly involved in improving social services for the needy, and more active in the work world as professionals and in business, the doctor's wife, as today, most often remained a nameless, faceless, and even voiceless person, only occasionally to be heard from as the once again remote "doctor's wife" of years ago.

Also, from *Medical Economics*, the article titled "Is There a Doctor in the House?" by "a doctor's wife" in 1929, and a series of six letters by the wife of a New England physician published in 1953 under the title "How to Be a Doctor's Wife!" by Lois Marlow (her pen name), both direct the wife's attention to covering for her tired, weary doctor-husband: find interesting ways to manage his leisure time; help him to develop a hobby; learn how to entertain; make a good impression for his patients; and abide by the rules (don't interfere, don't talk about patients, don't nag, don't be jealous). The list goes on and is much the same as those obligations still undertaken by the doctor's wife.

I love this from "The Doctor's Own Wife (His Fourth Investment)" by James B. McClinton in 1942: "Like an ointment in skin disease, the wife should sooth and stimulate." Or, "She may carve the goose, but she won't tell him how to carve in front of guests nor interrupt his story to finish it." And significantly, "It's the wife's job to know as much as he does. If by chance she knows more, she mustn't tell him" (pp. 472, 474). (I don't know what the other three investments are; presumably office equipment or medical instruments!)

The most popular article written on the subject was in *McCall's* magazine in 1969. It has been commonly referred to since. Its popularity was probably due to the author's willingness to talk candidly to the general public about life as a physician's wife. The article, "Never Marry a Doctor," was written by Jhan and June Robbins, who directly confront the doctor as poor husband material from the wife's perspective.

> You can't argue with a doctor . . . he thinks he knows it all.

> Let's face it, doctors often have serious problems about sex. Ask their wives.

> Lots of men would like to have an exciting and respectable absence from marriage. A doctor is one of the few who can.

> Marrying a doctor is like marrying a man who has spent six or eight years in a very good mental institution . . . you send nice boys to medical school, and they are never the same again. They get their brains washed out there. All they are taught is how to cope with illness, nothing about love and consideration for human beings.

> A girl's mother still gets exuberant when a medical student shows up on the doorstep and her father is visibly relaxed.

> Her main job is to admire him! He tunes out wife and children. They become faceless like his patients.

> The day-to-day life of doctors' wives is splintered with anxiety and confusion.

> They're jealous of . . . secretaries.

> Free care adds up to poor care or no care.

Etcetera, etcetera. The Robbins close by quoting a wife who says if your daughter marries a doctor, "there is no cause to jump for joy. She may well be happy. She will almost certainly be rich. But it's a very strenuous way to be rich and happy. I think there must be easier ways" (p. 127).

Thoughts shared in this historical perspective will be echoed in the forthcoming pages of this book.

E. P. Scarlett, in his article entitled "Doctor Out of Zebulun: The Doctor's Wife" reported in *Archives of Internal Medicine* in 1965, shared his astonishment that so little has been written on the subject. He scoured medical and "secular" sources. He wonders why it is "that in the vast ocean of commentary by and about doctors, there be such reticence, indeed almost a conspiracy of silence, about the physician's wife who—if we were to judge by medical annals at least—is most certainly the silent partner" (p. 351).

He suggests that one reason for the silence may be due to the total absorption of the doctor in his work. I would add to that the unwillingness of those thought to engage in the more serious, "meaningful" work of society to admit to the absolute necessity of the existence of the woman's role as the total supporter who enables him to succeed and to accomplish his role as provider! It was and is extremely difficult to look beyond stereotyped roles. To acknowledge her in this role would give power to her existence and perhaps allow that she too be able to follow her own path of achievement, if desired. If he recognizes her as a serious adjunct and provider to his success, his own achievement and power are both questioned and threatened.

Scarlett points out that even in modern fiction the doctor's wife is rarely showcased. Flaubert's *Madame Bovary* comes to mind as a lovely example in literature. Her unhappy marriage perhaps drove her to affairs with numerous other men. In Sinclair Lewis's *Main Street*, Carol Kennicott, a doctor's wife, may have been the first to voice the revolt of her role in society. She wanted to "lead an independent, purposeful and satisfying life." She found that happiness was prohibited in her dull, negative life. That was 1920 fiction.

Why is it, Scarlett asks, in "these days of rugged, realistic writing" that no one pays attention to the "handmaidens of medicine—the wives of medical heroes?" He continues, "Throughout history the doctor's wife has maintained a superb silence" (1965, p. 353). Why indeed?

More recently Lane Gerber, in his sensitive book, *Married to their Careers* (1983), describes the "macho" attitude common in medical training, which prizes hard work and self-denial. He points out that nowhere in their early years of school and residency do students hear mention of wives and families. Role models of medicine — the faculty, colleagues, and important MDs — by omission deny the existence of a wife or children. No one talks of life outside the hallowed halls of medicine. The word is reinforced every step of the way. The message is clear and inherited by generations of students: We are doctors, our work is important, and (implied) we do it all alone.

As I review the history of his wife's experience, then, I am not surprised by the silence on the subject of "my wife." The would-be physician learns to exclude thoughts or talk (especially talk) of his wife in his daily exchange with colleagues, and his wife learns to retreat into a quiet background. Separating personal life from the world of work, the men at work who do important things are discouraged from the distractions of talk of wives and family. Not only is she not acknowledged, but she is reinforced for not acknowledging herself.

Almost 30 years after Scarlett's admonishments about this unsung woman, I, too, remain perplexed by her silence and her willingness to fill the needs of her husband and his profession without regard to her self. In the last 10 years there has been increased reference to the physician's wife, albeit in medical literature or an occasional scholarly work. I might add that the increase in research has been spawned by the realization that physicians may have a higher incidence of impairment than the general population, i.e., alcohol abuse, self medication, depression, and suicide. Trying to evaluate reasons for these statistics has led researchers (mostly MDs) to look at the medical marriage, hence the wife is mentioned perfunctorily. This is also carefully kept within the confines of the medical profession. Psychiatrists speak of her in relation to her husband or as a clinical problem, detailing her depression or drug or alcohol abuse. Or she is called upon to assist her impaired physician husband, who is unlikely to take care of himself (Myers, 1988; Roy, 1985; Derdeyn, 1979).

Some researchers have tried looking at her status in society, comparing her to wives of attorneys or college professors. This research is promising since it helps to validate her existence as a productive participant in society, unequal to her male partner but with essential value nonetheless (Lorch and Crawford, 1978, 1981, 1983). Most of what appears, however, is rarely autobiographical and seldom biographical in nature. Rather, a researcher is hypothesizing about her and making assumptions about her needs, values, and experiences. We should not forget that the researcher, especially the psychiatrist, is most often male, or has been trained with an eye toward traditional male-oriented research findings and conclusions.

Carla Fine, in her 1981 book *Married to Medicine*, was the first author to showcase the life and experience of the physician's wife as told by the women themselves, to the dismay of some wives who disagreed with the author's focus on so much negativity inherent in the medical marriage.

To date, looking at the physician's wife's experience or hearing her words and feelings has been, at the least, uncomfortable or even undesirable. We have demonstrated overabundant interest in the male physician, glamorized him and his life, and maintained a glorified view of "the Doctor," while selectively and consciously keeping silent, and shutting off our curiosity about the woman who marries him. The doctor's wife remains uninteresting, shapeless, and voiceless.

The references to the doctor's wife we do find are limited to suggestions about her socially appropriate behaviors. What has and has not been disclosed about women married to doctors forms the basis for this book. I am indebted to the literature, though scant, and refer to it often. I question the authorship of some of the material written anonymously by "a physician's wife" in *Medical Economics*. My hunch is that the editors, all male in the 1920s, created this list of appropriate behaviors to perpetuate the ongoing saga of the ever-giving, subservient doctor's wife. The reality that these "appropriate" behaviors are still deemed appropriate today is frightening! Read on.

Chapter 1

Self-Esteem and Identity Anxiety: Once a Doctor's Wife, Always?

Reflections upon my first ordeal at a cocktail party for medical couples in Philadelphia, Pennsylvania still generate feelings of anger and sadness. Not once, but over and over again, women came up to me and asked about my husband's specialty. Then they all told me (without my prodding) their husband's title, specialty, staff position, type of daily work, and the important people with whom he worked, so that I might be sufficiently impressed. By the time I left that gathering, any sense I had of an inner identity was lost in the confusion of my now being a doctor's wife. What I didn't know then was what that scenario portended for the future. From that time 31 years ago to the present, the greatest single struggle in my marriage would be to hold on to my identity and to maintain my self-esteem as an individual.

I believe that whether or not the level of self-esteem is high upon entering into marriage with a physician, the nature of the relationship and the traditional values and paternalistic attitudes of the medical profession make it almost impossible for a wife to maintain her sense of self. The more women I spoke to, the more a common theme emerged and became reinforced. To speak from her own perspective with her own voice was almost impossible. It became apparent that it is extremely difficult, if not impossible, for the physician's wife to acknowledge her experiences without including her relationship to others, especially to her husband, his work, and their children. Self-worth and confidence, the ingredients necessary to feel good about ourselves and to feel a strong personal identity, are missing from the medical marriage where the nonphysician is a woman.

Linda Tschirhart Sanford and Mary Ellen Donovan's excellent book, *Women and Self Esteem*, defines five essentials for self-esteem, or the reputation we have with ourselves, which are imprinted in childhood: (1) Significance — the feeling that we matter, we are listened to, taken seriously, loved in ways that make us feel valued. (2) Competence — believing we can make things happen for ourselves in the world, having control over our behavior, being allowed to discover for ourselves through trial and error with the proper combination of guidance and support, being allowed to discover and strengthen our levels of competence. (3) Connectedness — balanced by our separation, feeling connected to but separate from others, knowing who we are, independent of other people, not alienated or cut off. (4) Realism — aware that no one is perfect and we all have flaws, acknowledging concrete information about how the world works, being realistic about ourselves and our possibilities. (5) Ethics and values — knowing what's right and wrong, establishing codes to live by which protect and guide in times of confusion (pp. 38-55).

Female children do not develop the essentials for self-esteem as easily as males do. We teach girls to be more dependent on others' opinions of them for their sense of worth. They often develop shaky levels of competence by not being allowed to venture forth and take risks for themselves with the guidance and safety they need. Female children are taught to be tightly connected and bonded to others, to be sensitive to the feelings and thoughts of others. They are not encouraged to view themselves as apart or individual. And finally, the realistic view required for high self-esteem is denied girl children. Either they are put on a pedestal or are not given enough information with which to make educated and thoughtful decisions. Things seem to happen as if by magic. They are either overprotected or are given unrealistic goals and information about themselves, i.e., exceptional at everything or not good enough at anything. Sometimes these messages are simultaneous, which totally confuses.

It is true that female children come into the world with a distorted view of themselves. Subtle and not so subtle messages tell them that men are more valued, more intelligent, more competent, more important. Our institutions reinforce these messages, including schools, churches, legal and political arenas, work places, and the world of medicine and health care.

Others have eloquently described reasons for women's lower self-esteem. The creation of "God in man's image" discussed in *Women and Self Esteem*, and then in an extraordinary book, *When God Was a Woman*, by Merlin Stone, describe the myth of Adam and Eve and original sin as underlying the present view that women are inferior and yet to be feared, and that view is used to maintain our oppression. *Him/Her/Self* by Peter G. Filene, an excellent overview of the changing roles of men and women in the last hundred years, traces the interconnectedness of the roles of women and their subsequent power and self-esteem, or lack thereof.

Freud influenced generations of mental health practitioners with his theories that women were overly sensitive incompetents who tended toward sexual fantasizing and overly dramatic demonstrations of their emotions or physical disturbances. These characteristics were thought to be unhealthy, undesirable, and unacceptable. He felt that women were basically imperfect and inferior men (having been born without a penis). Most of our sexually aggressive behaviors, he assumed, were because we wanted to be men — penis envy. If we felt sexual toward men, we supposedly really wanted to have our fathers, since our mothers had disappointed us by not having a penis, and if we were aggressive we were just copying a masculine response, a "masculinity complex," also to be like our fathers. We couldn't win either way. Some feminist scholars and neo-Freudian researchers and scholars have interpreted Freud's writings as implying that women were not only inferior to men, but also were rather confusing and confused, all because they were born without a penis. Any explanations for women's behavior were therefore totally traced to the effects of her missing this essential and reversed part of her anatomy (Eisler, 1987; Gilligan, 1982; Symonds, 1979; Freeman and Strean, 1987; Sagen 1988). Later theories were somewhat more sensitive to women, but even Jung, who was more generous in his views of women, thought women to be less creative and less able to be objective or take action than men. He too, then, ultimately saw women as inherently inferior to men (Bolen, 1985; Gilligan, 1982; Wehr, 1987; Greenspan, 1983). And so it went with psychological explanations for women's behavior. And so went and still goes our self-esteem. Religious, psychological, and physiological views have all reinforced women's imagined inherent weakness relative to men's supposed inherent strength. Throughout history women have been encouraged to be more logical, less sexual, more sexual, more expressive, less expressive, stronger, weaker, helpful, helpless, more intelligent, less intelligent, more sinful, redeemed from sin, dependent, independent, crazy, sane. Confused? That's the point.

For the purposes of this book and this section, the point also is that whether or not as children women were fortunate enough to gain self-confidence, assurance, competence, and an identity of their own — and I believe many women who marry doctors were (contrary to other research referred to later) — the marriage to a physician and his institution of medicine slowly, gradually ground away at initiative, power, self-control, and competence, and most importantly, diminished the wife's identity as an individual. To be successful in her role as doctor's wife and having her own identity are mutually exclusive. She is eventually unable to switch back from wife to person. She soon has no hat of her own. She sooner or later ends up with no own, no inner self, and ultimately with a diminished ability to control her own life and destiny.

I disagree with those who assume that it is only the traditional, subservient female who chooses to marry a physician, believing that her role will allow her to maintain and utilize her traditional values. The implication is that she is traditional and therefore wants to be kept in her place. Most women who marry doctors do so in the same way that any women marry — they fall in love and are innocent of the implications for their future, especially the future of their self-esteem and self-identity.

The role of doctor's wife is acceptable and even comfortable for some women; being supportive and helpful to their husband's professional and personal well-being is for these women fulfilling and gives them a great feeling of accomplishment. They do, however, risk a loss of pride in their own intellectual and creative capacities. What these women gain in being connected with and living vicariously through their marriage partner, they may lose in the lost sense of accomplishment and self-value derived from self-determination and an identity of their own.

Today we not only feel anxious about the question, "Is it all right to be a doctor's wife?" but we clearly feel anxious if we are "only" a doctor's wife. We ask, "Can I stay home and take care of home, children, and husband? Or should I be embarking on a career or developing personal potential?" Life as a doctor's wife makes the second question impossible to think about. The anxiety gets more powerful as we are more aware of the choices open to a woman in the late twentieth century. We may be anxious about not only our roles in the world, but as doctors' wives we are confused about whether we are indeed part of his world or separate. Where do we fit in? Clearly there exists an interdependency—we are simultaneously needed by him and dependent upon him—and we can lose ourselves in this maze. If we don't seek out ourselves, we may not experience identity anxiety. But parts of ourselves do creep out periodically, and the urge to peer out becomes stronger as our level of anxiety and confusion heightens.

You will see her obligations, experiences, and feelings taking on less and less of her, and more of him. This weakening of her self can and does cause confusion and anxiety, often not completely understood by her as she goes through the motions of her life.

SELF-ESTEEM AND IDENTITY

Who am I? A woman? A child?
What is my name? Am I old or young?
When is it my turn to live among the grown-ups?

To be a married lady like Sadie
    was the order of the day
Now it doesn't fill the bill.

Even marriage to a doctor doesn't tell me
who I am and how to be me.

Sadie, why didn't you say that marriage
takes away my identity,
makes me feel overpowered by someone else's
rules and regulations?

Is my pain mine or someone else's?
Is my joy mine or does it belong to him?
Did I say the right thing and behave the right way?
Who am I anyway? Who am I now?
Tell me before I die. Tell me.

Thinking of others first has been my game
If I continue will I miss
what — their praise
their respect?

Respect comes from the self first doesn't it?

But remember — I am not
the self escapes me. Only glimpses
on occasion.

Sometimes a glimmer of her shines through
and I can smirk approval
Then the guilt rises and is a disapproving
finger
You can't have a self. There's no time
no place for her in our home

Answer the phone, answer the door, there's more
there's more
Smile to all, make no mistakes.
Who are you? Who am I?

I am in the shadows of another
I fill him with love. I fill him with praise
If he approves of me I am full that is
enough in life to be grateful for

When is it my turn? What is my turn?
  Will I be? Am I? Is there more to
    this existence than his wife; his
    nurse; his counselor; his protector;
    his priest; his guardian; his angel?

The doctor is in. Can I be when he is in?
  Is there room here for a me or
when there is a we is the me invisible forever?

Chapter 2

My Mother's Fantasy:
My Daughter the Doctor's Wife

What could be so bad? He's never home, you have plenty of money, and people will always show you respect. — my mother, Anne H. Novak

I am my mother's pride and joy
I always was and always will be
she taught me all she knew
from the first time I sat on her knee

When you grow up you'll be a fine lady
someone will make you his wife
then I won't worry about you again
you'll be taken care of for life

For her the picture had to include
a man who has an MD
my mother's brothers and uncles
had the same sort of pedigree

She never knew a girl could learn
a girl could hold a stethoscope
a girl could use a speculum
or even design a microscope

Your husband will provide for you
take care of all your needs
a doctor is the best catch of the day
like some sweet fish from the seas.

Stop thinking about being creative
you'll have children that's enough
you'll sew, you'll cook, you'll macrame
then your family will judge your stuff

Put your energies into your home and kids
like I did and those before me
a doctor's wife is the envy of all
and that's exactly as it should be

He works hard, he's respected
he's smart and will make money too
you'll thank me some day—when you're old,
a doctor's wife is the envy of all
and that's exactly as it should be.

Mother, I hope you're proud as you can be
I did exactly as you said
I am a doctor's wife today and am still
trying to understand
what is it that you meant about
life married to an MD
that would be so safe, secure and enviable

Am I not the same girl underneath
no matter who resides with me?

It is practically certain that my mother's idea of a perfect career for her daughter was to be a doctor's wife. I say "practically" because I don't recall any direct language to that effect. Just innuendo or subtle statements like, "Look at Marsha Abramowitz [pseudonym], she's dating a doctor of philosophy," or "Did you hear that Rita Cohen is seeing a man who graduated first in his class at Pennsylvania's premedical school?" The words "doctor" and "medical" were imperative in describing potential husbands.

My mother did not have a college education. Her brothers did, but the women in her family, three sisters to be exact, had only finished high school or less. Her brother became a dentist, and her sisters married doctors, lawyers, or professors. My mother was committed to the second generation Jewish American ideal of higher education for men, preferably professional school, preferably medical school as an essential way of stepping through this life.

My grandfather (my mother's father) was a dentist. So what else could we expect?

Growing up in my mother's house (she ruled as if it was her house even though my father shared it with us) there was an air of the cultural, the intellectual, and the humorous. She played opera on the radio constantly. She read what she considered intellectual literature, the magazine sections of Sunday newspapers, or anything suggested on public radio as important reading of the day. Her greatest pride and joy was delighting in the whereabouts of her nephew and brother who were the family geniuses, one a renowned psychologist and the other a successful dentist.

Her reference to one genius or another I don't think was exaggerated; as it turned out, the family had intermarried cousins and enough inbreeding for a bona fide genius to be fairly common. Strange to me was the irony that only the boys and men displayed genius-level intelligence, while the girls and women were more likely to be "crazy:" "The girls on your father's side are all crazy," or "Ruthie must have gotten her brains from her grandmother," meaning the one on my father's side.

When I think of Golde and Tevya from *Fiddler on the Roof*, it brings an emblazoned image of my family to my consciousness. My father, a workaholic Philadelphia lawyer, always spoke as though he would have loved sitting in the synagogue all day to pray. When not at the office he was either sleeping at home, dreaming of being a rich man, or had a *Reader's Digest* condensed book in front of his nose.

My mother and her sisters were inseparable, physically, spiritually, and in the way they complained and worried about the futures of their children. Having suffered their ancestral uprooting through repeated stories and historical realities, ensuring security was uppermost in the minds of most Jewish households in the northeastern United States.

My mother and her sisters fretted incessantly about not having enough money to feed and clothe their children. While she was taking money from my father's pocket, she was deriding his ability to make our house payments. "Where will we get enough to help Aunt Ruth to get glasses for Joey?" She would wring her hands, but my wardrobe burgeoned with stylish new additions.

Inconsistency was the watchword for those times: tell strangers how smart my brothers were while telling my brothers how dumb they were; tell strangers how adorable I was, what a great dancer, so beautiful, etc., while telling me how embarrassed they were that I was so shy and timid. My home was the finest example of the mixed message to be found in the forties: "You're smart, but not as smart as your brothers. You can do what you want, but you better get married. Looks aren't all that's important, but be the prettiest in school. Talk intelligently, but not to the boys you're dating; they might be scared away if you're too brainy." My mother's favorite was, "Go to college, Esther. You need an education to fall back on." What was I falling from? We never talked about having a career. I still cannot figure out what my mother meant by "an education to fall back on."

To my mother and her sisters things happened by magic. The fish supplier's talents dramatically improved if the gefilte fish turned out perfectly for the Jewish holidays. Our phones were always burning with gossip among the sisters about how successful one of them felt if their child (one of my cousins) took the prescribed road in life. "Joey's teacher came to his senses and gave him a B in biology." There was magic in that. Not that Joey finally understood the work, but his teacher by some miracle could see straight that day.

If my father brought home a guest whose family knew of a nice pre-medical student, there was a real miracle to be preparing for, and burning up the telephone lines for days with advice, gossip, and planning among her sisters. My mother would be totally prepared to attract this unsuspecting guest, and by dinner's end she would not only have her daughter engaged to be married to this medical student, but might even be planning the wedding appointments.

She was a warm, gregarious, intelligent, witty (although sarcasm was her forté) woman. Her heritage and her beliefs made life quite erratic and interesting. Men were the providers, but were probably not to be taken too seriously—again an inconsistency for the times. Men were economically powerful and necessary, but in my house and in my aunts' homes, the women were to be reckoned with. They had the power over our minds and hearts. If mother wanted her daughter to marry a doctor, it would be done. If she wanted her son to be a doctor, it would be done, even if she had to feed and entertain the president of the medical school!

My mother's pet married couple were Aunt Charlotte and Uncle Benny. They were her cousin and my father's brother. Uncle Benny (you guessed it) was a family doctor. Again, magically, their life meant perfection and bliss to my mother. Every girl's dream he was not, but to Mother there were no dream men, only medical students.

She felt it a true blessing when I stopped dating the business student and lawyer and accepted a blind date with a medical student. She had arranged for her cousin to give my phone number to someone who knew of someone, etc., who was the perfect choice for me. I was unaware of these pre-arrangements at the time.

The phones buzzed off the hook. The sisters plotted, and I did meet Jerry, the naive fly in my mother's web. Looking back, it's impossible to determine if the romance was fueled by nature or mother's enthusiasm. Was I responding to true love or the hope of a Macy's charge card and a house in the suburbs? I suppose I'll never know how my mother's magic worked. At the time it was love for me. My mother would get her son-in-law the doctor. I was nineteen. Time was running out according to the Novak women (my mom and her sisters). I'd better see to it that this was serious.

Wedding plans, my Jewish mother's ultimate fantasy, would be realized.

Sadly, mother was ill throughout this time and would never attend what was certain to be the wedding of the year 1958. Two hundred people packed the synagogue, and all the women were green with envy and purple with pride. One of their own would be perpetuating the legacy of "My Daughter the Doctor's Wife."

When Jerry and I shared the details of our future with my mother, she was elated. Her job in life was completed. In her view of the world, my safety, security, and happiness were ensured (although I doubt if happiness was truly in her vocabulary). "What happiness?!" I can hear her say, "You'll have money. People will respect you. You'll be the doctor's wife." And I am certain to this day that when she died a few months thereafter, she died a fulfilled woman; her daughter had indeed married "a doctor!"

Chapter 3

Fringe Benefits:
Let's Look at the Bright Side

> I know being married to a doctor opens many doors to me. I ran for city council last term and won, I think because I've had a lot of exposure in the community as Brian's wife. — Rita

At the time of this writing, there are two state governors who are married to physicians. There are mayors, representatives, other women holding political office at the same time they are married to physicians. Not many, but a few. And perhaps this is accomplished more easily in the case of a physician's wife. Her role in his professional advancement leads her to volunteer work in the arts, education, and other areas of politics. Her contacts are enormous if she desires political work. Her organizational skills are honed and appropriate resources are tapped by knowing people with money; influence opens the otherwise closed door.

Penny, married to a very visible and respected surgeon for 22 years, decided to use her "pull and contacts to start a career in politics."

> I had done tremendous work in PTA and Junior League and League of Women Voters while my children were growing up. Then I was asked to run for a school board position. Everyone knew me. I won. After that it was so easy, and I love the interaction and hassles of political jobs. I was appointed to the planning commission. All these jobs led me to run for state representative from our district. I lost the first time, but next

election I know I'll win. Meanwhile I'm on the city council and work quite hard for the issues I believe are essential to our community.

My first experience was when I was asked to sit in for Brian at a board of directors meeting for the hospital board. One thing led to another. I've got so much experience now in our area, I'm a cinch to win the next election.

Do people refer to the fact that you're married to a physician?

Some do. They did more when I first worked for the school board. There was some jealousy and hostility. Some people accused me of using my influence to accomplish my political goals. I'm used to it now. Men use their influence all the time. Just because I married into it, I'm still entitled to take advantage of my opportunities. People probably accuse Elizabeth Dole of using her husband's influence to get her high posts in government. But in the final analysis you have to produce or you don't get reappointed or re-elected!

The essential ingredient to Penny's success is a supportive husband. Penny shared that Brian offered the right combination of interest, support, and willingness to step back from her limelight. She feels quite fortunate that he has been willing to pitch in at home and take over for her where necessary.

Connie and Laura went into business together. They opened a clothing store in a new shopping center in a mid-sized city. Both are married to physicians. Connie suggested that having the money and the connections from her husband's career afforded her this possibility.

Our husbands offered us the capital to start this business. I'm not sure if we could have borrowed the money on our own. Or, ironically, if we borrowed money it would only be possible because the banks know our husbands are good for it!

Gloria, a 36-year-old poet and artist, said:

> Being free to use my time as I liked and not having to work for a living was a great advantage in my life. . . . If Jonathon were not making the money, I could not have pursued my art career. We know it's hard to survive as an artist.

Most of the fringe benefits referred to are economic: traveling, having many possessions, schools for children, homes and furnishings that are materially exceptional and bring pride of ownership. In return for total support and dedication to their husband's time and career, the wife reaps many financial benefits: country club membership, charge cards, housekeepers, access to artistic and cultural interests and events, even an ability to be charitable. All of this can help self-esteem in a materialistic society.

The status benefits that are enjoyed by some wives cannot be overlooked.

> I love being fussed over in restaurants or at the theater. When I arrive I get deferential treatment. A warm and enthusiastic "Welcome, Mrs. _____. Will the doctor be joining you this evening?" I feel great, like a celebrity. Everyone knows us and appreciates Jack's work. I'd like to think I'm appreciated also, as his wife and companion.

> People offer us free tickets to shows and events all the time. We've gone on yachts and limousines and Leer jets that I would never get to see if I weren't married to Bill.

> I appreciate the rewards of Ted's profession. If it weren't for him, my sister would not have been cared for in an exclusive sanitarium for the last 40 years. She's been autistic since she was little, and when Ted and I got married he took on the responsibility of not only me, but Fran [her sister] as well.

> Doors are opened to me. I just use Dr. _____'s wife and people jump. "What can we do for you Mrs. _____?" We give a lot of money to various organizations in town and to our old alma mater. We sponsor underprivileged children in camp for the summer and try to help improve the lot of some of the homeless in our area. I feel fortunate to be able to help others.

I came up with these quotes from women when I asked in taped interviews: What do you think are the greatest fringe benefits of being married to a doctor? Most of those interviewed (about 90 percent) found at least one or two things that were benefits of marriage to a doctor. Not surprisingly, these were usually stated as those benefits most of us would view as positive: monetary rewards and respect from community members given to their husbands as "a doctor." The older women interviewed were generally more positive about the traditional benefits of security and prestige; 40 percent of the women over 45 years of age found many pluses in being married to a doctor. Those between 25 and 45 were less likely to attribute positives in their marriage to the fact that their husband was a doctor. Rather, they felt that the positives were due to his personality type. Only 25 percent of that group could attribute fringe benefits to the husband's being in medicine.

> Wherever we go everyone knows him, and we are given special treatment, especially if people have used him as their physician.

> He knows the meaning of all the medical terminology used in TV shows. Just kidding. He's obsessed with his responsibility for his patients. That makes me feel he's very loyal and dependable.

> I love being with a person who is called Dr. _____ by everyone in town. I feel special that I'm the one who actually goes home with him.

> Avoiding waiting lines, special treatment by celebrities, people's admiration, sometimes confusing my husband's identity with mine, but I get the goodies that way.

> Access to education, to foreign cultures while he's doing volunteer work in India or Pakistan. So I am learning and having experiences otherwise unavailable to me. My children grew up overseas while he practiced medicine there and we both did missionary work.

> I know a lot about medicine and health care in our country which I probably wouldn't be in touch with otherwise.

I've had the chance to meet interesting, educated people all over the world.

Memberships on committees and boards are so available I have to refuse occasionally. But I love having those opportunities. People think I'm smart, educated and informed because I'm Mrs. _____. I like it.

I love the automatic status whenever I'm introduced to a new group of people. "I'd like you to meet Mrs. _____. She's Dr. _____'s wife." Everyone seems to be impressed with that title. I know I am.

Having someone around to treat my children's scrapes and bruises and my illness is handy.

I have a husband who takes charge of everything, makes decisions quickly, and has great self-confidence. I feel secure and protected.

While Bill's alive I'll be taken care of.

I don't have to worry about details in our house. Tom does all the important stuff.

The biggest benefit is that I happen to still be in love with him after 38 years. I don't think being a physician has a whole lot to do with that!

We get fabulous gifts at Christmas time from other docs, payment for treatment during the year or referrals. That's always fun for the whole family.

Once in a while patients pay for service in trade or gifts. We get cabinets built or our walls papered. We even got a jacuzzi from a patient.

My husband is in the position to refer to many specialists, so we are guests at the most lavish parties constantly. Occasionally we're entertained on yachts, or at vacation villas. We are wined and dined, and I don't have to feel obligated to return the favors since _____ is the referring physician.

I never had to wait in doctors' offices when my children were ill or when I needed a check-up.

It's awkward and ironic to me that I can't think of many fringe benefits or reasons that make marriage to a doctor an especially positive experience. I married a doctor whom I fell in love with thinking that life would be charmed and special. I'm not sure that I didn't give up a great deal to be Mrs. Dr. _____.

The greatest fringe benefit that I can see is not having to fill out the health forms at a medical office when I'm ill. I get called right into the doctor's office and am very comfortable taking advantage of available medical treatment.

I live with an independent, successful man who can take care of himself. He is employable anywhere, well thought of in our town, has great integrity, is a good provider, and can diagnose problems of mine, my kids, and our entire extended families. We are all proud and grateful.

Personally, marriage to a doctor has given me time to be alone and mother my four boys full-time, if I desired, as they were growing up. My time with them was exceptional and rewarding. It felt right, and when I curled up and napped while they were asleep I was grateful for not having to leave them to go to work. I have also had to learn to be creative within my experience. It has also unquestionably increased my knowledge and interest in our health care system, and may have influenced my decision to work in the field of psychology and human relations.

Probably the greatest outgrowth of marriage to a physician is self-reliance. What begins as an overly dependent relationship can become a more healthy linking of two mutually independent and powerful people — with work, time and luck!

But there is a not so bright side.

MYTHS:
WHAT DID I EXPECT ANYWAY?

In my fantasy as a girl
I dreamed of life in a castle on the hill
surrounded by peonies, roses, and lilies of the valley

There would be music and light
and laughter and song
small children with smiling faces
Only small things would ever go wrong

The man and wife in my dreams
Were so intuned and respectful
Each valuing the other's opinion
Each revelling in the other's company

I expected to have a partner interested in many things
Curious about all of life's challenges
We could disagree at will and not be afraid
that the other would abandon or retreat

I expected faithfulness and honesty
and generosity beyond compare
A standard by which others would
measure if they dare

Ideally my dream man would be cool
calm and collected
His opinions would be sought by one and all
But neither his brains nor looks nor temperament
though admired by most
Would give him a second thought —
    nary a boast

Yes it's important to me to spend life with
    one who is never bothered by arrogance
    or self-centered immaturity

Playful yes — but never taking himself so seriously
    that all those around him must be
    careful and sensitive —

tip toeing around, fussing and fuming
for fear that this man's temper will be looming

A Doctor, a Doctor, such a sure thing
Smart and sensitive and trained to take care
I know my mother must be right
I'll never have to fear
Sickness or poverty or loneliness or
    disrespect or distrust
A Doctor, A Doctor is the only man
    with all the qualities I expect and want

He must know about people
they teach him in school
He has to like them
Or he'd be such a fool

Again and again the picture repeats
me and my Doctor
travel the world
Solving life's problems
While keeping ours sound

Any mother would be proud
if her daughter came home
and said, "I'm marrying a Doctor, Mama"
Never worry again — my future's secure
Doctors are so predictable, so reliable and so pure.

LIFE WITH DOCTOR

About Him and Life with Him:

Sharing in his work

Good knowledge of human behavior will help communication

Frugality

Generosity

He is a paragon of mental health

Wide range of interests

Exciting life together

Traveling

Fun loving partnership

Physical health taken care of

Emotional support

Actively involved father

Available when really important

I will be free of worries

No jealousy — no reason to be

Total trust

Accessible

Attentive

Brilliant

Humorous

Clever

Interesting

Enlightened

Loves reading

Keeps up with world events

Knows anatomy and physiology — great in bed

Caretaker — must be warm and interested in me

Bedside manner

Community minded

Open — not at all secretive

Gentle with children

Easygoing

Responsible

Omnipotent

Greatest catch of all!

Wait — things will be better when he's through his internship, residency, fellowship, first year of practice, etc., etc.

We'll see each other more

He'll be a better father

We'll take trips

He'll slow down

We'll talk more

WHAT'S SHE LIKE?
MYTHS FOR HER FROM SOCIETY

Secrecy

Mysterious — different from others

Spoiled

Empty headed

Special person

Self-sacrificing

Gets great medical care

Great sex life

Her husband's a great catch.

or: Her husband's a horrible catch.

He's too busy to fool around.

or: He's always having an affair with his nurse.

Lives in castle

Life so easy

No worries — free of them

Over protected

Passive

Helpless

Martyr — loves giving things up

Enjoys community service and volunteering

Chapter 4

Super Woman:
Her Job Description

No big deal—it's what my mother and grandmother did in their day! —Eleanor

Allow me to introduce Margie. She is 43 and has been married to a doctor for 18 years. Margie was born in a mid-sized town in Ohio where she was one of four children. She is uncomfortable recalling her early years, describing herself as the oldest child of parents who were not very supportive or communicative.

My father went from business to business until he finally settled on selling parts for use in plumbing. He did a fair amount of traveling, and while he was on the road my mother did bookkeeping and typing at home when she could. That was before computers, so I remember the kitchen table always filled with mother's papers, pencils, and erasers. Or sometimes after we were sound asleep—my sisters and brother— Mom would be pecking away at the typewriter at all hours. Actually my mother eventually taught me to type, for which I was grateful. But in those days we kids had to keep away from her things on the table. When meal time came Mother quickly and neatly removed her equipment to the cupboard so we could use the table for family eating.

Margie was responsible for helping run the house, and often had to parent her sisters and baby brother.

We had little in the way of luxuries. Our house was tiny but neat and clean. Although I do have vivid memories of kids in school ridiculing all of us who lived in that neighborhood, I wouldn't have known of the low status or unacceptable conditions if the others didn't pick on us. To me the house was adequate. Besides, I was busy with school, homework, child care, and housework so that my mother could do her typing.

There is a sense of pride in Margie's voice as she describes her ability to organize and care for her household. Her childhood responsibilities were good preparation for her future life in marriage.

I think women who choose to marry physicians know instinctively that they will be responsible for a great deal of the household from the beginning. I grew up with the belief that my job in life would be to take care of household management. First I did it for my mother and father. With that training I could move naturally and comfortably to another household and be in charge.

Margie finished high school and went to work in a business office doing filing and receptionist work. College was never an option, but with her eventual expertise in office work under her mother's close tutelage, Margie was competent and felt fulfilled in her work. She lived at home well into her twenties so that she could save money and continue to contribute to the household.

So at that time until I met my husband, Scott, I would get up in the morning, fix breakfast for everyone [her sisters and brother were from 6 to 10 years younger], go to work all day, come home and cook dinner, even help with homework for the other kids, maybe do laundry or cleaning. Whatever needed doing. By then my mother was really withdrawn from us, and my father stayed on the road for weeks at a time. Actually, when Scott and I met I was really ready to leave my parents' house and have one of my own. It was like mine but my sisters and brother were getting too old to really want to listen to me any more. Of course I had no clear idea of what marriage to a doctor would be, but Scott and I hit it off right away. Actually we met through one of the people I worked with. I was 25 and Scott was 28 and just ready to practice in internal medicine.

Margie is a beautiful, dark-haired, dark-eyed woman with a gentle expression which is electric when she smiles. She carries herself quite informally and has an easy way of speaking, as if she knows you'll understand what she's sharing. It's easy to understand how she could be called upon to be on numerous boards and committees. Her attitude of understated efficiency runs through her every word and action.

I spent two days following Margie to get a clear sense of her schedule. For me it was astonishing that beneath this slight, mild, unassuming person was a powerhouse of energy and accomplishment.

"Where to now?" I asked, hoping for a breather from a day of meetings, chauffeuring, phone calls, and people interrupting every time there was a peaceful moment. Margie was juggling her personal and household tasks—three children in school and their requirements; going to a conference for her youngest (his teacher was concerned about his inability to concentrate); her work with the League of Women Voters, of which she was now chairperson; her projects for a new business she and her partner were working on; working with computers and advertising; and her love of exercise which kept us involved in two swim classes and one aerobics class, which Margie attends every other day. She informed me of her pet project which was taking enormous time and energy—her commitment to bringing the Mothers Against Drunk Drivers awareness to the high school that her children would soon attend. This meant more political and social networking to fit into her life. Margie's skill at shifting from one activity to another, one group of people to another, and her superb problem solving and management techniques left me in awe.

After a day that put me in bed for an hour's nap, Margie then proceeded to put on a wonderful party for her husband's associates from the hospital. She told stories, shared recipes, wouldn't accept anyone's help in the kitchen, and did all this with aplomb and confidence. Her conversation was gay, charming, intelligent, and witty.

She looked extremely attractive and colorful and was undoubtedly enjoying the attention and devotion to her guests.

As far as I could tell, her children seemed mildly reserved but average. The 13-year-old boy with trouble concentrating in school was a delightful character. Margie encouraged his artistic ability and assumed the total responsibility for dealing with teachers, home-work, and parenting. Her phone never stopped ringing. Her appointment book was full. When I asked Margie if life with Scott was always like this, she unhesitatingly said, "Of course." It was clearly as though she thought all women lived like this.

After two days, I felt qualified to draw some conclusions. Margie is a woman of great inner strength and confidence. She doesn't share thoughts about whether life is good or not, but views life as a practical matter of doing whatever is necessary to accomplish the tasks at hand. She speaks of no personal ambitions. Even her own business, which she was excited about, was regarded as a practical matter, not something that required long and complicated insights and mysterious explanations. She and Scott seem natural, comfort-able, unsuspicious, and caring toward one another. They appear to have clear-cut roles and knowledge of the mechanism of their rela-tionship.

Margie is a pragmatic, earthy woman. She denies suffering from depression or melancholy. She is not a drinker, nor does she obsess about her weight or her looks. Her life is interesting and full of rich, new experiences. Her view of interpersonal relationships is envi-able. Although not the traditional overly concerned, nurturing fe-male, Margie displays an accessibility to her friends, colleagues, and husband and his associates.

I asked in many ways whether her schedule and demands were excessive or in any way uncomfortable, and she denied both. When I used the term "superwoman," she laughed.

> If I am superwoman, then all the women I know married to doctors must fit that description. None of my husband's part-ners' wives or my other friends married to physicians live any differently. Whether they work at home or outside in a profes-sion, they are busy and energetic like me.
>
> I can't even think of myself any other way. When I said yes

to Scott 18 years ago, I said yes to a job that would be a full-time responsibility. I was well trained long ago for making household decisions, doing the household books, making investment choices, coming up with entertainment ideas, cooking, cleaning, laundry — that's what I've always done.

I think Margie was surprised by the implication that her job was different or more responsible than any other woman's. To her, women are busy, strong, noncomplaining, effective, efficient, like she is, and like her mother was before her.

My mother was on her own most of the time. She was supportive of my father. She never complained. She was there for him and stood up for him to all who criticized. The only difference for me is that I have more "stuff" [I assume she's referring to things money can buy], and I was committed to being more in touch with my children rather than leave them to my oldest daughter like she did. My mother and I have never shared intimacies, you might say. So I don't know how she really felt about Dad's being gone and her being in charge. To me that's how it is. I guess I see myself as a partner in a business, the business of marriage and family. Scott never asks me about my job and I don't know much about his.

To describe mine, I'd say of any woman whose husband is out on the road a lot or who has to entertain his associates to promote his business that she's doing what I'm doing — cooking, shopping, cleaning, involved in community work, going to school, starting a business, raising kids, exercising, talking on the phone, chairing a meeting, changing a diaper, talking to the exchange, dealing with patients occasionally, reheating dinner, chauffering. It's all in a day's work.

She summarized her role efficiently while she blew dried her hair and changed her clothes to get ready for her meeting to introduce a prospective judge for election to voters in her hospital auxiliary.

The saying, "If you want something done, ask a busy person," comes to mind as I leave Margie's company. I now need a vacation, but Margie, I'm sure, will forge ahead and take life as it comes as a challenge, a demand, a reality.

To put the role of superwoman in historical perspective, I'd like to quote from an article that appeared in *Medical Economics* in February 1925, which described how a doctor's wife took over her husband's books. The article is entitled, "Are You Your Husband's Partner, Mrs. Doctor's Wife?" by Mrs. Charles E. Heider of Sutherland, Nebraska. In detailing how Mrs. Doctor's wife can render her husband assistance, she says he "needs someone to relieve him of this monotonous detail work [collection of accounts]" which he may be too busy to do (p. 17). She goes on to say she hated bookwork but someone needed to do it.

> Yes, Mrs. Doctor's wife. I do this and all of my housework, too, with the exception of my washing and ironing. And we have a baby not quite a year old whose robust health testifies that I do not neglect him either! Besides this, I manage to find time to attend and take part in our local women's club, to be guardian to a group of young Camp Fire girls, and to be a companion to my husband whenever we are fortunate to be allowed a few undisturbed hours together. To be sure, it often calls for special effort to get my bookwork all done and my statements out by the tenth of every month, but I do it. Many times, instead of reading or attempting a new book, I work late at night when my husband is out on a call and my little son sleeps. This month I have just completed and mailed about 250 statements, which represents many hours of work, and incidentally, several thousand dollars . . . and the best part of it all is, to me at least, that when the time comes I shall truly share in the accomplishment of our goal, for have I not been a partner? (p. 18)

Mrs. Heider in 1925 sounds remarkably like Margie in 1990.

Chapter 5

Fears and Insecurities

WHO'S IN THE WINGS AS MY UNDERSTUDY?

I am a new bride
What will happen now
Is there anything I should know
to keep my husband's glow?

It seems that I am grateful
to be chosen by this man
He is special among his peers
and I must deal with all my fears

He can't know what I am feeling
He'll think I'm insecure
unworthy to be his bride
a man of medicine is god to some
and needs an angel by his side

What if he sees me shaking
knows then that I'm afraid
New brides are for the taking
when Dr. Jones is what your named

I'll tell him I fear the future
I wonder what will be
I'll hope to god that he'll accept
the child still inside of me.

What if I really get sick and need constant care and attention? I can't face that—Frank is so distant and cool when I'm sick. Who will take care of me? —Mary Beth

Probably the thing I fear most is being upstaged by a younger woman who will gawk at and revere Roger so much more than I do. —A 42-year-old wife, married 20 years

I've always been afraid of not measuring up to the standards of Bobby's family. His father and grandfather are doctors and they're so formal, proper, and educated. I've always worried about whether his family approved of his choice in a wife. —A 35-year-old wife, married 12 years

What if Jerry realizes I'm a fraud. I trapped him into marriage 15 years ago because I couldn't stay poor any more and I knew marrying him would be a safe bet. —38-year-old mother of two children

My most scary thing is fitting in with the other doctors' wives. They seem so imposing and sure of themselves. I feel like a baby. —26-year-old wife newly married to 47-year-old physician

My biggest fear is what will happen when Joel dies. I'm totally unskilled. In this day and age I know it's stupid, but I've never worked outside the home and I am petrified about my future. —A 59-year-old wife, married for 37 years

I am always afraid. I'm afraid of aging, of being alone, of being left for another woman, of being boring, of not being sexy enough, not smart enough. I spend all my time trying to improve myself, going to classes, reading, talking to others who look so much greater. But the overriding fear since we got married has been waiting for the news that my husband has run off with one of his nurses. I guess that's why I've always knocked myself out to be the best cook, the most sexy, most glamorous, attentive wife I could be. —39-year-old wife, married 10 years. This is his second marriage.

My best friend and I both married physicians. Hers was in a different specialty, more prestigious. He's a surgeon and

John's a dermatologist. My biggest fear for years was that Tracy and I wouldn't stay friends. Her friendship has been at least as important to me as my relationship with John. But over the years as our husbands went into their own practices it's been harder to spend time as a foursome. There's a real feeling of importance that her husband flaunts over John. They can't talk about the same things, so Tracy and I try to carry the conservation the whole time we spend together. John's put pressure on me to drop the friendship with Tracy and Bill, but I can't do that. I'm afraid of losing her. She and I grew up together. The pull is always there. Our husbands have to come first and then our kids, but still, she's my real security in life and I love her so. If we split up I'd be devastated. — A 33-year-old wife of 12 years

I'm petrified that Arnold's drinking problem will affect his practice. I worry all the time. I cover for him with the exchange and the office whenever I can, but sometimes he goes out on an emergency really drunk and I'm terrified that he'll kill his patient, or himself on the way to or from the hospital. He doesn't want to take the problem seriously and always says I'm exaggerating. In fact, now if I bring it up at all he just gets furious at me. Most of the time I wait, frightened, by the phone for some horrible news about him. — A 29-year-old wife, married four years

This is hard to talk about, but I think my husband's been seeing another woman. He's been acting weird. Quiet and irritable one minute, and excited the next. He's been wanting to do things he never liked before, like dancing and listening to music. My father ran around on my mother and finally left me and my brothers for someone else. So I'm pretty sensitive to this. Plus I've been in therapy for a while and I'm trying to be strong and independent. If he's running around I've got to try to stop it or leave. I know that, but I'm afraid to confront the issue. I know this will mean divorce, and I promised myself that I'd stay married no matter what to raise my kids. I thought if I married a doctor from a stable family (no divorce on his side) I'd be safe and protected from what I went through as a child. There's no way I want to go home with my tail between my legs to my small town in Montana. — A 31-year-old wife of seven years

The fears and insecurities seem similar to those shared by women everywhere: Not smart enough, fearful of being left, apprehensive about physical appearance and aging, concerns with mothering, general competence, sexuality, and social status. Do I work outside the home or not? Do I feel guilt thinking about myself? Must I take care of ill parents? Should I be available to my spouse at all times? The list goes on. Do I take too many drugs? Do I talk too much? What do others think about me? Should I return to school — or am I too old. What if I have to raise these kids alone? I'm tired. I'm stressed. I can't complain. I'm lonely. On and on. But what's so different about these fears when they are felt by the physician's wife?

Perhaps the biggest difference is the denial, the inability to admit out loud that marriage and life with a doctor is filled with fears and insecurities. Remember, secrecy and confidentiality are so highly prized by the medical profession. The system as well as the cycle are maintained by the age-old credo: "Don't say anything to anyone not in the profession — they'll get the wrong idea." Also: "If we have troubles or problems we'll fix them ourselves." Or to the wife: "You don't have problems at all, it's in your head. Take a few days at the spa, go shopping, or take some Valium and you'll be fine."

Unable to share outside the rigidly defined system — be it family or the medical system — there is no way to truly address fears and insecurities with a sense of reality. It is handled only as the doctor husband sees it, and he tends to cover it up or gloss it over for himself, his wife, and his children. It is almost impossible to admit publicly to personal and/or family imperfections.

My personal deadly fear is not being heard or understood. When I had difficulty finding a publisher for this book, it triggered positive reinforcement for that fear. No one is interested; no one will listen; the public wants only the view that marriage to a physician is pure joy and altruism.

I dread being ill, either mentally or physically, and being ignored or cast aside by the public, "You're a doctor's wife—get cared for within the system." Just being an invisible extension of my husband and his colleagues (whether they are local or international) gives him full reign over my care. Thus no one can deal with my mental or physical troubles in an objective manner. This is a commonly held fear of women married to physicians (West, 1984).

I spend much time trying to be healthy—psychotherapy for my emotional state and fitness for my physical state. My choice of psychotherapist is not in the medical profession; I've never felt that I could get an objective interpersonal experience with an MD because there are too many preconceptions on his side and on mine. I have always needed someone who could view me as an individual and respect my fears and insecurities as my own, unhampered by the rigid and constricting views of psychiatry. The medical view toward emotional problems has been clinical, antifemale, patronizing, and authoritarian. My fear was that if I ever needed to be in that system, I would probably never get clear or objective enough support to return to emotional health. Frequently, doctors' wives who deal with the medically trained psychiatrist feel forced to deny fears or cover fears with medications or deadening psychiatric treatments whereby the perfunctory visits are acknowledged in a vague, almost ghostly manner. Regular, weekly, almost ritualistic, still she's often invisible.

The fears are misunderstood by many. The general public responds with, "What do you have to be afraid of? You've landed a doctor; you're set for life!" Her husband disregards her fears, and may humiliate her if she shares a fear that he may leave her for his young and gorgeous nurse. "Don't be ridiculous. Why would I do that? I don't even want to dignify your statement by talking about it!" And finally and most sadly, she often doesn't share with friends for fear that she'll be told, "I don't believe it." "But Bill just took care of my back sprain and he's so great," or "Why aren't you sleeping? Get Bill to prescribe something for you." One woman, paralyzed by agoraphobia who had been housebound for four years, tells of a "helpful" friend who kept coming over and saying she wouldn't tell anyone because it would ruin her husband's reputation!

The bond that marriage requires makes maintaining trust especially difficult in medical marriages. Obviously the wife of a physician wants and needs to trust that her husband the physician has her best interests at heart. He should not or would not intentionally undermine her or play on her most intimate fears and insecurities. However, and this is the big however, he is human, a man of many conflicts and fears of his own. To trust him alone with her fears can prove disastrous to her and to them both. Stoicism then becomes her constant companion. If stoicism doesn't hold, then she risks being told that she's complaining.

That explains my sense in interviews that women didn't want to share their innermost fears. Either they assumed I would ignore what they said, thereby invalidating their feelings, or I would view them as complaining unnecessarily and have no empathy with them, reinforcing their feelings of insecurity and discomfort.

> I'm most afraid of being honest about my feelings. I get so confused but don't really know exactly what to do about it or where to turn. Is it normal for me to have feelings like this? I have everything I could want. I'm totally taken care of and have a husband all my friends would kill for. But sometimes I'm overwhelmed with inadequacies. I worry about dumb things, like not being a good enough wife and mother. I have feelings about Ron running off with someone he works with and just leaving me and the kids with nothing. I know it's silly, but I'm not getting any younger, and neither is Ron. We don't talk much and I just can't ever be sure if I'm okay to him, if he still wants to be here with me. Oh, I guess that's stupid! — A 43-year-old wife of 17 years and mother of five children

With all the self-help books and television shows enlarging our connections with the outside world, taking care of us and our marriages, giving us permission to share our fears, why are these physicians' wives so isolated and still so reticent about revealing themselves?

It's severely difficult to exhibit fears, inadequacies, and insecurities when in a position of value and respect. Either others delight in your insecurities or deny them. We are made to feel guilty for our fears, stupid for our fears, or we are told we have nothing at all to worry about.

Clearly fear of losing our husbands the doctors and our eventual financial support to other women appears to be the most commonly verbalized, honest statement about our feelings. Remember if the doctor's wife is afraid of being supplanted by a younger, better, prettier, or more compliant woman and has been using most of her energy to support her husband's career and social life, is it no wonder that fear of her supporting herself when and if abandoned is a reality? What will she do? How will she provide for herself and her children when not within the framework of her medical marriage? It's likely that she has not developed a sense of her strengths, abilities, or entitlements separate from her husband's career and family needs. The fear, then, is perpetuated as she retains her overconnection to her husband's position and isolates herself from the world outside the medical community.

I wonder what the greatest fantasy is about confronting our fears. Will they come true? Will he actually run off with his nurse as women married to doctors have been told for generations, and which has been true for generations? Or will no one believe us if we confront our fears, allowing our humiliation and invalidation to tell us we were right to deny ourselves and keep as quiet as possible? Or worse yet, will we be considered crazy and then pay the consequences by ultimately being put away, physically or on medications, so that we lose our freedoms?

None of the alternatives appeal. So wives of doctors had better continue to play by the rules and ignore what really frightens them. Keep up the picture of health and happiness, and take care of the doctors — their public awaits.

Chapter 6

Waiting and Accommodating: He Should Be Home Soon!

You'll get used to it. Get a hot plate and learn to make reheatable casseroles. —Toni

WAITING

The dinner's cold
the children are bathed
the light is getting dim
My question once again
is when are you getting in?

Your mother called
Your sister's sick
Your father's feeling fine.

Can you come to the phone
or should I tell them
you'll call when you have time?

Last week I cried
This week I tried
Next week I just don't know.

If you don't come home soon
if you don't eat dinner on time
if once more I wait and anticipate
I may just give up and die.

There are few professionals who have to be on call to their profession with the regularity and dedication of the physician. Part of the mystique of medical care is the concept of patient/hospital/medical school first and the personal life of the doctor second or last.

I know you are wondering about the plumber or electrician. The power is out or the pipes have leaked and the water is contaminated. Isn't that the same as the doctor on call? I doubt it! The plumber's wife doesn't compete with life and death, nor does the electrician's wife. Today the computer wizard must be on call to bring up a destroyed system, or a company of 15,000 employees may lose a week's hard work on the crippled technical system. Still, no one will die or be paralyzed for life. Machines can be replaced, but not people! And the plumber, electrician, or computer technologist can send in a substitute for himself. The physician feels he must be the one to go to take care of his patient. He is God's messenger, God's repairman, and his wife must sit by quietly like his guardian angel, unobtrusive and uncomplaining until his return to the gates of heaven where he will be nurtured and replenished for his next important mission.

How does the guardian angel feel when her life is always interrupted and constantly on hold, submerged completely beneath the importance and intensity of his work's demands? How is it to wait and accommodate with such regularity that she doesn't even realize that her existence may be unusual or at least not similar to that of other married women?

When I asked others about the issue of waiting, I heard many ways in which women accommodated to a life of waiting. "Bring your own car to social events so you won't be stuck without a ride home or so that you can be on time," was a repeated discovery and practical solution to a husband's on-call dilemma. That seems to be the healthiest way to avoid the subjugation of waiting for someone else.

Stopping at the hospital and waiting in the car while my husband checks on especially ill patients has become second nature to our married life. I am still furious if we have shared a lovely, quiet evening of dinner and good company, and on the way home Jerry says, "I hope you don't mind if I stop at the hospital to check on So and So. I'm worried about him." It causes tension every time. I think to myself, reality time again, the nice evening is blotted quickly from his mind. It's back to Esther second, patients first. He could take me home so I can be angry and hurt in peace while he checks on his patient. "But we pass right by the hospital," he has said so many times. "I won't be long," he pleads. "If it takes me longer than ten minutes you can yell at me," he continues. What am I to do? It's only ten minutes. He's assured me that ten minutes of my time after all these years is extremely unimportant. The patient is so much more valuable and essential than ten minutes of me seething quietly in the car in the parking lot of the emergency room. I say, "I'd rather be driven home if you don't mind." He hesitates. He looks at me almost completely nonbelieving, with a look of cold steel in his eyes. "Is it possible that you said to drive you home when this is such a simple request? I would do it if the situation were reversed," he thinks to himself, or sometimes says aloud. But the situation is never reversed. My work is never so important or never is such that you cannot be driven home first — I think to myself.

Over and over again he wins. I cannot begin to compete with the patient so sick and helpless. He needs me now, and me and my time and my wishes and desires and needs are truly less worthy no matter how it may seem to me. The hooker here is that to argue the point reinforces the sense that I am being petty and small and unworthy while he — the doctor — is magnanimous, valuable, almost holy in his self-righteous aura. After all, he had a lovely evening too, so he says. He would much rather forget about his work, but duty calls. "Who is duty?" I have said to myself numerous times over the years. Duty dressed in the white of purity, duty who lives in the shadows of all doctors' lives and within the homes of all doctors' wives as a constant reminder of how good the doctor is and how unworthy his wife!

Duty was under the sheets as women described interrupted sexual intimacies with their husbands who abruptly shifted gears and cooly remarked, "I'll be back soon as I can," when their beepers went off or the hospital called with a supposed emergency.

If duty calls the doctor, what does duty say to his wife? Be patient and understanding. Don't scream in frustration; remember what happened the last time you screamed when you were about to have an orgasm and the beeper went off instead of your clitoris. Tears came to your eyes from frustration and rage and disappointment instead of sexual and emotional fulfillment and satisfaction. When you screamed at the doctor and let out your rage about having to wait again rather than hold it in dutifully, what happened? He yelled back at the top of his lungs, "Do you think I like this? Do you think I want to leave now? I don't! But I have to go! Mrs. Cohen is in pain. Her ulcer is acting up again. Her blood pressure shot up. I have to go. I have to go!" he screams back, almost out of control.

"Now look at what I've done," you think to yourself. I've upset the doctor. He won't be able to perform his duty to Mrs. Cohen. She'll get sicker or even die this time, and it will be my fault for yelling and keeping the doctor at home. My fault. I'd better catalogue this moment. The frustration and rage, and the excrutiating guilt. I know now I won't yell my experience again no matter what. Duty wins out. I'll wait quietly and patiently while the doctor, my husband, gets dressed, leaves the house, dutifully does his job, takes care of and hopefully cures Mrs. Cohen. I'll wait. You'll wait. She'll wait. Again and again.

And with the waiting comes the accommodating. Both, as I have said, are so ingrained in a woman's life that the admission of it as different, unusual, or even a sacrifice on her part is not something easily admitted by doctors' wives. Here is a typical story revealed by a woman seen in my office. Lee, in her early thirties, mother of two lovely daughters, born and living on the East Coast, tells:

> My husband called to say he would be out with some of his friends (male) but would be bringing them home for dessert in awhile; would I get something nice for them, he'd be there soon?

This woman is remarkably assertive; her female role models were outspoken Jewish women who expected to get their way when it was important to them. She continues:

My husband had been having dinner with his friends, which was okay, but the request for dessert at the last minute didn't sit well with me. However, I went to the bakery and bought eclairs and made coffee, and began waiting. One and one-half hours after expected arrival time, and after I put the girls to bed, Charlie called again. He had stopped for drinks but would be there any minute. Two hours after that in walks Charlie, alone, none of the guys. He says hello (no apology or anything, as if he forgot his request in the first place), and I threw the eclairs in his face!

She was proud of herself and furious at Charlie.

Charlie, however, is not a doctor. He is in business in hardware. I question whether a doctor's wife would ever throw something at the doctor because he was late, plans were changed, or she was inconvenienced. The example of Charlie was used to describe usual feelings of infuriation at being kept waiting after being told to provide a service for a husband and his friends. Even if the request was made politely, some women find it incredibly presumptuous and no longer part of their job as wife and partner.

Contrarily, doctors' wives assume that accommodation to their husband's profession is expected and even a privilege. Cassandra, an attractive, 28-year-old executive secretary in the fashion business who has been married to a doctor for four years, explains:

I wouldn't dream of complaining about Will's regular lateness and unpredictability. Early in our relationship at a meeting of the wives' auxiliary I asked the others what they do about it, and the consensus was "Reheat the food," "Get a hot plate," "Take your own car to parties," "Tell the kids, 'Daddy's a doctor. They're always late to things. He'll get here when he can.'" I implied that sometimes it's annoying and I got no sympathy, only "You had better get used to it if you want to stay married!" I realized that while I was growing up in my mother's and father's house, my father was quite considerate of my mother's role as mother and wife, and rarely caused tension by lateness or asking her to entertain his clients (he was a salesman). But now I, as a doctor's wife, was to conform to the views of these other doctor's wives, who were united in the expectation that it comes with the territory.

"Don't take it personally," is the engraved message that accompanies the wedding to a doctor. So burnt dinner is just the beginning. Entertaining alone is frequent. Watching children's activities alone, taking yourself to the theater, to parties, to the doctor, to the hospital to have your operation, all are a continued part of accommodating. It may even be necessary to bring dinner to him at the hospital or office, to have the kids go there to see him, to bring his visiting parents to the emergency room for a chance to see him, and eat in the hospital cafeteria. These are not uncommon occurrences in medical families.

If you have an important opening or business meeting, don't expect your husband to attend, for there will be less disappointment when he's late or doesn't attend at all.

Part of the job description of a doctor's wife is to wait patiently or make other arrangements. Too bad who's upset or disturbed by this; it's important to repress upset feelings and find practical alternatives. Otherwise, it's possible to be a bitter, impatient, critical, constantly petty, complaining woman, and the doctor probably will make his wife feel guilty for not having fulfilled her job description well. He threatens (overtly or covertly) to replace her with a more suitable wife.

What appears to underlie this waiting and accommodating is the clear message that the doctor's time is most important and valuable. Have you noticed how all people will graciously accept a doctor's tardiness? No one expresses anger or disappointment when he enters a room, party, or meeting late. Rather, he is greeted with reverence and great curiosity as to his latest conquest in the world of medicine. He is given blanket acceptance for behaviors considered rude and inconsiderate in other mortal beings. Who else can get up in the middle of an important meeting and just walk out? No one needs to know or say more than, "He's a doctor," and that lets him off the hook of normally expected social consideration. As doctors' wives, we are to be the most compliant and accommodating. With the marriage vows, we agreed to tolerate these social inconveniences. We are also constantly reminded that our time is not worthy of the same consideration as his. We can presumably make the necessary adjustments in our lives to favor his ill-appointed schedule. No one blinks an eye at our arranging and rearranging the family, the home, and our outside work to fit into the doctor's more important demands. Each time we try to overrule or break with tradition, the guilt, the force of years of history in medicine, and male domination is overpowering.

Chapter 7

Loneliness and Isolation: Does Being Alone Always Mean Being Lonely?

I recall with melancholy the wonderful times we spent together while we were dating and we were both students together.

— Sarah

Sarah implies a joy in the companionship of her husband when they were students together. Her reference to the memory in a state of melancholy implies awareness of the loss of his companionship. Alone, detached, separate, isolated, unaccompanied, solitary, lonesome, forlorn, secluded, and remote are all familiar words when referring to a lonely state of being.

The dictionary definition of "lone" is companionless; solitary; a *lone* tree; isolated; unfrequented; sequestered, lonely. "Lonely" is defined as without companions, lone, characterized by aloneness; solitary; lonely existence, dejected by the awareness of being alone. "Let alone" is described among other definitions as to refrain from interfering with [someone]. Alone emphasizes isolation from others and does not imply unhappiness. Lonely adds to isolation the painful consciousness of it (from the *American Heritage Dictionary of English Language*).

In Natalie Rogers's book *Emerging Woman: A Decade of Midlife Transitions*, she speaks of two images, of two forms of loneliness. First: "separation and loss; death, tragedy, uprootedness, divorce, rejection, separation from loved ones, abandonment." These have been spoken of and written about in many forms. We are more

articulate about the concrete forms of loss in our lives and the loneliness derived from them.

But Rogers continues in her second image: "being ignored or
misunderstood by important others, being listened to but not heard,
feeling misunderstood, misinterpreted, not connecting in a relationship" (p. 74). Having knowledge or experience that no one else
seems to understand.

In my office and in my experience with women's groups I have
shared with others this second devastating experience. I agree with
Rogers that little is written or known about the experience of that
kind of isolation, the kind women describe over and over as being
felt, even in the company of others. The familiar sense of being
alone in a room teeming with people, but feeling excruciatingly
detached and separate from the others and perhaps from the experience itself, is more common than one might think.

I'm not sure we have the words to describe the desolation of
living with another human being in close proximity, for years sometimes, and yet feeling lonely.

In Sarah's case, when she met Troy they were young, vital people excited about their lives and studies. Sarah was 27, in graduate
school, studying marine biology, and Troy was in first year medical
training.

> I met Troy in a physiology class I was taking at the _____
> School of Science and Medicine. We would work on our stud-
> ies together. We were attracted to each other almost instantly.
> I loved my work and was especially turned on to the fact that
> Troy was so enthusiastic about his. Our time together was in-
> tellectually stimulating as well as very romantic in those days.
> Originally I was planning to become a marine veterinarian, but
> when Troy and I became serious his medical training seemed
> to come first. Once we decided to marry I couldn't go on to vet
> school. One of us had to stay home to help the other. At least
> that's how it was for us. In subtle and not so subtle ways more
> and more of my energy was drawn away from my work and
> studies into helping Troy with his. I started typing papers for
> him and doing some of his research work. I'm not even sure
> today (this was ten years ago) how all that slipped away from

me. I can't recall us ever sitting down and deciding that I would put off school for a while till Troy finished. It just happened. Our time together after that class in physiology was just too important to me to continue in classes of my own. I loved Troy's company, so if he had time to see me, I made time for him even if it meant not going to my classes or preparing my work. So soon I was not a student any more, but I was Troy's wife.

The trouble was once he left school and went on to residency training our initial bond, intellectual curiosity, and excitement died. We weren't studying together. He was studying and I was pampering him. He expected me to be home for him and have meals and laundry and do research and typing for him, but he stopped talking about the projects or the work he was doing. And I had nothing to share except what went on at the supermarket! Yuk, how boring I must have been to him. Oh well, soon I decided a baby would be a good idea. The only trouble was I couldn't get pregnant. So now not only didn't I have much of Troy, but I was alone without a child.

So what's so different about Sarah compared to other wives who have busy husbands and who want to fill their time, who perhaps want a child to help them feel useful, less empty, less lonely?

It's hard to put my finger on it. Troy was happy in his work. He'd fulfilled a dream of his and his family's—he became a doctor. I was there with him. I helped him almost every step of the way. For a time that was enough for me, to see his joy and pleasure of his accomplishments. I felt he helped me to feel like an important, even essential, part of his success. But in little ways his medical studies began excluding me. He said I couldn't come to a meeting with other residents. He soon suggested that I do the research for his papers at another local medical library. I noticed my name was never on any of his work and he stopped telling people at social gatherings of my contribution to his work. What did that all mean? I didn't even notice it for a while.

Medicine is a tough task master. I was spending more and

more of my evenings alone. He'd come home and stay for dinner and then say he had an exciting case at the hospital to look in on. His chief resident expected him to be there at all hours, even on weekends. Our connection was severing. Even at parties the sense of disconnection was apparent. Now Troy was Doctor _____, not just a regular guy who I met in school and fell in love with. Sometimes I felt like he was embarrassed by me. He stopped introducing me to people he was impressed with. It was as if he had some image of himself as a physician and the higher up he got in his specialty training the lower I got in his eyes. I, of course, felt it was me. I tried to get involved, read more about his work, read more about the world, get involved in auxiliary work, charity work. Whatever the doctor's wife is supposed to do, I did.

But the wall was too rigid now. I wasn't getting pregnant and he was becoming more engrossed in his new life and identity as a lung specialist. As he worked with the biggest names in his field, I became more and more isolated.

Did you think about getting help or returning to school?

Sure. I tried to get Troy to come into counseling so we could relearn our communication. He refused. "Psychiatry's a crock!" he'd say. "You go if you want. I'm fine the way things are." How could I go back to school? I had lost nine years, out of the trenches for nine years, depressed, didn't know who I was any more. It never dawned on me that this wouldn't get fixed, that it wasn't just a fluke or even a product of in my imagination.

The hardest part is to explain to someone what's going on with me. They look at our life. Troy's a big lung specialist now. We go to the expected events. We put on the appropriate show of proper doctor and wife. I even seem okay to other people, I guess. So that's what gets confusing to me. The other wives describe the same things: isolation, disconnection, not feeling important or understood at times, the embarrassment of not knowing where their husband is most of the time, or what he's doing. The worst is the lump in my throat when other people envy my situation. What situation? Who am I anyway? The other wives don't seem to need understanding. They say, "Get used to it. That's what a doctor is like. So be quiet and be grateful." He's not expected to be anything but taken care of and admired so that he does his work. What does that mean to me? My soul is hurting. My spirit dies a little more every day that he listens to me try to explain my loneliness and my feelings. I don't really exist as a person any more. He listens and says, "I don't understand what's so upsetting to you. I've provided a good life. I've worked like a dog. What's wrong with you? Why are you getting angry and upset?"

The inner sense of isolation felt by a doctor's wife can be unbearable. She can't understand it herself. There are few out there to explain the experience.

I have felt despair at times in my life. I've been troubled by the thought that my experience is different from what others feel, and plagued by the sense of failure when surrounded by others who smile and express gaiety when I'm feeling empty inside. This kind of loneliness seems to be spiritual, one in which my core has been bruised. All the time I thought that I was independent, rearing children alone, interacting with a few adults, managing a house alone. I was under the false assumption that I was strong—to be a doctor's wife, they tell us how strong we must be. Take care of it all. Find things to do to interest yourself. The independence—I don't need anyone else—which is fostered especially for those of us who marry medical men, is an out and out lie. I am not independent. I am lonely and dependent. If I were truly independent, the closeness would be a pleasure, and solitude a spiritual joy in finding and connecting to my inner core, my strong inner being. But for me the loss of my self, the insecurity of my self, the continuous doubting of my self has increased my dependence, not my independence.

I am not speaking here of the existential awareness of our ultimate aloneness, the shock that radiates through each one of us as we realize our trip through life and death is a separate experience. I am referring rather to the terror of a fearful, helpless child, a child whose very survival depends on another.

If I had been able to achieve and accomplish for myself, not just for others, if had I been valued as a productive member of society, if had I been able to support myself economically, then the approval of others would be less essential to my existence. When we live vicariously through another or others and we lose self-pride and self-fulfillment, we experience disconnection, disunity, unacceptance, devaluation, isolation, smallness. We return to that childlike dependence on others for our survival. The tinier we feel, the more fearful our aloneness grows. A doctor's wife is alone often. She is unable to trust her own resources; her inner strength does not grow, but diminishes. She is also tiny in the eyes of the world around her. She may then experience a loneliness that is indescribable. While she is nurturing and providing for her husband's needs, hers go unrecognized and unspoken, unspeakable even to her. She experiences the painful consciousness of isolation — true loneliness.

SECRECY AND OVERPROTECTIVENESS:
WHOM DO I TELL?

It's so lonely up here on the hill
  No one understands my life
I project a picture to the outside world
  free of worry; free of pain and strife.

As the years go by I realize
  that I am doomed by isolation
Others don't care that I am human
  I see and feel and hurt as they.

When I try to share my thoughts and feelings
  others look on in horror
You have nothing to complain about
  your husband's a doctor.

We see your maid, your country club
  your exceptional castle on the hill
We know you play tennis and golf all day
Oh if we had your life, Oh to have your life
  they all say.

Soon I'm filled with secrets unable to share
  Even the women who have lived my
    life are quiet.

What are we hiding? Is it from ourselves
  or from the world?
They tell us we're lucky. We're the chosen
  few.

Like the Jews who suffer, are prejudiced
  against, hated and misunderstood.

So do we suffer alone and lonely in our
ivory towers   Ignored

Keeping secrets from ourselves and others becomes

our key to survival.
To tell the truth threatens our security
the hand that feeds is not to be bitten.

So we keep the mystery, to describe the
humanity, frailty, and sensitivity would
be to demystify.

Can we bring god down from his pedestal?
Or should we raise ourselves up to his?
Struggle, struggle with the meaning of it all.

Secrets. He's angry, he's hateful, he's arrogant,
I'm lonely, I'm tired, I'm sad,
the children don't know him at all.

More secrets — He loves another woman, I love
another man, he's afraid, I'm afraid.
Perhaps he's not god, perhaps he needs
me more than I need him.

What if the world finds out that medicine
is an art and not a science?
If they know that he's helpless at home
helpless without his nurse
without the hospital to protect
his image?

What of me?
Can I say I almost left him seventeen times
Went home to mother half that many
I use too much Valium
am smoking and drinking all the time
Have thought of suicide often when
he disappointed me for another
emergency?

What of me?
Can they hear how he beat us last
night in a fit of rage after working

on OB all day?
We fight about money more than the
  poor people do.
My spirit is shattering
My life is a shell
  Who can I tell? Who can I tell?

MYTH OF SECRECY AND MYSTERY

Secrecy

                                    Unrealistic demands and
        Mysterious body of knowledge   expectations

                Club of medicine   Miraculous healing

                        Isolation

                                    Public dependent on
                                    healers (MDs) for health

Eventually

Mistake of death,
not healed.
What, not God?

        Malpractice   Insecurity   More and tighter
                                 and doubts   secrecy

        Rage

            Disenchanted   Pressure for
                                 peer review   Greater, more
                                               complicated technical
        Could lose job   knowledge

                                               Special

Myth that death is curable by physicians. If not, if doctors are indeed people, we all are indeed capable of death.

Politics and economics of avoidance of death, rather than of life and living.

Chapter 8

Social Expectations:
Use the Correct Fork Please

It's unnerving to go to your first party at the surgical chief's house and feel envy and pride that you too will have all these things someday, all the while knowing the whole thing is just a calculated game. Just play by the rules and you're in. — Carol

More than other professions, medicine requires inside referrals for survival (Lorch and Crawford, 1983; Gerber 1983; Myers 1988). In the army a wife knows that she will soon be transferred to another post. The executive's wife may be an executive herself. Not the doctor's wife. She usually has enlisted in her career for life, and society demands that she stay in her job for the duration.

For Rita, preparing another coffee to welcome new doctors' wives was always a pleasure. She spent years collecting the newest appointments for her table: a matching coffee set of lovely silver, crystal cake dishes, some of her mother's special china in an exquisite cherry cabinet that was probably passed from generation to generation. I watched Rita's deft hands pour the coffee and place a home baked pastry onto a gold-rimmed pastry plate. She asked me if I wanted cream or sugar, and my years as an army doctor's wife flashed before me. In those days in North Carolina and Georgia, I always used the presence of my children to avoid these social obligations. Those were my first real experiences with proper wifely graces: pouring tea, light conversation about which army post will be next, inquiring about her husband's specialty. The army as an officer's wife was wonderful training for what could be a life as a doctor's wife.

I recall that officers' wives also thought of themselves as career wives. Somehow their social comportment reflected their husbands' success in the battalion. Why all the high alcoholism and depression among army officers' wives? For the identical reasons that doctors' wives have high alcoholism and depression.

To live a social role in order to improve one's own self-esteem and position, and to succeed is in itself quite demanding, but to live it for another and never own the self-esteem or rewards is quite another issue.

Rita described her disillusionment with social propriety. She laughed when sharing the "real" people underneath the tea and crumpets. At 43 Rita had suffered from depression and had been hospitalized twice. Her lively face belied the anguish she must have been hiding.

> It's always been so hard to know if I'm doing the right thing. My mother-in-law pushes all my buttons. Since her son's the doctor she's expected me to further his career in any way possible. I wish someone would have told me when I was younger that a doctor's wife requires nerves of steel to survive the demands. It's exhausting to be perfect all the time. Generally the public would be shocked to see what happens when no one's looking. I have begun resorting to opening Larry's [husband] personal mail and tearing up invitations. It got so sickening having to send formal notes of thank you or regret, or worse yet speak to the hostess in person with regret or acceptances to parties. I'm sick of politeness for his image. I feel the contempt of the other wives now because we don't go to social functions like we should. First my depressions kept us home. Now after years of therapy I realize I don't have to be depressed to avoid things. I don't go.

Rita's inability to do anything but tear up personal mail directed to her husband touched me. She felt she was forced to take matters into her own hands, no matter how indirectly, and regardless of the injury to her pride.

The repeated descriptions of wearing two faces, one for the public and one in private, are haunting. The social role is so strong and so unrealistic that these women feel like great liars and deceivers of society.

> Every time I'm polite in public as the doctor's wife I have a cold chill that someone will find me out. Maybe they overheard me yelling at my youngest child or cursing at the noise and ineffectiveness of the piano tuner in my house. If only you could hear me rail at another disappointment.

If we keep in mind that it is only recently in our history that the status of the physician has been so high, it might put the role of his wife into better perspective. The medical profession came into its own in the later part of the nineteenth century with the Industrial Revolution. Suffice it to say that before the upsurge of status and power of the American Medical Association and medical education in this country, only a few physicians catering to wealthy clientele were lucky enough to be considered upper crust. The profession was not cohesive in the nineteenth century. Competition was fierce, knowledge of medicine was poor and inexact, and generally it was not so great to say your child was going to be a doctor. Poor publicity, infighting among the ranks of health care givers, and nonprofessionalization made it a scary line of work.

Twentieth century professionalism, plus scientific discovery, greater understanding about the cause of diseases, and the great moneys of the rich being put toward research and education have elevated the status of medicine to godliness (Duffy, 1976; Ehrenreich and English, 1978).

As far as I can tell, this would mean that the position of the doctor's wife as a career choice, with the subsequent status and role responsibilities, has been a twentieth century phenomenon. With greater professionalism of medicine has come greater "professionalism" of the doctor's wife.

Until this century lawyers and ministers had much greater status. Therefore, even though we know women were not becoming lawyers and ministers, their status as wives of those men in those fields was accrued through marriage. Consequently, to be a minister's wife held the attendant role responsibilities and the awe of the community. Status and power for women had to come predominantly from their connection to their husband's position in society, as women have not been privy to the same opportunities. Since status in a society does come from education and economic reward and women have been denied access to both, they relied on "status by proxy," as I like to call it. To be a physician's wife today the status by proxy is there, but it is a double-edged sword.

Today her role requires social aplomb. Continuous entertaining for her husband's colleagues is essential for him to get referrals and maintain good will in his medical community (Lorch and Crawford, 1983). His profession may be the only one in which the wife has to devote himself totally to ensure his greater success. Since World War II, choosing to be a doctor's wife has meant making that role one's conscious career.

Using the correct fork is the tip of the iceberg. If we look at how pressured she is to perform her role, to meet time demands, to put herself second, and to perform according to the social rules of her husband's profession, we can imagine the conflicts. Witness: to maintain or improve her status, a doctor's wife must help to ensure her husband's success in his field. If she does a poor job, he will conceivably be looked down upon by his colleagues. To fail to see her role as essential would be to reduce her chances for success and status. We see the cycle of living through one's husband as a vicarious success. Is it only vicarious?

So when I went from home to home and was overwhelmed by fabulous decor and absolutely perfect tea and coffee service, it should not have been so surprising to me. I have always resisted social imposition. My response to using the right fork would be to serve Oriental food and have to use chopsticks. Dressing appropriately to entertain or be entertained by other physicians' wives only causes me to add to my wardrobe of funky, outlandish designs. My rebellious nature cannot be contained. Perhaps if I had realized that doctor's wifery really is considered a full-time career involving proper etiquette for dress, entertaining, cultural interests and involvement, and vacation behavior and destinations, I would certainly have insisted on wages and the ensuing status.

It is well known that a significant percentage of physicians drop their first wives who put them through medical school if it is perceived they come from the wrong side of the tracks. Marrying their high school sweethearts often ends in disaster because the social responsibilities of a rising young physician require knowledge of the right voice, the right dinner conversations, the right table settings, the right flowers, the right menu, and the right guest list (Gerber, 1983; Fine, 1981).

To be proper by choice is one way a society function complements its members. Rampant rage and disrespect would be devastating to its members. However, stringent role requirements with no outlet for letting down is inhuman. Doctors' wives feel the heat of these expectations. Whenever I go to the hairdressers I feel a performance is being conducted for my audience. I am painfully aware that the audience isn't truly interested in me for myself. I'm a curiosity—the doctor's wife. How does she cross her leg under the dryer? How does she look in rollers? Does she chew gum? Worse yet, does she fall asleep under the dryer?

Always alert to criticism, we who marry physicians have to strut the stage and perform according to someone else's script. If people heard the dirty jokes that I know, the sexual fantasies shared by us among ourselves, the personal eccentricities, would they be shocked? Would they care?

I'm afraid that keeping up appearances serves to protect from something scarier than mere disapproval. I'm truly afraid that appearances hide the truth that women married to doctors don't even show up at all. Appearances hide the reality of blankness. Appearances give me a job to do and make me feel somehow important. Take away my appearance and you may take away all I have.

Chapter 9

Perfectionism:
Do We Both Have to Be Perfect?

> I'm getting better, but still, under stress I start cleaning the
> house over and over. — Teresa

In *Women and Self Esteem*, Sanford and Donovan have identified
perfectionism as a trap encountered by women in our society. They
devote a chapter to the effects of our need to be perfect and how that
keeps us in a cycle of lowered self-esteem (1984).

I can recall the first time someone asked me if I was a perfectionist. "Who me? Are you crazy? I'm the sloppiest person I know. I
hate to keep things neat. The more things are piled up the happier I
am!" You can always tell which side of the bed Jerry sleeps on. His
is neat as a pin. Mine is chaos! His side of the closet is orderly.
Mine always needs a research director to find anything.

What I didn't realize then was that even though house cleaning or
desk tops are not my forté, I could still be considered a perfectionist. Outer neatness and order aside, my psyche was begging for
perfection. If I could only do this better, or if I could be smarter,
funnier, better at math, a better mother, a more perfect cook and
hostess . . . In fact, whatever was important to me or reflected my
sense of worth should be better, or ideally, should be perfect. I
never felt that what I did or could do would ever be as good as what
Jerry did. I didn't realize then that other women experienced their
lives similarly.

As stated before, one of the requirements of Mrs. MD is competence. The doctor is a perfectionist, and this trait was a necessity for
completing medical school. As his wife, Mrs. Doctor needs to be
almost one step ahead of her husband. As he tends patients, she,

remember, tends to him and his family. She keeps the wheels turning and oiled in all areas of their personal life.

Perhaps her choice of a medical student or a doctor tells us that she believes her need for security is greater than other women's. Her strong need for protection from physical harm as well as her needs to be accepted and acceptable in society have guided her choice. But will choosing to be a doctor's wife give her the sense of security and protection that she requires? Knowing that financial and status needs will be met, the requirement that she live up to her part of an unspoken bargain doesn't seem too unreasonable in exchange. To be available personally and to present a picture of perfect family life to the outside world is all that her MD husband usually requires of her.

She becomes perfect wife, hostess, mother, social organizer, charity worker, friend, secretary, business manager, house manager, decorator, teacher, fashion expert; above all, she is perfect at putting her own needs last! Her temper and emotions must be in check at all times. Her feelings appear perfectly controlled, her losses ignored, her feelings of jealousy jealously guarded, her loneliness perfectly shut down, and her self-esteem perfectly low at all times. Underneath her cool, competent exterior the doctor's wife is certain that she could do better, that she is really never quite perfect. She can handle another job, another set of responsibilities, and perhaps then she'll be perfect.

Sheila, an extremely beautiful woman with fair hair flowing down her back, green eyes, and the most striking skin I'd ever seen, said the following when I asked her if she would describe herself as a perfectionist:

> Do you think I'm a perfectionist if I have everyone remove his or her shoes at our front door before entering our home? I guess I am. I don't have anything out of order. I clean all the time and never think it is quite clean enough. I think I get worse as I get older. Now I can't stand anyone to come to my house until I've cleaned thoroughly. And I've gotten more critical of how I look and how my children look and behave. My thought is always — that's good, but you can do even better. I do catering sometimes for parties, but it's getting harder

for me to work with anyone else. They say I'm too particular and demanding. I get migraine headaches a lot. They're worse now, too. My counselor says that if I could relax and let go a little my headaches would probably be less frequent. It's hard. My life's generally demanding and I'm on view a lot to the people Stacy works with. I have to be exceptionally charming and witty after a day of carting kids all over. Also, Stacy seems pretty picky about how I look and behave. I guess it rubs off. The trouble is that no matter how other people feel or what their reaction is to me — "Sheila does a fabulous job!" or "Sheila, you're so lucky to be so talented," or "Sheila, aren't you proud of your kids?" — I smile, say thanks sometimes, and then tell myself that's bull (pardon the vulgarity), they're just saying that! I really don't understand why I'm like this. But the more I do, the more I take on, the more I seem to doubt myself. To tell you the truth, I'm not sure I can judge what my capabilities are. My standards for myself are so out of whack!

To be a doctor's wife in our society is to wear the banner of ultimate insecurity. She is reminded always of her imperfection. She could help more, be kinder, nicer, better, funnier, smarter, less guilty, less angry, less critical. In short, she could work harder at achieving perfection, ultimately to try to measure up to her husband's standards of perfection. He's the expert, the doctor, the god. If he is the slightest bit critical of his wife, then she must begin again, looking for other ways to please him and to right the imperfect situation.

Since her husband deals with trying to live up to his profession's unreasonable standards of perfection every moment of every day, he may (and often does) utilize his wife (and children) to prove his strength. In other words, they are the buffers of his world. In order to cool his heels and replenish his strength and confidence to go out and slay the medical dragons, his wife provides a theoretical dumping ground. She may be forced to receive the brunt of his constant criticism and disapproval at the end of his day of never achieving but always attempting perfection, yet on some level he truly believes in his capacity to be perfect. The doctor forces his insecurity on his wife.

Why is dinner late? Why haven't you finished the project I asked you to do for me? Why are Johnny's grades only B's? You have overdrawn the bank account? My suit is wrinkled! Our telephones are ringing wrong! The fan belt broke in the car. Your dress is green — you know green reminds me of my mother! Can't you clear the table faster than that? Did you pay the electric bills? Why did you fire the housekeeper? Can't you see the curtains are fading? The music is too loud. My boss's wife said your hors d'oeuvres were cold last Saturday. I'll be home late tonight so keep dinner waiting. You forgot to give me a message last night. Where are my blue argyles? And so on.

She feels pressured the more he picks at her. Her anxiety goes up in response to the implication that life in her home is not perfect. Often the process is disguised or is played out through other family members. It happens unconsciously and unwittingly. Everyone is affected.

"I now know perfectionism is problematic in our household," says Sandra, 36 years old, married for 12 years, mother of four daughters.

> I didn't realize what effects I was having on everyone until my second child, Jolene, began having trouble in school. Her teachers say she makes herself sick trying to be right all the time. She gets all A's, but if she gets a B+ she stays home from school for two days with pains in her stomach. This girl is only eight years old. But her older sister gets great grades and is quick and bright. She gets praised for it constantly in school and everywhere. The kids know we want them to do their best, but to get sick at eight! I feel terrible, and worry about her constantly now.

> *Are you thinking you're at fault here?*

> Well, I guess so, since I'm the only parent here with the girls. It's pretty much my job. I know they want to please us, but I consider myself the parent. Jack only sees them for very short

periods. So what she does, how she behaves, and how she feels must reflect on my parenting skills.

She's done something wrong. She tries to clean more, decorate more, be on time more, keep the kids in line more, have better parties, and better conversation, read better books, be more self-less, and more giving — in short, make life better for her husband the doctor! He must be able to do his job perfectly. She's ultimately responsible for that! Or so she truly believes. And so he makes her believe. When he's been successful, it was due to his hard work and brilliance. When he's failed in some way, it is always his wife's fault and responsibility!

If he doesn't get enough sleep, it's because she couldn't keep the kids quiet! If he's cross or irritable, she probably wanted to make love when he had more serious life and death problems on his mind. When he yells at his nurse, his wife probably asked him to help with Johnny's homework last night. How dare she!

Perfection is a trap, a steel trap. Medical school turns young, eager idealists into compulsive perfectionists who get tremendous work loads and ever constant readiness for more work from those who went through the program. The spouses of these well-trained perfectionists live with the disease of perfectionism, and in order to relieve their own tension and feel acceptable, they too become more perfectionistic. Fight fire with fire. If he complains or criticizes, I will correct my errors. He must know what's right; he's a doctor, everyone respects him. He makes the bulk of the money here. I should try harder to please him and make his life a little easier.

Unfortunately, being a perfectionist poisons our self-esteem. We can be perfectionists but we can never achieve perfection! So there's a built-in system for failure implied in that system. We become perfect at being perfectionists — that is, we continue to fail and try harder to be perfect! Try, fail, feel guilty and try again, fail again, get depressed, etc. The difference between the doctor and his wife is that she rarely feels supported or experiences only a fleeting sense of accomplishment. She more often sees her imperfections in a magnified, overall sense (global, as Sanford and Donovan view it [1984]). Even as a great household manager or competent parent she cannot put her strengths into perspective if she is always measured against her doctor husband. He's paid well, highly praised, and respected for his accomplishments. He can get support and applause daily in every area of society for who he is. She has to keep looking for ways to overcome her imperfection. He is a doctor and a man. If all else fails today, tomorrow will be all right. Society supports and reinforces his efforts. Society ignores her and criticizes her failures!

For her, today's failure, no matter how small, can be devastating. Her self-esteem doesn't have the cement foundation required to get her through the inevitable less-than-perfect outcomes. She hears criticism and generalizes it to feed an overwhelming sense of low esteem. Setting the table wrong can be enough to set off a chain reaction of negative messages about her worth as a human being. Pretty shaky stuff. And it appears the longer she is in the situation of living with such a revered member of society, the harder it is for her to feel worthy. While he is told he'll get another chance in tomorrow's surgery, or that the patient would have died anyway, she is told her failure is her fault, and inherently she is bad.

Perfectionism is one way the cycle continues. In its attempt to relieve anxiety and insecurity, it eventually causes depression and failure. Since she can never be perfect, the more she tries and fails and the less secure her sense of her own abilities, the more other people want her to be perfect, the more she attempts to make it true. Ultimately she withdraws in a deep sense of despair and depression at having failed to live up to the requirements of her job as a good doctor's wife. "Dr. Jones' wife does this so much better," she may believe, and that feels even worse.

A combination of forces in marriage to a male medical professional makes solid self-esteem almost impossible. Never will society view your job, your talent, your motivation, your feelings as highly as that of a physician.

Even if perfection is possible — and it is not — a perfect doctor's wife will not equal her mate in influence and power under any circumstances. An imperfect male doctor will always have greater value than his imperfect female spouse. She then is doomed to being second class and valued less, if noticed at all.

MARTYRDOM AND SACRIFICE:
THY GUILT IS OVERFLOWING

I was raised on guilt
Upon awakening it was in the air
For breakfast it was next to the cereal bowl
All through the day it was as close as
    my touch.

Next to guilt, sacrifice went hand in hand
If I didn't eat my cereal
the starving Europeans would be in more pain
If I balked at practicing the piano
I was quickly reminded how much my parents gave up
    so I could learn to play.

It hurts now to recall the things my
Mother did sacrifice for us
She never went to school past high
She never wrote her book
Or sang her songs of freedom
Or danced on the stage of life.

My father sacrificed his time with us
to work outside the home
He gave up fun and games
to provide us with clothing and shelter.

They didn't laugh hysterically together
Life was too hard
and there was too much to feel guilty about.

It's okay, I'll stay home with the children
I'll miss the concert this time
the children are more important
than my soul and feeding it with music.

It's okay, said he. The children need
new coats and books for school
I won't go fishing this time

take the money and give it to them
My pleasure can wait till next time.

Guilt, Martyrdom and Sacrifice
A way of life for us
Jewish, East Coast, second generation
We had to atone for a lot
All the Jews who suffered and died before us
All who had less than we
I learned that nothing comes easily
Nothing is taken for granted.

What I didn't realize is that
Women were better at martyrdom than men
We were told to sacrifice so that
Our men might succeed.
If we denied ourselves and helped to provide
then we could survive as silent
sacrificing partners in life's not so
    funny joke.

If I sacrificed and became a martyr
In my marriage then I was called
    a masochist
My mother was never called that
She was like Joan of Arc in all her glory.

If I employed tactics to
make people feel guilty and beholden to me
I was called passive aggressive or
    angry or hostile or something unseemly
My mother was never called that
She was holy in all her glory.

I don't really understand
I thought I learned well
to sacrifice my self, my inner being
so that those around me would flourish
I only looked downtrodden sometimes
I only reminded everyone of my trials on occasion.

Where did I go wrong?
I feel a failure somehow
I was raised on guilt and martyrdom
and infused with sacrifice as if by blood
and yet as I grow older
it is less appreciated
It is seen as unhealthy and manipulative.

Where did I go wrong?
No one pays homage to me properly
all the times and hours I gave up
the refusals to accept what was my due
I thought it would make people happy
to know what sacrifices I made.

Actually it hasn't really made me happy
Nor has it explained the mysteries of the world
The fact that some have and some have not
Is the same as it was for my parents
None of our forfeiture changed a thing.

Except perhaps a brief but powerful sense of
    being above it all
As if we could protect ourselves
From the centuries of assault
By guarding our pleasures with the pain of
momentary martyrdom.

Chapter 10

Jealousy:
Where Has My Ambition Gone?

I see how much being a doctor has helped Tim. He's got confidence and social awareness he'd never have had without people calling him "Doctor." Lucky him. — Rosemary

Among the many interesting women I interviewed one stands out as I consider the jealousy factor. We met a few times over a period of six months, alternating between her home and various local restaurants where we shared luncheon or afternoon tea. She was intrigued with the idea for my book, but always qualified her responses with how healthy her relationship was and that without great respect and good communication between a couple, a relationship will never work.

Tanya, now 44 years old, was brought up in a strict Germanic home. Her parents and grandparents came here to escape Hitler's oppressive politics when Tanya was very young. She was reared in an environment where education was valued above all else. At the time she and her future husband met, Tanya was teaching at the medical school where Grant was studying to become a specialist in neurosurgery.

While Grant was in medical school, Tanya continued her studies toward a PhD in biochemistry and worked. When they married she was 27. She became pregnant fairly soon and stopped her own career pursuits. "After my first pregnancy, I quit my studies and until now never looked back at exchanging my doctoral studies for marriage to a doctor." She shared the difficulties of long, long years of Grant's surgical preparation and training. He didn't work as a physician until well into his mid-thirties. Eventually they had three children: two sons and one daughter. During our interviews she often switched from talking about her husband to her children, but had difficulty focusing on herself. "Children of physicians have it very hard because their parents expect so much of them. Just like my parents expected so much of me, I suppose," she said.

While teaching at the prestigious medical school in the midwest, Tanya was awed by the caliber of students she encountered. Her husband "was one of the brightest."

> They had to be so dedicated and work almost inhumanly to keep up with their studies. We fell in love and have shared our love of hard work, learning, and achievement, and I guess we've passed it on to our kids because they are very active and accomplished people also.

The long years of Grant's training were "terribly lonely and stressful" for her, raising small children and no longer having her own connection with academics. "But we always talked things out," she continued. "I was so in awe of what Grant was doing and have always felt that he and his life were so exciting that it kept me going." Repeatedly during our talks Tanya referred to their life together as "a partnership." His education and residency and fellowship were referred to consistently as "ours." "We could never have withstood those grueling training years were it not for our commitment and good communication."

Tanya had clearly put aside her dream of a major scientific discovery of her own, almost without awareness of the dream's disappearance. It had escaped unbeknownst to her. Her focus consciously changed to her husband's career and her children's lives. She denied stifling her own ambition, and she also unqualifiably denied being jealous or envious of Grant's ability to finish studies and become a very successful physician. She is aware of her support of him and feels that she contributed greatly to his success. Once they settled into their home community and Grant began practicing, she utilized her great skills at entertaining and organizing, became involved in Junior League, the women's medical auxiliary, and has been on numerous boards to improve the community's access to artistic and other cultural events.

Tanya describes herself as a perfectionist and a "true super-woman." She continued:

> What people in the late '80s are calling superwoman I have been, I guess, since I married Grant, especially while I was in school, teaching, supporting Grant through his training, nursing kids, helping to establish his career, and maintain my activities in the community as they were necessary. I don't understand what the women are complaining about — all doctors' wives take on a big load, especially while they have to financially support the doctor and the kids till he finishes his training.
>
> Only recently have I become obviously restless. I just restored a wonderful old home and decorated it for Grant to use as his new office.

She shared that biochemistry, architecture, and interior design were all areas of study for her as a student.

As we talked I observed the all too familiar tears filling her eyes. She cited distress with one of her teenage children, overwork, and less availability of her husband as causes.

> I need a smooth running household. In fact, I have always gone to great lengths to keep it that way. I guess I need to manipulate my life better so that I feel less drained and stressed.

After some time for reflection, Tanya shares that she can never talk to anyone, "Even my parents. No one understands."

This woman, on her way to a double PhD, obviously extremely intelligent and ambitious as a young woman, continues to express her ambition and creativity through support and at times even total organization of her husband's career. Freud might have called it sublimation — denial of her own needs and vicariously living them through another.

Not until her mid-life, when her children are almost grown, is she getting restless and inexplicably frustrated with life. Enthusiasm for her husband's success and activities is waning, and she doesn't understand her restlessness. Try as she might, creative efforts through her husband's work are no longer as exciting as they were. She cannot allow herself to feel jealousy; rather, she still describes what she experiences as "awe of doctors—the time they commit and the intelligence they require."

"What about your intelligence?" I ask.

> It doesn't feel very important or valuable right now. Oh, I know it was there. I kept up with my colleagues when I taught in the medical school. But I have been away from the books for a long, long time.

Tanya never admitted to feelings of regret for her stilted career. She never even thought that those years of encouragement and "partnership" in her husband's career could have been utilized to further her career, and she may even have forgotten about the possibility of making an exciting scientific discovery or two on her own.

Other women were able to express jealousy, even rage, at the redirection or loss of their personal ambition. Women of my generation stated that the choice was clear—one's ambitions were nurtured vicariously. I never entertained the idea of my becoming a doctor or lawyer (my father's profession, you will recall). I was discouraged from becoming a secretary by my mother, who felt that office work was a demeaning profession. And yet that same mother, for whom only teaching and nursing would do for a woman, thought marriage to a doctor was great! Now it's funny: to be my husband's secretary, cook, and laundress was quite respectable in her mind. To be a secretary, earning wages, involved as a producer to the economy, was not respectable. I never learned to type because of that attitude! But I digress. However, my mother was a perfect example of a woman whose ambitions were choked off and killed without her even knowing it. In similar ways her marriage to a lawyer was for her the only viable fulfillment of her ambition.

But my mother never went to college. What of this class of women; the wives of physicians, who have gone to college and often have graduate educations? What of their ambitions?

In their excellent book, *Between Women*, Eichenbaum and Orbach (1989) suggest using jealousy to signal the want of our own to which we are not attending. If we feel envy of what another has, rather than ignoring these feelings or deriding ourselves for the experience, we should use the chance to discuss them, clear the air, and then use the information to figure out what buttons are being pushed. Why are we reacting so strongly? Because we probably inherently know that we too would like the achievement, success, power and creative expression of those of whom we are jealous.

The jealousies between women married to physicians are the feelings that keep the women from comfortably sharing with one another. The feelings are strong but at times inexplicable. I contend that those envies and jealousies are a displaced frustration among women who are unable to truly express their own creative impulses. Until very recently, they have been unable to achieve economic success in a society which values contributing to the economy, not just consuming (Holmstrom 1973; Fowlkes 1980). The jealousy among each other tends to mask the personal difficulty of facing the underlying envy of the men for whom all their energy has been spent.

Younger wives coming from college and postgraduate schools and medical schools are more apt to fulfill personal ambitions for achievement. They will try harder to arrange their lives with physician husbands so that they too can pursue their chosen professions. But try as they may, they are by no means choosing an easy route.

Olivia, a medical student herself and newly married to a resident, describes her dilemma:

> My mother gave up a career as a singer and actress to raise us and to take care of my father, who was a pediatrician. I am terrified of losing my sense of direction like she did. Would you believe that she said that to her it was enough to see my brother and I become something? She said she wasn't a great singer anyway and her acting left a lot to be desired. My mother gave up! She became a wimp under my father's thumb. If he called or snapped his fingers, she jumped. Jealous? She never said she was jealous of my father, his freedom, his earnings, his prestige; but I think she saw herself as his shadow anyway. Why be jealous of your shadow?
>
> For me, always feeling sorry for the authority my father had

over her and the kids and observing how what he worked for in
medicine always seemed so much more important than what
we wanted—I knew when I was ten years old there was no
way I wasn't going to be a doctor. Girl or not, female or not.
Years of school. I didn't care. I became obsessed with what I
thought was associated with being a doctor! I experienced my
mother's jealousy and ambition for her, I guess. If a man can
do it and have it, so can a woman, I thought. To me, being a
doctor was power and prestige, making decisions for oneself
and following whatever internal drives were calling. You
know, my mother even stopped singing after a while. I remember when I was tiny she sang to us all the time. Later the
music stopped. Well, my music won't stop.

My marriage to Travis caught me by surprise. A doctor,
another doctor in my house! But I'm hoping to be his equal. I
won't have to envy his success or accomplishments; I'll be
contributing my own and receiving recognition for them. He's
aware of my attitudes and he's aware of the generation in
which we are living. Both people can, should, and do work
outside the home if they choose.

At this point I was about ready to let Olivia sit down and write
this book. She was fiery, excited, and committed to making her life
fuller than her mother's. The "deadening" of her mother wasn't to
be her future. She continued:

My mother's generation gave up. Her friends consoled themselves by buying more or taking pills or drinking at the golf
course. When Travis and I disagree we talk or yell until we
both feel resolved. We will take turns with household work,
and child rearing when that time comes. I do not intend to
work part-time in pediatrics like the other women doctors I
know in my class. Or if I have to cut my hours, so will Travis
cut his, or this won't work!

Olivia made me uncomfortable with her lack of empathy for her
mother. Or for women who could not achieve the equality that she
hoped for. She didn't seem to be aware that the choice was not there
for her mother like it is for her. For her mother, as for Tanya, whom

we heard from earlier, personal ambition was a characteristic frequently unknown to women, or at least unacceptable in their
psyches.

Generations of women were derided and punished for acting on
personal ambition. The most her mother and her mother's friends
could hope to achieve was the personal satisfaction of making a
good home and, if lucky, to rear healthy, stable children. Their
sense of accomplishment was to come only from how much they
gave and how well they supported the men in their lives. To do
otherwise was selfish, unwomanly, and very threatening to their
survival.

So jealousy was and still is a difficult emotion for us. If to be
womanly is to nurture and give to our men, their success is our
reward. In a world where doing a good job and being rewarded for
it gives us great personal satisfaction; where up until recently and
even today doctors' wives are not allowed the privilege of working
for pay because of their husbands' earning power; and where their
work has been unpaid support and promotion of his career and care
of his home and family and hence his personal satisfaction — what in
the world do we have to be jealous about? Nothing, unless of course
what Olivia is enjoying: the freedom to choose!

Chapter 11

Kids, Who Remembers the Color of Your Father's Eyes?*

THE CHILD BLOSSOMS ANYWAY

How does the flower grow
from a mere seedling put in the earth
the magic there bewilders me

Is there a difference between flowers
and children
Would the seed sprout if it were stepped on
    trounced stomped and battered
Watered some and then forgotten
    I doubt it.

Would the seed sprout if all it felt were
    sounds of anger, bitterness and hate
Flowers are gentle and delicate — they require
    the combination of sunshine, rain and food
they need shelter from harsh storms and
    flooding
they need protection from too much
    sunlight and heat

Their time of blossom is short to us but
        ever so radiant
Just like a child's — if we choose to see it

---

*I have included the chapter on children in this section as the reality in male physician medical families is that children are the mother/wife's experience.

Food, sunshine and water
  not harsh storms of criticism
 or the intense heat of an angry hand.

Children grow more like cactus, starthistle   ,
            or chickory
they grow in spite of us
with proper care or without
Suddenly they've blossomed right before our eyes

If the water was only there sometimes
and the light and food withheld or
    not generously given
if they never knew what it was to trust
and their world was unsteady around them.

The color of their blooms may be pale
the sound of their voice may quiver
Bitterness may be in their heart
and sadness fill their spirit

But unlike the flower, the child grows to adulthood
    even when conditions were wanting
His body survives almost anything
We just don't know about his soul

A flower withers and dies when physical needs are
            unmet
A child is strong of skin
She holds out for another day
    hoping for care and understanding

To be a child is to put all one's being into
            the arms of grown-ups
to trust that grown-ups know her
vulnerability and will protect and cherish it.

If unwatered, unfed and uncared for
the child still grows, looking

searching for those things not forthcoming
    for answers to why

Was it me — did I not deserve the
        nourishment
    What did I do?

Perhaps the flower is lucky. I suspect
    it doesn't know why it has thorns
        or petals
    or may have grown unlike the others.

A child soon becomes a grown-up and thinks and wonders
Not understanding makes him
    continue the cycle
Not knowing makes her ill and weak

But they both grow up
and they both continue to need
        water, sunshine and food
            protection and love
    Always.

If you were to ask my four sons what it is like to grow up in a
doctor's house, they would probably shrug their very large shoulders, smirk, and say they could see no difference between their
house and anyone else's. Growing up in a New Jersey suburb, their
life seemed much like the neighbors and the friends they acquired
over 16 years in a very typical middle-class suburb on the bus route
to New York City.

Other fathers they knew took the bus very early in the mornings
and commuted to Manhattan to do whatever their business was —
stockbroker, real estate appraiser, company executive. Those fathers came home in droves by train, or in our neighborhood, most
arrived at 6:30 or so by bus. In fact, the men often walked from the
bus stop together in a two- or three-block radius from the station to
their respective houses. So from a child's perspective, growing up
in the suburbs meant only women around during the daylight hours,
and then the march of men when the evening settled on the country-

side, the latter all carrying briefcases and the *New York Times* of the day, or perhaps the *Wall Street Journal*. Those fathers said good-bye to each other as they reached their respective houses and suddenly would disappear inside the front doors. The only time they were seen before the early morning trek to the bus was if it was summer and the grass needed cutting or their sons were playing ball in the streets and they needed an umpire or someone to pitch.

In those days there was one man at home before dark. Mr. Green. He worked a night shift. That household was unusual in the neighborhood. Mrs. Green worked as a secretary during the day and Mr. Green worked in a factory at night. He actually reared his three children. In fact my children always wondered whether he ever slept. He managed to be around any time they wanted to play with one of the Green children. If anyone was hurt or got into trouble, Mr. Green was close at hand to bring everything under control, even if it meant a very unpleasant reprimand for one of my boys. It was predictable and perhaps comfortable because of that.

My children's father was the same as other fathers in not being at home during the daylight hours. Then there were differences. He carried a black bag instead of a briefcase. To the boys, their father was the one who took care of any problem when they were hurt or sick. Not only did he not take a bus to work, but he took a car, a bike, or occasionally walked. Then he was an unusual person. Exercise was important to him before the world recognized the importance of keeping fit.

My boys recall trips to their father's office with a mixture of delight, impatience, and trepidation, depending of course on the reason for the trip. Their favorite part about the office was what they referred to as "the doctor supplies." They often took home reams of bandages, cotton balls, tongue depressors, and gauze squares. In fact the younger children became experts at making unusual buildings and unrecognizable artifacts with medical supplies.

There were, however, trips for medical check-ups. Getting shots was always a horrendous experience. Each boy handled the ordeal according to his personality. But none, whether brave, squeamish, stoic, or vociferous, ever got used to being dragged into Daddy's office for a shot that was deemed appropriate by the doctor himself.

At times I took them to the office to see their father as a way of increasing our already limited exposure to him and myself. If we showed up on the steps or the waiting room of the office, perhaps that would speed up Dad's work day and quicken his pace so that we could get on with the business of being parents and have an enjoyable time together with our sons.

The kids again responded according to their personalities. One might fret nervously about being in the same office where only days before he'd had pain inflicted upon him, and another would play with equipment or supplies and amuse himself innocently and happily until we were all ready to leave. Another probably asked questions incessantly about the office, and tried to follow his dad around and inhale all the information about doctoring that he could handle or his dad could tolerate. The other child may have been impatient and bored at having nothing to do there without his friends, or perhaps he brought homework or interesting reading to entertain himself during what may have turned out to be an excruciatingly long wait.

Their dad would keep popping his head into their place of safekeeping to say, "Hello," and "It won't be long." I suspect he also was keeping track of the potential damage his boys were doing to the office. There was always a sense that Jerry's partners were ogres, and even though they all had children of their own, they were unable to understand the anticipated behaviors of four healthy boys. Somehow our sons were to behave themselves in Dad's office, respect the important supplies, and keep their voices down in the waiting room or in the back offices because someone was sick and couldn't be disturbed.

Then there were the white coats and white uniforms on the doctors and nurses in the office. They were frightening to my children, maybe more than to others whose fathers weren't in the business. Not only did the uniforms mean a painful experience, but to children of physicians they meant that extraordinarily good behavior was essential or they would be thought of poorly, or worse, their father would soon return and threaten something frightening.

To a doctor's child a threat of, "I'll take you to the doctor," or "You'll get a shot if you don't behave," is not even necessary. In fact I always cringed when other mothers used those words in or out of a doctor's office to keep their children's behavior under control.

What a cruel way to threaten a child, I mumbled to myself. Little did I realize that my children didn't need to hear the words. To them there was always the possibility that real or imagined debts would be repaid by some painful treatment in the office of their father, the doctor. I can only begin to imagine how often they blamed their own behaviors or thoughts when they were receiving routine medical treatment. They must have concluded that they were terrible people or they wouldn't need this medicine or these shots.

The other side of their very thorough medical care is the reality that it was a sure way of seeing and interacting with their dad. Today, even 3,000 miles away and in their late twenties, if there is something physically troubling any one of these young men or their partners, they call their dad for help.

They saw neighbors bring sickness or accidents to our home, and watched their dad take charge. They saw a heroism and a respect from other adults that other people's fathers were not receiving. Yet, once one of my boys said that he wished his father could throw a baseball like Rick's father. Another questioned why his dad didn't have time to be a scout leader.

From my perspective the word of my children's father was so authoritarian and so final that none of us questioned it. A physician develops a style of interacting, an air of knowing, that no one dares question. He needs that attitude to get his patients to follow his treatment orders. Consequently he brings that air of no questioning and definitiveness home to his children. If Dad says it's so, then there is no room for inquiry or other possibilities.

My father was a lawyer, an articulator, yet I can recall bantering and debating issues or openly disagreeing with a thought or theory of his. We laughed about that often. I'm not certain my children had that privilege. If Jerry gave an opinion or stated a proposal, it was interpreted as a directive and was not often necessary to repeat.

Things which involved the entire family were done Jerry's way. Getting ready for trips was a traumatic time which the kids still joke about. It was called "Dad's trip mode." They describe him as assuming another personality: nervous, list obsessed, and tyrannical with instructions until we reached our destination.

The children actually became quite astute at picking up personal idiosyncrasies of their father and me. They said generally that their father required much more accommodation than I. Probably as in other families of the day, I was the primary caretaker and could be easily persuaded or influenced. Their dad, however, spent little time with them in their waking hours, and what time they had was serious, not to be tampered with by experimentation or joviality. Actually since they and he have matured, they find much more time for relaxation and frivolity.

So what does it mean to have a doctor for a father? Some quotes from children six to 18 years of age:

> Whenever I'm hurt, my dad brings home the medicine to fix me.

> My dad goes on emergencies and takes care of people.

> He can't come to father-son night. He's in the hospital, helping somebody.

> My mom taught me to play soccer. My dad was too busy.

> My dad is strong and he knows a lot of stuff. People call him all the time.

> We never talked about personal things, just about when my health was involved.

> Other kids got to spend Saturdays with their dad. Mine always was making rounds.

> I remember falling down in my backyard from our jungle gym. My shoulder was killing me and I was trying not to cry. My mom called my dad from the office. He said to bring me right in, and we drove fast. I was hurting so bad. Mom was singing to me in the car. When we got to the office Dad's nurse, Sally, talked nice to me and put me up on a table. Then Dad came in in his white jacket with his name tag on his pocket. He talked quietly, patted my head and wrapped my shoulder with tape. Soon the pain went away and he gave me a toy airplane. I knew then my Dad would always be there to fix me and to fix anything I ever needed.

> Being a doctor's son is fine, except people expect you to be perfect. No drinking, no drugs, always look nice, good

grades. "You're Dr. Jones's boy, aren't you?" they say. I'm proud, but also annoyed. I'm not Dr. Jones's boy. I'm Allen Jones. If I want to be a trouble maker or a singer or go out with three girls at once or yell at a teacher or fail a test or be a race car driver, that's me, Allen Jones. I didn't ask to be a doctor's son. Sometimes I really think being a regular guy's son would have been so much easier. Nobody special. I wouldn't have to be so perfect all the time. I could be a river guide or a pre-school teacher or a bee keeper, and no one would say, "Oh, did you hear Dr. Jones's son is a nothing? How awful for the doctor and his wife. Allen wants to raise bees.

One of my more poignant interviews was with a woman in her forties who had been married 23 years and had three children. Her youngest daughter had become embroiled in the drug scene in early high school years.

My experience with Carolyn and drugs was so unexpected and so devastating I'll need counseling for years. I thought that a doctor's kids would be immune to this kind of hardship. My husband ignored the problem, all the warning signs. To be honest, he wasn't around enough to see behavior changes. Our oldest son was a great student, straight A's, valedictorian, an excellent athlete, handsome, beautiful girlfriend — the envy of all parents. The middle girl was quiet but also lovely. She and her younger sister didn't get along. But Nancy didn't complain or notice anything peculiar about Carolyn until she started taking things from her room. Nancy's clothes and books started disappearing. We got Nancy a lock for her door. Soon Nancy started reporting Carolyn's misdemeanors to me. They even became physical toward each other. Two teenagers, big, healthy girls, and they were physically abusive to one another. I started to talk to Joel [husband] about Carolyn. Her grades dropped. She stopped talking to me. She started banging in doors, ranting uncontrollably at odd times. She wasn't eating or sleeping right. Joel said, "She's a teenager. Ignore her." When the school called five or six times and said Carolyn hadn't shown up, I got scared. I insisted that Joel come to the school counselor. He didn't back me up at the interview. He said I was overreacting, that Carolyn was a great kid, a little rambunctious, but wasn't that normal for a teenager? The counselor directed us toward books on teenage drug use and told us what signs to look for. Joel yelled at the counselor. "Don't you think I'd know if my child were on drugs?" he said. I almost died of humiliation.

This woman (Marion) continued to explain her later education in drug use and abuse among high school students. She went on to educate her community. All the while her daughter's rehabilitation was painful and devastating to her own marriage. Her husband's denial and sense of failure was almost irreparable.

Our relationship with our children had been such that I was in charge of all the practical details — how they looked, their social graces, who they played with, what music they liked, and what books they read. Joel depended on me to be in charge of those things. When Nancy and Carolyn started hitting each other, I was to fix that. When he finally understood that Carolyn was using marijuana and cocaine, he was so horrified and somehow felt I had let him down. He said he had done his job as provider all these years, but he thought I failed as mother to those kids. We're in counseling together. Carolyn's in therapy.

I hope we can heal. At least we can talk about this now. And I'm now realizing that it takes both people to parent children.

Generally the medical profession doesn't encourage parenting on the part of physicians. They parent patients. There is little left for their own children. Only when the children have grown do they realize what they have missed along the way.

Male children who appear to be especially at risk for trouble later grow to be overachievers or underachievers with doubts about their competence. In a telephone communication with a psychologist married to a physician, she shared her fears from her clinical practice in a large medical hospital on the East coast:

I'm really concerned for the children. What I'm seeing more and more is children of doctors in emotional stress, especially boys — anxious, fearful, unable to cope. They are overly concerned about living up to their father's standards and may be too emotionally attached to their mothers. Many have reported physical abuse by their fathers in early childhood and can't deal with that realization as adults. They had the heavy burden of responsibility at home, and see their fathers as unavailable, quick-tempered men, and see their mothers as their only safety between themselves and their father. (Scolaro-Moser, 1989)

Since this is not a treatise in growing up in a physician's house, suffice it to say that often children of physicians are perfectionists, overburdened with responsibility, and overly involved and protective of their mothers or the parent who cares for them. They often feel it impossible to live up to the image of their father the doctor, and are likely to spend their lives either trying to prove their value in whatever job/profession/field they enter, or choosing the profession of medicine themselves, thus continuing the spiral of helping others but not caring for themselves (Derdeyn, 1979; Konner, 1987, Myers, 1988).

MY SON'S BRUSH WITH MEDICINE

During the writing of this book one of my sons was diagnosed as having ulcerative colitis. To me the entire process is worth documenting for posterity. It somehow sheds a poignant light on the plight of the medical family and our painful detachment from realistic feelings. (To protect their privacy, I have changed the names of my son and his partner.)

About one year ago, after some weeks of stomach and intestinal distress (which I would call gas in the lower stomach), Mitchell's partner, Sarah, started calling me and sharing her fears that Mitch should talk to someone about his pains. He was having some diarrhea and was telling her all about these changes in his body, but characteristic of Mitch, he was very reticent to speak to anyone else, especially his father, about his worries.

I guess six or eight weeks went by with Mitch trying different diets and exercise to control his symptoms. It should be noted that around this time Mitch was studying for his comprehensive exams in graduate school and truly thought that once the tests were over the physical distress would leave. He is the type of person who keeps personal feelings very much to himself. He's usually very playful and fun loving; pain is the last thing to which he would attend.

Previous to this Mitch was never concerned or really aware of his body. He is strong, quite handsome, and built sturdily. Until he started losing some hair—which had formerly been thick and black—he, like most young people I suppose, took his health and strength for granted. He is a bit of a perfectionist though, and losing his hair was the first shock to his invulnerable youth. It proved to be the first of more than one change that Mitch would experience about his body and sense of himself.

As if hair loss at 24 wasn't bad enough, threatening his sense of youth, strength, and virility, the symptoms in his colon and intestines would not go away. No amount of denial, diet change, or exercise would spare him the constant distress of diarrhea and bloating. His pants wouldn't close on his previously tight, muscular stomach. He started wearing elastic across the waistband. Still, there was no communication with his father the doctor, who was usually consulted in cases of other household members' health problems.

I started worrying. But I, too, always deferred to Jerry about health questions. I told him what Sarah's concerns were, and Jerry felt he should wait to hear from Mitch. They were playing cat and mouse, each not wanting to make a "big deal" out of these symptoms. Jerry was saying, "Stay out of it." In so many words, "Don't make a sissy out of him," or, "Perhaps if I don't call him he won't really be sick." Mitch was saying, "I'll handle this myself. It's just that I've been eating a more healthy diet, all fruits and vegetables, my body is adjusting." For weeks it was just Sarah and me worrying about Mitch's health. She would call me and say, "I'm scared. Mitch's sick and tells me he's worried, but he won't say anything to his dad or you."

Pesky as I can be, I finally let go of my fear of meddling and talked to both Mitch and Jerry, got them together, and said,

"Talk." Still they needed an interpreter. Mitch would make light of his worries and symptoms, and Jerry would make even lighter of his reaction. However, there was one symptom that could not be ignored — blood in the stools. This was the very symptom that we had heard Jerry ask others about on the phone for years during our dinner hour. At that time it got so that it was a family joke. No more. Now this was a symptom one of our own children was experiencing, and judging by the tone of Jerry's voice, this could be serious.

However, the very peculiar part of all this was that Jerry looked serious, pensive, anguished, but he wasn't talking to us. Nothing. Just, "Mitch, you need to get some tests. Take these stool cards and follow the directions and send in stool samples to my office soon."

"What could be wrong?" I asked, frightened and curious at the same time. I had no knowledge of what "blood in stools" could mean. Totally naive, I expected my husband the doctor to tell me what could be going on. He was immovable, withdrawn, and continued to be silent.

I pressed, "Could he have an ulcer?"

"Yes, maybe. But if it's not . . . " Then he shut up again.

I, of course, was getting aggravated with the mystery and the silence, and the feeling that I was deliberately being patronized and shut out and avoided whenever I pressed further. Finally, "We better talk to Dr. Stone [not real name]. Mitch needs a specialist. I can't take care of him myself," Jerry concluded.

Father and son decided (with respect for father's ultimate judgment on the subject of health care) that Mitch should come to our town for diagnosis and treatment. Yes, there were doctors at the university, but it would be better to come to this more reputable medical center.

Tests were begun: x-rays of colon and intestines, sigmoidoscopic exams — all very rude intrusions into a 24-year-old body. These are humiliating, not-spoken-about exams, probing into dark holes and places that refined people like to pretend don't exist. I have since become aware that colon diseases, including cancer of the colon, probably go undiagnosed and untreated because of our shame and humiliation about that part of our bodies. The anus, rectum, and feces are so loathsome and dirty to us that to have regularly scheduled check-ups and stool sample checks touch our unconscious repulsion and make it impossible to carry through.

I believe now that embarrassment and revulsion horrified Mitch and kept him in a state of denial about his condition. It's not easy to talk about our excretions, especially if in the household we had always covered our own feelings with derogatory humor when patients called with similar symptoms.

Mitch probably would have dealt with other symptoms like headaches. Those are so much more respectable. But to say that, yes, he saw blood in his feces, was both terrifying and embarrassing, a potentially deadly combination. In fact it was the acknowledgment of blood in the stools that provoked Jerry to get Mitch to the proper diagnostician.

Still, no word to me, no matter how I prodded into the meaning of this all. I colluded, terrified for my son and myself. I didn't look up the possible causes for his symptoms. I could have asked another physician or gone to the library. I was frozen. None of us were talking.

The x-rays were complete. The tests over. We went to Dr. Stone's office. Jerry, myself, Mitch, and Sarah all marched in together. Dr. Stone, looking quite solemn and distant, immediately handed Mitch a book entitled *Krone's Disease and Diseases of the Colon* and sat down. "You will not die from this disease," he said. He pointed to his colorful picture of the anatomy and showed us the affected areas of Mitch's body. He continued, "We will keep in touch and I'll want to know your symptoms."

Stunned, we all sat immobilized. What does this all mean, I wondered. No one ever mentioned colitis to me. Ulcer, possibly. That was bad enough. But what is colitis? What do you mean he won't die? What will he have to live with? I wondered.

We were still quiet, waiting. Some reassurance was surely in order, some explanation to a 24-year-old who now is considered defective, imperfect, and afflicted with an embarrassing antisocial condition that keeps him in the bathroom a good part of the day, smelling up the apartment, and who is feeling levels of humiliation and self loathing as a result.

Finally I couldn't keep quiet any more. "Can you do something for him? Isn't there some medicine? And how long? One or two weeks until the medicine works?'' I cried in desperation.

"We have medicines which we can try. They work in 30 percent, but on 66 percent or so percent of the population *there is no cure*. We can only experiment with help for the symptoms." He continued cooly, clinically, "You will probably not have to be hospitalized or probably won't need a colostomy." What? Again indescribably horrified, I chimed in. This doctor, without ever talking to Mitch in his life, had quoted statistics, horror stories, and the worst case scenario about the potential for Mitch's body and future. He had taken all of our hope away and left us speechless, no questions to ask, no thoughts or possibilities to pursue!

"Are there any other questions?" he continued.

To my astonishment, my husband, Jerry the doctor, was stone silent. My savior, Mitch's protector, our connection to God when it comes to our health care, spoke not a word. Just sitting there, I thought at the time, he's colluding with the specialist to keep us in the dark.

Later I realized Jerry could not deal with the diagnosis. He was totally denying the fact of his son's illness and future with a chronic disease. We were all devastated and so into our own selfish responses that Mitch, who is so reserved anyway, was almost overlooked in the picture. He asked some questions about medication. He and Dr. Stone, so alike in their clinical approach to statistics (Mitch is a computer scientist, quite analytically minded), quietly decided on a schedule of medication to start with. "And if the symptoms get very bad we can put you on high doses of steroids. Let's first see how you do on the sulfa drug."

That was the first of what was to be many semisatisfying communications between Mitch, Dr. Stone, our family, and Jerry. Because Mitch was allergic to the sulfa medication, suffering violent headaches, fever, and rashes, that was no longer a possible way to control the colitis. It had been the most hopeful choice for treating the chronic condition. The search would continue for a control. We learned that no one understands the cause of the illness and there is no cure — from the book, I might add; no information was forthcoming from the physician, either specialist or father-doctor. Silence, brooding, and noncommunication were the modus operandi.

Mitch has undergone testing with three different medications in over a year, none with satisfactory results. That is to say, if one symptom is deviated, a side effect such as headache, weakness, acne, depression, or agitation is so overpowering that diarrhea seems a tolerable alternative.

Since that first visit to the specialist's office, our family has rallied to assist Mitch. Spending hours in the libraries of major universities and medical hospitals, Mitch's brothers have tried to get updated information, experimental or otherwise, on this previously unknown to us condition. Mitch has since then taken charge of his illness to a greater extent. When I recall the look on his face that first night at home with only a book to explain what could be a future with colitis, the despair, confusion, and sadness remain as vivid in my memory as if it were today.

It took Jerry months to begin to talk about the colitis, the treatment, the feelings of hopelessness and impotence he was experiencing.

Sarah spent hours talking about the fears she had about Mitch and her relationship to him. She was used to being the one getting the attention. She relied on Mitch to be strong and healthy to carry much of the load in their relationship. Now she would have to look beyond herself and her feelings to attend Mitch and provide support and courage if she could.

Mitch's self-concept is still at risk. He is still studying for qualifying exams at school. He is still not apt to comfortably share information about himself and his feelings and the experience of his life.

We are more adjusted to the idea of colitis today than one year ago. Still, I am poignantly aware of how easy it is to become a disease once labeled as its victim. I cry inside when I see how hard it is to forget that for Mitch he is no longer taking his body for granted. True, he now deals with Dr. Stone himself and with the university health center in his town for treatment. He keeps up with the latest available research materials. He questions everything about medications, side effects, diet, and has begun to see that he can have some power and control over his body, his health, and his medical care. He is more at ease now, back to having fun. When not feeling particularly ill, he plays, and the glint in his eye has returned.

He loves to call me with information that might be suitable for this book, like, "Mom, listen to this. At the Health Center at school the doctor I was talking to about getting medicine up here didn't realize I could hear her phone conversation as she spoke to a colleague. She said, 'This young man needs the medication but his case is further complicated by the fact that his specialist is in M-ville, and also his father is a doctor!'" Mitch continued to explain that she was agitated and showed great consternation in her voice, as if the father-doctor connection was to be a real trial in this case.

To my son's credit, his spirit, patience, and general well-being have allowed him to rise above the tribulations of his bout with "the medicine" and our reactions. He has put up with confusion, fear, mystery, cold and distant communications, hopelessness, and powerlessness, all from the usually powerful, all-knowing profession. He has watched his father and me in combat, in denial, in collusion, and later in painful but supportive communication about his illness. He has struggled to change his view of his body, his health care and maintenance, his self-image, and his relationship to Sarah. As a family, we frantically feed him information of varying degrees of usefulness from whatever sources are available — self-help, visualization, meditation, holistic treatments — all in opposition to Jerry's training and professional alignment, and against our training as a traditional medical family. To his credit Mitch has put up with our conflicts and gone on to discover for himself the strengths and weaknesses in the present system of health care. He is well aware that he is both privileged and prejudiced as a doctor's son.

Mitch has helped me to better define some personal issues with the medical profession and the medical marriage and family. There were moments in my horror of the detachment of Dr. Stone on the first, second, and third visits (when Mitch finally insisted that he be in charge and that he no longer wanted an entire family in the doctor's office with him) when I saw Dr. Stone's bewilderment and despair. He shared in a moment of true humanity when I said, "Will [first name is traditional to use as a doctor's wife], what do you usually offer to families and patients with colitis?" and he responded, "Esther, I don't really know what to offer them. In fact I should probably talk to a counselor about how frustrating this job can be sometimes." What an admission, I thought.

As I re-read this, I recognize my detachment revealed in the choice of words and my clinical recall. The pain of a mother's never-ending sense of responsibility to her child is still hard to face. In spite of my rage at the profession to which I have been married for 30 years, neither I nor my son are immune to illness and despair. My poem expresses my feelings more easily.

MY CHILD IS SICK

Anyone who ever heard the cry
   of a wounded bird
Knows the agony of a child who's ill.

What they can't know is the mother's view
   inside her gut is wrenched
with helpless and blinding impotence.

I was blessed with children
strong of will and body.
Never did I fear beyond my capacity
that they would not be well.

Measles, mumps and chicken pox
took them one by one.
Even an ear drum poked through
but I knew in time he'd heal.

All in their turn grew big and strong
keen of eye and mind
but then my placid calm blew up
in a storm I could not survive.

An illness struck unknown to me
for which I was told there is no cure.
A young man with his whole life ahead.
I'm not certain we will all endure.

Selfish of me to worry
about how I would survive the news.
He was feeling the pains and taking the pills
yet my cries were louder than his.

How often I questioned the sense of it all.
Why not give me a chronic disease?
Why a young man with all of life's joys
in front of him yet to be spent?

Was there no protection from something so raw
his insides churning, burning and red.
Inflamed, they said, just like my heart
    when they told me the news.

My rage would not be contained.
How dare my boy be the one.
He's innocent in all this,
a fun-loving, brilliant, jovial son.

It's not possible for him to be sick.
Of what am I really afraid?
Does his illness make me look bad?
Am I to blame, responsible somehow?

Is he not perfect, after all?
Am I powerless to help him adjust?
Does he want or need my help?
Or is my silent love enough?

What does he really think
struck at age twenty-four
worried now about his health
thoughts that never touched him before?

Yes he talks of it now.
He's not so shy.
Yes he feels better, no he's not going to die.

Pills maybe forever
Forever reminded of human frailty
Forever to see that no matter how perfect
How taken for granted

No matter how hard I try to take the pain away
The ache when he looks pale or tired,
It has to be his health, his body, his will
His struggle to survive.

We are, after all, alone
Though a mother's bond is so intense
The cord so tightly wound.
No matter how I try to reconcile,
My son's illness is my own.

Perhaps there was something to be learned from this cruel touch of fate. I got to put into action some of the communication and partnership techniques that I am advocating. I revealed honest concern and fears to Jerry, Mitch, Dr. Stone, and Sarah throughout this experience.

We go on. We try. We ask. We learn, and hopefully we change and affect those around us in ways that can improve life for all concerned.

Chapter 12

When I Am Ill:
A Shoemaker's Child

Doesn't being married to a doctor take the scariness out of being sick? —from a friend working out with me in a fitness class.

When I'm ill, it's important that I be able to complain, feel a little sorry for myself, worry, be afraid, ask questions, and be waited on hand and foot. As these needs were ignored by Jerry, glossed over and made light of, I attributed his coolness to "sick people overload." "After a day of dealing with the world's unhealthy, who wants to come home and care for a sick wife?" I thought.

The logical assumption is that a doctor is the best person to have on hand when one is ill. He is around illness and pain all the time. Nevertheless, when there is sickness at home, the hat of professionalism, detachment, and diagnostician remains. The notion of his caring for his family members is at once threatening, frightening, and maybe intolerable.

Through the years I realized that doctoring is different from nursing, and never the twain shall meet when it comes to the doctor's family. Nurturing, comforting, plumping pillows, and making chicken soup are nursing tasks. Doctoring tasks are investigating symptoms, making diagnoses, and prescribing medication. The soft, feeling aspects of health care are foreign to doctors. Early medical training teaches by implication that these methods are unscientific, inadequate, and beneath professional dignity, and, very incidentally, "feminine" tasks.

The code of professional ethics is unclear and inconsistent when family members are at stake. Sometimes it is acceptable for the doctor to treat his family, but if the diagnosis is uncertain or the illness out of his specialty, off the patient goes to a colleague. As a doctor's wife, when I'm ill I'm never sure if I'm his wife or a patient. Perhaps then, I'm both.

Inside medical circles it is an accepted fact that doctors are the worst patients. Jerry is both charming and alarming when he's sick. He was diagnosed with pneumonia in our first year of marriage. I discovered he needed 24-hour care from me, his mother, and all the professionals at his disposal. I was worried and unsure of my nursing abilities. His fears about his health and illness (as a medical student) were highly demanding, and his health condition had greater importance than any other illness in our household. I did not understand that for years.

During times of personal illness I developed a built-in radar system; if a symptom rears its ugly head (runny nose, sneezing), I instinctively know the response from Jerry will be, "Take an aspirin," or if there's no fever, "Drink liquids and go to bed." If I have a stomach pain, baking soda sipped slowly pops into my head. "Don't go on about it, be brief," he seems to say, "and then forget it."

I learned to be my own doctor and nurse, which has its merits considering today's focus on holistic health and being in charge of one's body. Nevertheless, needing warmth and advice from the highly trained expert and receiving cool detachment instead was crushing. I was sent to another doctor whenever there were questions — "I can't be objective about my own family." That too was frightening and unsatisfactory, and was the beginning of my treatment as an object by strangers in the field of medicine.

Women agreed most (over 80 percent of those interviewed) on the subject of their health care. I can see Elaine, an energetic woman in her thirties, mother of two, married 12 years. We came to the subject of how it feels when she's ill, and after some deliberate thought or digging for a repressed concept, she said:

> That is something I don't even like to think about. After all, Rick is in gynecology, so something other than that area is not his domain. But I can't go to him for OB or GYN [obstetric or gynecological] care either. [Presumed unprofessional or un-

ethical to treat your wife.] And any other health care problem he is uncomfortable with. . . . I hate to get sick. Actually, I'm afraid to death to get sick. It's more like I have to protect him when I'm sick. So it's a lot better to ignore my feelings or nurse myself back. What if I ever really have a terrible disease and need him? I don't want to think about it.

I am reminded of the threatening sense that I and other doctors' wives suffer with personal illness. There is a proper protocol. Behaving a certain way is acceptable: no crying, no display of fear or anguish over one's well-being, no questioning of *any* physician's word.

Joan, in her second marriage, just had a severe bout with possible breast cancer. She held back tears and was terribly anxious when describing the details of her trauma:

> Walter deals with the sick and the almost dead every day of his life. He wouldn't take me seriously when I expressed fear about a lump in my left breast. "Don't disturb me now. We'll talk about it later," was his answer. I'd heard so much understanding from him when talking to other doctors or during phone calls to his patients . . . real concern, feeling. Everyone loves him because he's so caring.

She became more agitated and angry, and as she spoke, veins were popping in her neck. She seemed self-conscious and surprised by the extent of her feelings. She continued:

> I finally made an appointment with Walt's colleague, behind his back, feeling scared and guilty to be overriding his opinion, but I was a wreck! Maybe it was nothing, but it is my breast and a lump is a lump. I had to have the lump removed and biopsied, and all the time Walt pretended that I was overreacting, "being a baby!" I felt rotten, so worried about hurting his ego as a doctor, going over his head, and all the time knowing my life could be in danger. There was no cancer, thank goodness, but now I'm so hurt and shocked that I won't trust Walt for a long while. He won't talk about it and he acts as if I've done the whole thing to purposely humiliate him in

front of his co-doctors. That was six months ago. We both keep quiet about it now.

For those of us who thought we'd have easy access to health care, reality sets in quickly and quietly.

In an excellent article by Gilly West entitled, "Doctors' Wives: Poor Little Rich Girls of American medicine," the author describes the hazards of being ill when married to a physician. In her interviews, West discovered that wives are considered malingering or "a crock" until proven "sick" (p. 287). One of the big problems West illuminated was the husband overriding the treating physician's prescriptions, by ignoring, belittling, or actually prescribing other treatment for his wife.

My favorite personal scenario is the trip to another doctor's office for my regular gynecological exam. I go to see the doctor Jerry recommends. When I get to the office and fill out the patient form, my husband's name and profession are included. "Oh, Mrs. Nitzberg, we'll be right with you," says the saccharine receptionist. With a waiting room of people, they call me immediately into the back to wait in an examining room. At that moment I feel both embarrassed by the privilege that gets me in ahead of everyone else, yet relieved that I don't have to wait like the regular population.

The nurses are patronizing. A doctor's wife, it seems, is to be outwardly respected and inwardly reviled and envied. So I pick up the complicated messages and as usual try to put the nurses and the office personnel at ease. I have to be likeable. It's important to me that they realize I'm a regular person. However, in so doing, I feel uncomfortable showing weakness or vulnerability and tend to joke about being afraid of the examination, the findings, or the entire experience. What they don't realize is the visit to the doctor is probably more mysterious and frightening to me than to anyone. I successfully block out my trepidations and go through the ordeal like a good sport.

Having waited undressed for what seems like hours—even though I've been pulled from the outside waiting room as a courtesy to my husband—inside, in the examining room, I wait interminably. When the doctor enters, he begins with small talk, "I hear you and Jerry went . . . How are you?" But no time is left to answer. He examines me. I'm fine. And he'll call Jerry right away with the results. Humiliating—I'm not there at all—a piece of flesh, no mind, no spirit. What about my feelings? What about my thoughts? "Have Jerry call me if there are any problems," he concludes. I'm stunned! I dress again, try to deny the whole experience, act adorable and cheerful to the staff and extremely grateful to the doctor. You see, I also don't pay for this visit (professional courtesy, as it's known in the field). I'm indebted for all of their generosity, even though I truly feel my treatment was perfunctory, and in fact, given with suppressed hostility.

Later, at home, Jerry treats my visit indifferently and maintains the mystery by saying that he'll speak to my doctor about the findings.

Many doctors have said, "You're a great patient, Esther." The birth of four babies, and always the doctor boasts proudly to Jerry that I'm a fabulous patient. I never felt that there was any other choice. Do it that way or look bad for myself and my husband. "Don't ever make trouble. Don't humiliate."

Professional courtesy means no charge or a reduced charge to families of doctors. We all know that I'm not paying, so unconsciously the service I get doesn't have to be the same as for paying patients. This is reminiscent of the reverse discrimination of the welfare patient. In subtle ways the anger of office personnel and the doctor for not getting paid in full for services rendered is taken out on the patient—me. If the patient is a doctor's wife, the treating doctor ultimately answers to the patient's husband (West, 1984).

There is a saying among doctors that if something is to go wrong it will be with a doctor's wife. So everyone is on edge. What are the ramifications of that philosophy for the wife? She enters the office or the hospital knowing she's more likely to have something go wrong. The doctor, nurses, and her husband are all on guard. A self-fulfilling prophecy?

My first baby, Jimmy (now 30), was born totally unattended in the labor room at Lying Inn Hospital, University of Pennsylvania, Philadelphia. He literally popped out onto the bed while I was dazed by medication. No one was with me at the time. As if it were yesterday, I recall the fear, even while I was under sedation, that Jimmy would fall onto the floor and be killed. Jerry was horrified, as was the obstetrician (now dead), who was apologetic and embarrassed. (Though the implication was that this was that this was not so surprising for a doctor's wife!) The code between the doctors was silence. They tried to make light of it. Fortunately, Jimmy was a strong, healthy baby and I was fine. Only now have I allowed myself to relive the distress of those moments. I remained passive and handed over the problem to Jerry, this, after all, was his profession, he'd know what to do.

My own experience might seem coincidental, but I've found through my interviews that similar stories of doctors' wives and their health care are numerous. Jennifer, married to her second husband, describes going to her doctor for a problem with vaginal bleeding, and to her astonishment:

> He told me to forget about it, just have a hysterectomy and I won't be bothered or inconvenienced by this ever again. "Your troubles will be over." Then he said that when he married his present wife, she had been having bothersome cramps and annoying female symptoms for some time. "I simply arranged for her to have a hysterectomy and now that's that!" I was horrified. That poor girl didn't have a chance; once she married Herb [Jennifer's gynecologist] she was at his mercy, medically speaking. Can you imagine a hysterectomy as a wedding present?

Jennifer knew I was writing this book and had hurriedly called me with this piece of her experience.

The reports continue to fill my files: wives afraid to obtain second opinions or question or show the slightest doubt of their husbands' word; the insecurity that comes with little knowledge of the body; information kept at bay; mystery perpetuated; special treatment available; medications readily handed out.

Carol and Patrice, sisters, both married to doctors, agreed to meet with me for lunch. Lunch went into dinner as we became engrossed in our shared experiences. Their simultaneous realizations surprised them. Carol said:

> It seems easier to get all the medications I want, but not so easy to have emotional support when I'm not feeling well.

Patrice added:

> Sometimes I'm convinced that the best way I can get David's attention is to say I'm sick. He asks for some symptoms and gets some medicine for me at the office or drugstore. In a day or two, he checks up by asking how I feel, or says, "You look a lot better today," and that's that. I could have, in fact I do have, the best stocked medicine cabinet anywhere — tranquilizers, pain pills, antihistamines for allergies, lotions for rashes, anything you could want. The truth is, I want David to talk to me and care. That's all.

Women have undergone extensive plastic surgery because it's readily available; either they're married to a surgeon, or a good friend is returning a favor. In contrast are those wives who would elect plastic surgery but feel that they can't undergo any without their husbands' approval and blessings. Either way, making an independent, unbiased choice doesn't seem possible for the doctor's wife. She is conditioned to please or consider someone other than herself.

Emotional aches and pains also are couched in oppression. Communicating feelings of sadness, confusion, and hurt to a doctor-husband is virtually impossible. First the feelings are ignored or minimized; then he expresses more annoyance than understanding. Out of desperation he suggests his wife see a psychiatrist. After all, he doesn't understand, but the sooner it gets fixed the better, so perhaps his friend Joe, the psychiatrist he knew in medical school, can repair her.

Anita was troubled by discontent and confusion for years. She cried easily, seemed angry but unable to face it. She came to my office after seeing three psychiatrists. Her husband of 16 years was also confused. Why didn't she like going to see the psychiatrists? After one visit with them both in my office, I gleaned this from him:

> I can't understand her moods. One minute she's fine, then she's yelling at me. We've ruled out hormones and physical problems. What can I do? I thought Dr. J. [the psychiatrist last seen] would give her something to get her back under control.

Anita said:

> When I go to a psychiatrist they automatically suggest medicine, don't really look at me or listen to me, and make me feel like I'm a real sickie. That's the way Hank [husband] makes me feel—like I'm not okay and he is. If I would take a pill everything would be fine. He could keep working till all hours and I'd stay quiet and be fine.

After a while it was apparent that Anita and Hank had problems common among medical couples. It was not just her problem, but a difficulty in the marriage itself.

How often is the wife sent off to be cured? In the case of the doctor's wife, if she sees another doctor for her care, she may be going from the frying pan into the fire. Or if she and her husband do attend counseling sessions together in a psychiatrist's office, it is likely that the doctor-husband and psychiatrist attempt to preserve the dignity of the values they both hold dear. Unemotionally, silently, logically, they unconsciously collude to medicate her and keep her in the dark. She is overpowered by the presence of men wearing the robes of Hippocrates.

West concludes her research by stating that doctors' wives pay a high price in adjusting to their poor medical care:

> They pay in missed diagnoses . . . feast or famine care . . . and in sacrificing the rights of ordinary patients to choose their doctor, to be informed of the results of tests and reports, and to withhold consent to surgical procedures. (p. 293)

So we have the extremes. On one side is the doctor's wife who is overabsorbed by her health and well-being. She can communicate and feel close to her husband only through his life's work—medicine. She is overtreated, overmedicated, has more surgery than she needs, and spends her time in one or another doctor's office. She is then known as a hypochondriac—obsessed with aches and pains and fearful that disease is present when in reality it is not.

The other end of the spectrum is the doctor's wife who shuns medical care and treatment altogether. She has learned that complaining about her health gets little or no reaction from her husband.

There is no warmth, tender loving care, extra pillow, or flowers to cheer her and help with healing. She totally despises the possibility of disease, perhaps to the detriment of her health. Never going for treatment or delaying it until the last possible moment, she risks her life.

Either option insists that the doctor's wife be silent and compliant. She lives with the threat of being divorced or shunned by their peers and friends in medicine. Whereas the public can now question their health care with the threat of lawsuit or insist on a more equitable voice in their treatment, the doctor's wife is doomed to follow the doctor's prescription to the letter. She is certain her life depends on it.

THE UNDENIABLE MID-LIFE D's

Oh no,
I think something
strange is upon us
Suddenly life is no
longer bright, shiny and cheerful

Last year
at this time
we were feeling fine
looking forward to our future
excited, anticipating what lie ahead

Suddenly
without warning
the big D hit home
Despair, Depression, Disappointment
Disillusionment, Discombobulation and Disgust

What a shock
We never ever talked
about these things before
feelings welling up inside
Instead we went about our lives unscathed

Abruptly
without warning
without a proper sign
we're weeping, irritable, restless

Or angry, destructive and impulsive

Can't cope
Can't cope at all
What do we do now?
Change jobs, change wives
move far away, buy a boat

Is this it?
the mid-life blues
Where did the kids go?
Our parents are back home
We're aging as fast as we can

Oh my God
this is horrible
We're totally unprepared
If we had only known the half
of this insult to our otherwise staid existence

Don't Dare
Delude our Dream
Disenchantment, Despondency, Denial
Dread, we're not at all ready
to give into Despair or especially contemplate Death.

Chapter 13

Electronic Intrusions:
Enemy #1, the Telephone —
Love It or Leave It

Did I marry a man or a telephone? — Alyssa

I went into marriage starry-eyed, naive, hopeful, and ignorant. It never occurred to me that Alexander Graham Bell's invention would profoundly affect the rest of my life.

The telephone was a part of life when I was growing up. My father, a lawyer, got calls at home. My brothers and I loved talking to friends, as teenagers especially, and my mother was a telephone addict. She had such a large family that I remember her with the phone permanently adhered to her right ear. She used the phone to plan her social life, solve family problems, tell jokes and stories, keep the home organized, and generally to connect with the outside world.

My early view of the telephone was unbiased and quite positive. It was a purveyor of fun, used for friendship. Good news or cheer was almost always on the other end of the line. We even ordered groceries by phone. I had no reason to be suspicious of that familiar instrument.

Once I married, all that changed. A while ago I finally admitted that I have come to hate the intrusive object. In our house, the telephone has a life and psyche of its own. Sometimes I think I should ask it when to have dinner ready, when to talk or be silent, and when I'll get sleep, or if I should forget about it and just wake up and go for a walk instead.

I thought that having babies was tough. You know — three or four feedings in the middle of the night, the constant screaming until the frustrated, hungry, or irritable infant is attended. That only lasted three or four months. Then, I thought, the conditioned response which I had to the slightest snickering from the baby could subside; my sleep could not be restored to six, seven, or even eight hours of uninterrupted silence. Not so at all. The telephone in the bedroom definitely had a life of its own. It reminds me now of the man-eating plant in *Little Shop of Horrors.* "Answer me! Answer me!" it says at any ungodly hour.

A doctor's wife develops a special view of the telephone. There's a love/hate relationship. Their bread and butter depends on the doctor's accessibility to his patients (his telephone exchange or answering service). At first it's even exciting when the phone rings. Perhaps he is getting some business; the more business he gets the more money there is for the food, clothing, and shelter; his job provides for his family. But, there is incessant inconvenience. We feel that if it is for the doctor; everyone has to be quiet. The conversation about someone's sickness is serious stuff. We (children and wife) learn that reverence is required when the doctor is on the phone with one of his patients or colleagues.

When Jerry first began practicing and the phone calls were coming every other night at all hours, and quite regularly, I began having strange reactions. Our bedroom was small and I always worried that the babies would wake up if disturbed. Once, when it rang at least 15 times and Jerry slept through it, I lay there unwilling to wake him, thinking, "This is your baby, Jerry; you have to feed it!" All the while my stomach churned, worried for Jerry, the patient, and me. I needed my sleep to care for the kids.

Should the wife be supportive, polite, even a telephone receptionist for the doctor? To what lengths should she go to enhance his career? Repeatedly I mumbled, grumbled, and rolled over when the phone rang during my sleep, waiting impatiently for Jerry to answer. He slept more soundly at the time; the babies had trained me to respond to night sounds.

I recall times when Jerry picked up the receiver and in that dreamy, half-asleep, half-awake state, said something incoherent, then hung up. Two minutes later the phone would ring again, and again (I surmised by his response) he was asked the same question.

This was scary. What if there was a real emergency and his orders over the phone were crucial? I felt anguish and then guilt, and then removed myself from any responsibility. After all, he was the doctor. He would handle the confusion, embarrassment, or whatever the telephone call ultimately meant.

Secretarial skills, diplomatic skills, and covering for the doctor are necessary tools that wives develop and at which they become quite proficient. The telephone teaches us soon enough. The phone rings when we're home alone or with the kids; we answer it, take a message, or get an inquisition at the other end of the line.

Mild intimidation stirs when taking complicated messages of medical jargon that are spewed forth irrespective of my level of comprehension. I feel responsibility—what if I get it wrong, forget something crucial to someone's life? It's hard to describe the flood of emotions felt when someone is badgering me on the other end of the wire.

"Where is Doctor N? He said he'd be available. When will he be home? Are you sure he's not around somewhere?" The latter is my favorite. Are they implying I'm stupid or do they assume I'm complying in a scheme of deception?

In our house we now joke about the telephone conversations that occur during our dinner. Why is it that as we sit down to eat a sumptuous meal the phone rings, Jerry picks it up, and before we know it words like diarrhea, vomiting, and mucus are filling the atmosphere? The conversation might go as follows:

"Hello. Yes, this is Dr. Nitzberg. How was your trip? Yes, hmm . . . any blood or pus in your stools? Uh huh."

Meanwhile, my youngest son, Eric, looks down at his wonderful zucchini and cheese casserole and gags! I look over at him and roll my eyes in complete understanding.

"Passing a lot of gas? Are the stools well formed? Any unusual odors? Well, sounds okay. It can probably wait until morning . . ."

And so on. We call that our classic anal anecdote! Other specialties have their own forms of dinner-distracting vocabularies, such as pityriasis rosea, vestibular ataxia, laryngotracheoscopes, biopsies, and such. Only wives in nursing or health-related fields are undisturbed by those words bouncing through the telephone wires during dinner.

This discussion would not be complete if the pager, beeper, or small square thing hooked on the doctor's belt was not addressed. It is intimately tied to the telephone, a definite symbiotic relationship. Doctors' wives have emotions yet untapped regarding those little buzzing, beeping, or now even quietly vibrating electronic wonders.

There are those who fight fire with fire, stay on the phone for hours hoping to combat the incessant ringing for the doctor. Remember, however, today the beeper can go off and interrupt her attempts at revenge. Her husband comes into the room, taps her on the shoulder, and says, "I was just paged." That means she'd better get off right away or he'll pull the plug. Subversive hospital members regularly have the operator break through the line. There is no real safety from interruptions, emergency or otherwise. The telephone company always responds to the words, "Paging Dr. Nitzberg."

Medical families now deal with this by keeping two or three phone lines: for the doctor, his wife, and perhaps the children. It is the most peaceful solution.

The telephone is seen as competition for the doctor's time, affection, and concentration. There is jealousy and anger at the intrusion. How abruptly conversations stop, thoughts and feelings are forgotten, when the phone rings. "Put it off again until later," he says. She will. But chances are she won't remember, or she'll be asleep when the next opportunity arises to resurrect discussion.

Enter the pager. Now any time of their lives — in the theater, at the kids' basketball game, at a party, days off, early morning, late at night — the doctor can be beeped, reached, disturbed, beckoned by the medical powers that be. People turn around in the theater and respond to the beeping. In the restaurant all the patrons know he's an important person. Life and death may be in the balance. The doctors themselves are the first to admit that most of the interruptions could wait. His wife is either proud that she's married to this beeper carrier (they did get a great table at the restaurant because he's a doctor), or is frustrated and embarrassed because all this attention is spotlighted on him, thus her. She may make jokes, excuses, stutter a little. Someone has to cover with their friends while he answers the page. She smiles and changes the subject. She knows that people around her are jealous, resentful, impressed, and curious about the interruption. When the doctor returns, questions focus on the medical emergency, and the wife, who may have been engaged in an interesting conversation of her own, is overshadowed.

The vibrating pagers are the newest and most technologically advanced. Now in the middle of a conversation, Jerry gets up totally out of context, unexpectedly, and leaves the room. "What happened?" I inquire. "Oh, I forgot to tell you, my pager went off," he says. My anger level rises dangerously. I always wonder what it was that I did or said to induce this irrational, unpredictable behavior. Rather extreme, considering we were just admiring travel brochures.

Thank heaven pagers are now being used by people in other professions. I will say they seem to wear the pagers with pride, and great respect; I suspect they hope that they'll be mistaken for doctors!

Our latest debate centers around obtaining an answering machine. I am fighting this. My allergy to the telephone makes me quite adamant in my refusal to connect another box that will give me messages. More intrusions. I could, however, leave my own messages on the answering machine: "Welcome to General Hospital. Call later for the continuing saga of the Nitzbergs."

CAN HE HEAR ME?

There goes the telephone
Answer it—it's for you
Mrs. Jones swallowed a toothpick
Mr. Smith can't see straight

Pick up the telephone
They know you're here
Tell them how to fix it
Tell them dear, tell them dear.

When I am hurting
Who should I ask for help?

You're already on the telephone
No matter — I will probably get well.

Why do I think you're listening
Your ear's always stuck to the phone
Why do I think you'll hear me
No matter — I will probably be fine

Wait, Wait, Do I see your eyes on me?
Can it be?
Can it be?

Do I have your attention now?
Let me see
Let me see

There goes the telephone
once again it rings
once again my heart drops
as the telephone sings.

Mrs. Jones tell my husband
Mr. Smith if you would
tell my husband I miss him.
I guess he never understood.

PART II:
HER EXPERIENCE
WITH HER HUSBAND

Chapter 14

Repression and Denial:
If I Have Everything,
Why Do I Feel Like This?

The greatest difficulty in presenting the physician's wife has been to cleanly divide the wife's interpersonal issues from those between herself, her husband, and the society at large. In this section I have focused more directly on her interaction with her husband.

I have concluded that an underlying theme between the wife of a physician and her husband is denial, a conscious or unconscious repression and refusal to believe feelings and thoughts occurring in everyday life, as well as those from the more distant past. Likely, small emotional distress and/or great pains will be ignored or tucked away, never to be heard from again it is hoped.

This process of suppression is insidious, especially for the wives. As mentioned before, denial and repression are defenses either already utilized comfortably by a new doctor or developed through medical training and practice, perhaps to protect the practitioners from feeling the potential pain in their work. But it is impossible to turn these defenses on and off at will. Soon they are integrated into the personality, and eventually are brought home to the wife and children.

I would add here that in my counseling I am aware that men generally are more apt to deny their feelings, and value more concrete fact assessment in a given situation. Traditionally it has been more acceptable for women to contact and express inner feelings, and they are undoubtedly better practiced and skilled than men.

What of the doctor's wife? As a woman she is likely more comfortable with feelings and their expression. She may enter a marriage with the range of available emotional expressions and be able to reach her innermost feelings. Or she may be more reserved, reared in a family where to express one's real feelings was too dangerous and somehow disapproved. These women, of course, share the full range of personality traits and means of expression.

Once married, however, the man of the house is likely to encourage a rigid style of interaction. His profession requires logical thinking, and traditionally he wants a peaceful, supportive, pleasant retreat from his overwrought experience in the harsh world of the hospital when he comes home. This view has been described eloquently in *For Her Own Good* (Erhenreich and English, 1978), where this view of women providing a retreat for men and their world of the marketplace is called "sexual romanticism." Home is the refuge for men, and women are the consolation for his lonely quest as economic man (p. 23). This recalls the nineteenth century view of women who had to be emotional, intuitive, and were thought incapable of quantitative reasoning. All the human qualities, including her childlike or "puppy" qualities (p. 25), rather than economic ones, are attributed to the doctor's wife.

So if her job is to make life comfortable for the doctor, she is clearly not to raise her voice, be angry, gruff, show hostility, or express negativity in any form. Gradually, after being chastised for one or two incidents of hollering and throwing an object as a means of being understood, listened to, and heard, the pattern of feelings denial and experience of repression becomes more acceptable. I vividly recall throwing an old yellow slipper of mine across the room amidst confused and frightened small children and a husband who seemed bewildered by my response. In fact, my family remembers the incident and calls it to my attention as the family joke. I became humiliated at the time and learned that free expression of my feelings caused truly negative consequences—fright for my children, humiliation for me, and from my husband, confusion and disapproval.

I learned well that it was too painful to really be myself, at least the me that could be spontaneous, excitable, and emotionally unpredictable. Over time I controlled my emotions, not realizing what was happening. The disapproval of my reacting so freely was a powerful deadener. Other wives described a change from their earlier selves. There was a consensus that unbeknownst to us we lost our feeling selves to a more controlled state of being.

The result may be a chronic state of depression, or an unspoken rage at not being understood, or even an underlying questioning: "If everything is as perfect and controlled as it seems on the surface, why do I feel like this?" Doubting her own experiences and responses, she soon may say, "I guess things are fine. I'm just restless or I'm making up my murmurings of discomfort. After all, I have things, a house, lovely furnishings, wardrobe, wonderful children, a respected husband who provides me with anything I want. It must be in my imagination that all is not well." She and her husband don't talk about it since long ago the implied rules eliminated sharing negative apprehensions. He keeps his fears and doubts to himself, and so must she. Or when she is there to listen and comfort him if he does open up to her, she gets little back if she dares open up to him. He needs her to be comforting and emotionally supportive. She learns to keep her inner world to herself and instead appears to be a bulwark of strength for him and her children.

The denial and repression become imagining and doubting. Socialized to gain complete satisfaction by being a good caretaker, she persists in pushing back her self. The further back she goes, the less it hurts or confuses. So she thinks. She may drink more, or take chemicals more. She may withdraw from friends and life, all the while thinking she's doing something wrong. To all the world her life's a model of propriety and the positive aspects of the American dream for a woman.

We will look at how the interaction of Mrs. and Dr. promotes denial and repression by the nature and demands of the rigid roles required in their traditional medical marriage.

MORE MYTHS

When I grow up and marry
I'll be careful who I choose
Even in today's world
there is ever so much to lose.

Someone smart and solid
Interesting and fun
Who cares about what I do
Who's not so apt to run.

A father for my children
If that's what we both want
to guide, inspire and involve
himself in the daily carryings on.

My sights are set on a lover,
a provider, a teacher and a friend
a man whom others look up to
a true partner in the end.

Equality within our household
Equality within our bed
Taking time with one another
keeps our relationship in good stead.

If I marry a doctor,
a lawyer or the like
Others will know I'm worthy
and have captured myself a prize.

Prize what, is the question
Is he like no other man
Will there be more safety and security
Will there be more joy at hand?

"Sure," I think to myself
I've heard for many years now
to insure my peace and happiness

a doctor will provide me
with protection guaranteed.

A doctor if he's your husband
makes sure that for you all's well
After all he's the ultimate humanitarian
So I've always heard tell.

Someone who cares for others
must make a great partner in life
Selfless, interested, loving
Caring less even for himself than for his
    wife.

Chapter 15

Sex and Intimacy:
Don't Turn on the Lights

> At least our sex life will be great; he knows all the ins and outs
> of the human body! — Toni, a 36-year-old married eight years

Or so most of us thought when we married doctors. With delight
I recall the 36-year-old Phylliss, mother of two boys, married for 14
years:

> Our sex life is fabulous. We connected almost immediately
> that way. Both of us love to play in bed. We make up games
> and try almost anything once! Sex for me is the closest time
> we have. It's the best way we communicate!

Or Carol, mother of three, married six years (this is her second
marriage), who said:

> Sex is what saves us from all the other stress in our lives. Even
> when we don't get to see each other for days, we know that
> when we get together in bed everything else disappears and
> life is good. It keeps us close, and our bedroom is where we
> catch up on everything! In my last marriage, I had given up on
> sex altogether, so it was important to me to be able to talk
> about it with Ron from the beginning. We feel blessed to be
> compatible that way.

It was fun to watch her talk with so much animation and enthusiasm, with an almost childlike spontaneity.

Though the percentage was small, some women stated that they
have a satisfying and even delightful sexual relationship. They

141

beamed when the issue of sex came up in our interviews. "That's never been a problem. I love sex and so does my husband. We're not afraid to talk about it, experiment, get a baby-sitter for the kids, have 'nooners' or matinees, as they used to be called, or we understand if one of us wants to wait until later." These women were in the minority.

More often, when I asked, "How would you describe your sex life?" or, "What about intimacy?" the answer was stereotypical: "Intimacy to my husband [the doctor] is intercourse. That's it." Over and over again, the "wham, bam, thank you, ma'am" saying was thrown in my face. Sure sex is fine — when we have it — not too interesting, unimaginative, and somewhat boring.

"Don't turn on the lights" refers to my observations and impressions that it's difficult for doctors to let go of their inhibitions about sexuality. Trained to be in control and maintain composure and detachment to do their work, physicians learn to guard themselves. Letting go and relaxing, essential for enjoyable sex, becomes a challenge. Physicians do not take personal pleasure without conflict and discomfort. Having learned to withhold immediate gratification for future goals definitely spills into the bedroom. So we have the usual sexual impulses and desires combined with guilt and distress when experiencing enjoyment, a provocative combination within a sexual relationship. Add to that an attraction to a woman who is often his opposite. She may be expressive, feeling, spontaneous, and very sensory oriented, thereby causing more conflict and ambivalence.

How does this translate to the couple, and the wife in particular?

Sexual intercourse may occur frequently and may be the most intimate time in a medical marriage. But women are disappointed, and describe an emptiness that even frequent intercourse doesn't fill. Doctors are compulsive, another trait necessary to complete medical school. That means that they may also be obsessive about sex, i.e., think about it all the time, fantasize about it ad infinitum. But while his enjoyment may be the intercourse and ejaculation process itself, albeit combined with guilt at enjoying himself, for his wife sex is too quick and uninteresting or unarousing, and therefore ultimately frustrating.

Monica, 42, married 16 years, said with delightful candor:

I didn't realize what to expect from sexuality or intimacy. I loved my husband and felt quite sexy as a young newlywed. We couldn't keep our hands off of each other in those days. However, I didn't realize that Howard's quick ejaculation was not the only way that it could have happened. It became an acceptable part of our relationship in bed. We'd get sexy, huggy (we were so cute), and hop into bed, and before I knew it the consummation was over. Having masturbated since girlhood, I could orgasm. But I was too ignorant and shy to say to Howard, "Isn't there more to this? Could we take our time? Perhaps I could be manually stimulated for my pleasure."

I remember when sexual self-help books started becoming popular. I, being the more avid reader, reported all the details to Howard. *The 'G' Spot, Female Sexuality, The Joy of Sex, Human Sexual Inadequacy*. His repeated and steadfast thought was that since people have had sex for years and that it was a natural biological phenomenon ("The animals have been doing it for years without the advice of specialists!"), there isn't anything that a doctor didn't either learn in school or couldn't do naturally! Conversation over! However, I will admit that I had fun reading!

A classic example of this naive trust came early in my own marriage. We only had Jimmy, our oldest, at the time. We were getting ready for bed and were relieved that Jimmy was quiet at last; he loved being up till all hours. In a high, lighthearted, humorous environment, the question of penis size came up in conversation, probably inspired by something I'd heard or read, and I asked Jerry if there was a difference in the size of penises. After all, I was a '50s woman and I had had no other lovers and the men's locker room was off limits to me. I can remember the expression on his face— astonishment that I could question his knowledge. Jerry flatly, with great authority, said not to worry, that when erect all penises are the same. I took that as the medical gospel. For years, in my naiveté, I thought the outrageous descriptions in literature might be true. Do some men really attain giant erections which are much more fulfilling in bed, or not? Current scientific literature has not corroborated Jerry's statement. Penises do come in all shapes and sizes, and some are capable of great feats of length and hardness (Hite, 1981, 1987; Barbach, 1975). The point is, when Jerry made the statement, so confident, so final, there was no reason to even question him. His expression of calm, cool knowing is one that still frightens me at times. The attitude of scientific, medical authority overflows even into this aspect of our lives together.

We developed a style that he found quite satisfying, mostly initiated by him, but over the years I began to feel anger and inequality in bed. It became perfunctory for a while, actually until I went back to school for my master's degree in psychology and luckily took some human sexuality courses. Then I began having a lot more fun. We both felt somewhat less inhibited and more experimental. That was great for me, as I was reaching what we now know as my sexual peak, in my thirties.

More grist for my confusion mill arose on the subject of vibrators. Would that be fun? Maybe my sex life would improve. Insecure, trusting, and innocent that I was, I talked to Jerry about it. I had visions of the two of us shopping in magazines or x-rated stores for the perfect vibrator!

"What do you think?" I asked. He rationalized, somewhat shyly, somewhat confidently, that there's no need for a vibrator — he would take care of it. Besides, he wasn't about to be replaced by an electronic device. I still don't have one. I felt embarrassed, and dumb, for even thinking about it. Eventually I felt too uncomfortable and sneaky to get one for myself without his knowledge and approval.

Later, in the seminar on human sexuality that Jerry and I both attended professionally, Lonnie Garfield Barbach, author of *For Yourself: The Fulfillment of Female Sexuality*, talked about women freely enjoying their bodies. "Use a vibrator with pleasure," she said. It still seemed that Ms. Barbach couldn't be right. Jerry the doctor should really know and be right about anything to do with my body.

I always worried about not being sexy enough, and not having mutual orgasms during intercourse. Jerry always said he enjoyed our sexual relationship. "It's perfect." I was missing something, but as time went on, even as a counselor I struggled, unable to pinpoint my dissatisfaction and the reasons for feelings of disappointment. I now see the built-in problem of marriage to an "expert." I never trusted my own instincts and my body's responses. I believed Jerry's words and denied my self.

How many other doctors' wives keep quiet about their unmet needs in the bedroom? Women most often talk about their husbands going right for their breasts or vagina or buttocks. This is the signal to have sexual intercourse. Although they admit it is not romantic or enticing, they feel powerless to take any responsibility for changing the pattern.

Even today, inundated with information about how to improve our sex lives, statistics show that women are loathe to ask for what they want or need in the bedroom (Hite, 1987). As doctors' wives, we soon learn that to talk or ask means to question the authority of the expert. We repress our communications.

As she denies her frustration, becoming more and more withdrawn, even "frigid" (a label used by professionals to describe a woman's lack of sexual desire), in reality she is probably uninspired, unaroused by her inexperienced or insensitive sexual partner. But then she feels even more guilty.

Bea, a 34-year-old married for 13 years, was quiet for a moment when asked, "How would you rate your sexual relationship?" then began:

> I'm not sure how I feel about our sex life. I always thought I was the cold, disinterested sexual partner. It seems that somewhere along the way I got turned off to Joe's overtures and awkward advances. So now, rather than be rejected or humiliated, I just freeze up. In fact I don't even think I really feel sexual any more. It's too upsetting to even try to face it. . . . I thought since I didn't respond right or when I was supposed to that I was a failure, an unsexy person. So now I don't like to even think about it.

At this point we were both uncomfortable. She was sad, teary, and I recognized the signs of confusion for her, myself, and others.

How can they talk to someone about these frustrations? He or she wants more or less sex, more or less foreplay or afterplay, more romance or hugging not leading directly to intercourse. But like so many couples, they don't express it to each other. The difference with the medical couple is that he is in the profession of healing and bodies—we assume that he knows anatomy and physiology, so he must know sexuality! To see a professional counselor, sex therapist, or another physician about these problems is unthinkable! Eventually, unable to face the pain of doubts and insecurity, feelings are totally submerged and denied so that over the years they no longer seem to exist.

The intimacy, which consisted mainly of sexual intercourse and talking about the children and maybe his busy schedule and hard day, is now reduced to automatic occasional intercourse. As intercourse occurs less and less, so may talk about the kids and business.

A more obvious reason for inadequate sex in medical households is the schedule and demands of the doctor. It's almost impossible to entice, cajole, or in any way inspire an exhausted, overextended, responsible, God-like person when he doesn't wish it to happen.

And there are the telephone or beeper interruptions that make concentrating on intimacy, sex, and romance almost impossible. The wife begins to feel that anything else comes before her pleasure. Mrs. Jones's appendectomy has to be more important than achieving an orgasm tonight or just cuddling to promote intimacy. And the wife knows she must concede to Mrs. Jones. So the doctor leaves his bedroom. He feels some frustration, but duty calls. He gets his strokes at the office, hospital, or from Mrs. Jones's successful operation and gratitude. Mrs. Doctor, on the other hand, is left at home with unresolved confusion. If she feels angry, the guilt overcomes her. "How can I feel anger? He had to go to the office. His work outside the home is much more important than my sex life. He may be saving a life!" The guilt-anguish cycle rears its ugly head.

It is striking that both doctor and Mrs. have the feeling that there is no choice. When duty calls, he listens no matter what the cost to their personal life. It would shake up the system, the myth of indispensability, a conditioned paralysis to behave otherwise. A chance for some intimacy between them is lost again and she may masturbate for her pleasure, but still she may feel alone, inadequate, guilty, angry, and confused.

Courses on human sexuality have only recently been offered in medical schools. Today it is ludicrous to imagine anatomy and physiology without human sexuality. But even with that addition, doctors' wives feel that their husbands remain aloof, detached, and not very spontaneous with sexuality.

So the doctor wins! He's repressed, rigid, compulsive, and orderly in the bedroom, and so she must be to have any closeness with him. I have been told that some men withdraw altogether and women live for years with no sex, no touching, and therefore little chance for any intimacy. Florence, a 35-year-old with four children, seemed relieved and thankful to have a chance to talk about it when asked about sex. With tears in her eyes, she described:

> We've been married for 14 years. Sex was great before we married. He wanted to make love all the time. Then something clicked off. After we married, he lost interest. I had to start begging him to come to bed. He doesn't hug me. He's not demonstrative anyway, but boy, he sure seemed to like sex early on. Now we've had sex about six times in the last four years. We don't even sleep in the same room anymore. If I ever suggest or hint at my disappointment, he gets furious, breaks out in a sweat, then shuts down and walks away. I feel like I'm being punished for something and he won't even talk about it! He just goes to his room, and that's it! I don't know what to do. I've tried sexy nighties, screaming, crying — everything. What else is there? I've worried that Owen had some medical problem or an emotional one, but whenever I suggested this to him he became infuriated. He said that he would certainly know if he had a medical problem. The emotional part he won't even address. My biggest problem is that I don't know if I want to spend the rest of my life like this. I'm young. We enjoy other parts of our life together. Isn't it a waste!

Florence had this bottled up so long, her secret. I tried to be empathetic and supportive. I suggested counseling, and she responded, "He won't go." It seemed that though it was painful for her to share there was a huge weight lifted from her narrow shoulders. While her husband's pride kept him from asking for outside help and he struggled with feelings of failure and humiliation, Florence kept quiet and lived inside her shell of guilt, blame, frustration, and anger.

Karen, a 29-year-old married for six years, shared:

> I was physically abused and sexually molested by my father while I was growing up. I've only recently begun to deal with the issues that left me with. It helps to explain my reluctance to relax and be comfortable with sex in my marriage. At first Richard couldn't understand my attitude. I was terrified to be intimate. Certain kinds of touching made me sick to my stomach. But I felt I had to tolerate Richard's advances. So I closed my eyes and waited for him to finish. I would pretend I was somewhere else or emotionally detach from the whole thing. After a few years of this and hoping for less and less sex, Richard finally insisted that I was not normal and I should get help. By then I was shaking if he touched me in a way that I knew meant he wanted intercourse. My father forced me as a small child for five years to have intercourse with him until my younger sister was his next victim. I stopped being sexual completely till I met Richard. I was 21 and had never been with anyone but my father. Richard seemed really safe to me. He was in med school, and I trusted that he wouldn't hurt me like my father did.

Karen has been in counseling for three years and has great insight into her fear of sexuality and intimacy. She and Richard are working together on their relationship. Although it is not Karen's fault, nor should she be labeled abnormal (as Richard stated), she is more fortunate than most that Richard is both patient and caring enough to work through this with her.

In contrast are reports of "kinky" behavior, or what was formerly thought to be fetishism and sexual obsessions. (Let us not forget what a doctor considers kinky or a fetish may be his wife's undressing in front of him in broad daylight.) This is great when both partners mutually agree and mutually enjoy. A friend said she and her doctor husband really enjoy triple x-rated movies together. It turns them both on. She thinks that he, as a psychiatrist, is more open to experimental, extemporaneous sex. Others shared feelings of intimidation and control by the "body expert." The husband sets up the scenario and demands that she perform sexually to fulfill his compulsive fantasy, without regard or sensitivity to her desires and experience.

Ellen, 35, in her second marriage of six years, shared:

> Personally I was turned off or even repulsed by some of Daniel's sexual fantasies. He wanted me to be violent and rage at him before he could get excited. I was never comfortable with that. He insisted that I really hurt him. Or sometimes he'd get our dog or cat involved and want me to hurt them. I'd get nauseated, but I tried to please Daniel. After reading a lot of books, I realized it was all right for me to do what I wanted, or not, in bed. I forced Daniel into counseling for help with our sex life. But I was afraid for a long time.

Again we see the double bind for the doctor's wife. If she doesn't go along with his sexual demands and fantasies, he may leave her for someone else. Besides, he's the doctor, the expert. He knows how two people are to be sexually satisfied together. If she expresses discomfort or plainly is not aroused or excited by the same fantasies, then she ends up feeling inadequate and unsexual. Her self-esteem is lowered and she may close down the whole sexual side of her being, feeling unrespected, belittled, and ignored.

The final part of the catch-22 is that if she tells anyone, she looks bad and she has the problem. She blames herself. Worse yet, it threatens the doctor's professionalism. She feels disloyal; secrecy is the contract, not betrayal. Again, these are the myths that keep problems in a vicious, unhealing cycle.

The confusion, anger, fear, and ultimate denial and repression in these women leave little room for the fulfillment of their intimacy needs. On the contrary, they contribute to their loneliness and isolation.

Chapter 16

Affairs:
It Takes Two

I thought my affair was the best way to avoid fighting, but really a good fight could have improved our marriage one hundred percent. — Valerie

Whether to call this section "Affairs of the Heart" or "Business Affairs" was a question. It was always thought doctors were so busy that love affairs were the last order of their busy schedules. In fact, the lonely, ignored wife at home was thought to be prey to the traveling salesman or the tennis or golf instructor who would take advantage of her frustration and money to become her part-time lover.

With the picture of a serious, hard-working doctor comes to mind the image of one who fits an affair into his day like a business appointment; scheduled, compulsively attended, having someone else, like the proverbial executive secretary, send flowers or buy gifts, unbeknownst to his wife. It is no secret that physicians have embarked on this secret life, keeping it well separated from their family life (Konner, 1987; Gerber, 1983).

The most familiar scenario is a sweet and attentive nurse or other health professional constantly available and admiring of the larger-than-life physician. She flirts, or he flirts. It doesn't matter who starts it. Or neither flirt but rather find that proximity has drawn them together. Konner talks about how the excitement and danger of an emergency surgical case with doctor and nurse working side by side can feed the sexual and romantic juices of the healers (1987). Before they know it they are sexually involved and, if everyone plays by the rules that require discretion, an affair can go on between these two for years. It's fun, it's convenient. It's mutually satisfying, and there are no strings attached. And, as the tradition goes, the wife's the last to know.

The physician even more than most other married men has the opportunity, the money, the prestige, and the availability of many willing partners to conduct affairs, either serially or ongoing. It has been a code of medical ethics for physicians to cover these indiscretions for one another. In addition, the entire medical community, whether it be hospital, academic, or private office personnel, will protect the doctor from being found out by his wife, family, and patients. He believes that if kept secret from his wife, he's not hurting anyone. He is supported in his belief by our view of women as sexual conquests.

The hours away from home, whether for meetings, emergencies, or the usual long work load, make discreet trips out of the house simple.

I never even suspected that Steven was fooling around. He would come home late and tired all the time. He would get calls to go to the hospital at night or on weekends all the time. He'd get up and leave parties or the theater, and I never thought that was unusual. It wasn't for him. We made love in a regular way two or three times a week. I enjoyed it, and I thought Steven did. We have three kids who Steven adores but only gets to spend an occasional weekend with. This residency stuff is exhausting and time consuming. I'm busy with the kids. They're two, five, and six, so I've got my hands full. . . . Well, I've spoken to the other residents' wives. They occasionally gossip about doctors and affairs with nurses. I thought that's ludicrous. Steven's so tired all the time who'd want to have an affair with him? Or how could he anyway? Plus, I always thought if your sex life was pretty good and you got along okay you wouldn't look anywhere else. I went to hospital auxiliary teas. And we'd have the residents and interns over, or go to the other staff members' houses once in a while. Inadvertently I stumbled into a room during a hospital party and saw Steven passionately kissing a nurse from his service. I was devastated. How stupid — right there where any-

one could walk in on them. He made all kinds of excuses. "I
was drinking too much," "She pushed herself on me," whatever he could come up with. I went home, packed my stuff,
the kids' stuff, took them out of bed, dressed them, and left. I
went home to my parents' house in Michigan. The humiliation
of it! All the hospital people knew about Steven's escapades.
Even some of the other doctors' wives said they knew, but
their husbands made them swear to secrecy! Can you imagine?
I was the last to find out! Right under my nose. He'd be shack-
ing up with her and then come home and make love to me. Or
worse yet, tell me how terribly exhausted he was. No wonder—exhausted trying to keep two women happy at once!
What absolutely baffles me is the unscrupulous behavior of
that nurse! She knows he's married and has three kids. She
knew we hardly get to see each other.

Well, my family and Steven have tried to tell me I'm overreacting. "Boys will be boys, you know." Maybe so, but so
will girls, and I can't live with someone who can't resist temp-
tation out there and who I have to worry about for the rest of
my life—will he be faithful or will someone always be able to
charm him away? Actually I don't know who to blame. Him
for betraying me and the kids? Her for her availability? Or the
system for making it so easy to pull that kind of behavior behind my back? And all the times the hospital secretaries were
so sweet to me, "I'm sorry Mrs. _____, Dr. is in with an
emergency C-section," or "He's in a patient's room," or "In
a meeting with the chief," or bull. He was probably screwing
nurse _____.

This 27-year-old woman married Steven, her first love, at the age
of 19, and had her three children fairly soon. They were high school
sweethearts, he knowing he would be a doctor, she knowing she
would be his wife. Her reaction was a common one, but she went
on to divorce Steven. No amount of reassurance or excuses could
convince her that their commitment could ever be renegotiated. Her
trust was broken as was her heart. It took her by such surprise, and
in her naive innocence she was irreversibly traumatized. She had
always felt that what they had was special, unlike the other, gos-

siped-about medical couples. She felt invulnerable to the accessibility and secret code of ethics and double standards that make affairs easy for the physician.

My interviews also included many women who were nurses married to physicians. Their view of the closed hospital system of protection and secret knowledge, and of a double-standard inner culture, is from the inside.

Clarissa was on the other side of the picture.

The nurses used to all say, "God, I'd never want to marry a doctor." We'd laugh about all the shenanigans and adultery. We most often felt sorry for the wives, although secretly a lot of us wanted to be in their shoes. On the one hand the doctors were gross, arrogant, bossy tyrants, especially to nurses. We knew how horrible they could be. Sweet as sugar to patients, and obnoxious to us or behind the patients' backs. We also hear the jokes and humiliating comments doctors make about their wives, like, "Boy, I can't wait to get home to _____. Another really exciting evening of cards or TV!" or "That bitch. She wants me to watch the kids tonight while she goes to her women's group!" We hear them complain about how much money their wives spend or how frigid they were. It's like football locker room stuff, I guess. Between the doctors. Put down their wives all the time. I guess they put down us nurses too when we can't hear them.

Well, even knowing that, I personally found some of the doctors attractive and exciting. The older ones especially. They drive Porsches, wear fabulous clothes, have everyone waiting on them hand and foot. It's exciting to me. I had my eye on the top surgeon in the hospital. I know he had a rotten home life. They all seem to, if you can believe what they say, anyway. So when I was assigned to his case I was ecstatic. One thing lead to another, and we fell in love. I know it helped that I was always there to listen to his sad life story—how lonely he was, how his wife ignored him and only wanted his money. I admired him, and he loved it! We went together for four years and finally I convinced him it was either me or her. What he doesn't know is that after a while I probably would have kept having the affair because it was enough for me. He bought me everything. He paid for a great apartment for me, near the hospital, and we spent a lot of our free time there. I would have kept it up, but I guess he couldn't live with the situation, and finally divorced his wife.

Now I'm the wife, and that's another story. I'm paranoid about him seeing someone else! If he's late, I'm suspicious. I try to work with him as much as possible, to keep an eye on him. We've been married three years. I hope I can relax soon. Maybe I'll never relax about that since I know what really goes on.

It's as if the life at work (including sexual activities) is so separate from home life that even normal guilt feelings are denied. Clarissa said, "The nurses always joked about doctors being good for one thing — getting laid!" She went on to add:

We felt no guilt about our lives with doctors. They didn't seem to feel guilt either. That's the way the hospital life is. But once you're married into it the feelings change. Suddenly I'm petrified it's me who's being cheated on, not the one cheating. Suddenly I see the missing guilt and remorse. Why don't they feel guilty?

Perhaps the standards and expectations of the social culture of hospital and medicine with constant emergencies, life saving, split-second decisions, long hours, great connectedness between personnel — the true interdependence and partnership that happens between doctors and nurses — increases the tension and sexual energy between them. If it is socially acceptable to act on these feelings between consenting adults, and if they are able to treat the feelings as purely sexual or sensual, and if the experience is only momentary, with no expectations for future involvements, then perhaps guilt is not an issue. If felt, it is absolved — diminished by the rules, implied or expressed, of the social system. Others offer assurances that these feelings and actions are okay, so no one in the system judges or speaks out of turn.

Once removed from that safe, accepting, almost provoking environment to the very different realm of the home and family, that same woman, who was sexually and romantically available at the hospital, may react differently because her behavior is reinforced differently.

Affairs are by no means limited to the doctor. His wife does have affairs. But my sense is that he has affairs from convenience, and it's acceptable in his male-dominated medical culture. His are a mere distraction. To him the women are play toys at work, an ego booster for his already over-attended-to ego, another notch in his belt which is not only tolerated by his peers but protected and encouraged. The nurses in that milieu are expected to feel and act on the same values. His wife, a more traditionally housebound person, has an affair to make a heavy statement about her marriage. Once married, she has less ease within the system of the family and home front in carrying on an affair, whether she is a health professional, homemaker, or other. She does not have a social system from which to cover or hide her activities. She is often extremely secretive; perhaps no one knows, or only her best friend knows. She is not adding notches to her belt. Unlike her male counterpart, she is not letting her colleagues know how wonderful, powerful, and attractive she is, or how arrogant, or that even while married with children she can openly defy the system while her peers not only cover for her, but applaud.

Women having affairs with physicians in the work place — the medical helpers, personnel who are after all doing subservient work to the male physicians — are seen as the temptresses. As I reported earlier, I became aware of my personal anxieties: about the nurse who sets out to betray another woman and steal her husband. That fear of the "Jezebel" working with my husband and luring him away was deeply entrenched and reinforced in my personal history. She is the sinner, after all, not the doctor who agreed to enter into the liaison. Nor is he often blamed for pursuing the woman. Rather he is seen as innocently captured and tempted into sin, much like Eve tempted Adam in the Garden of Eden, causing the loss of paradise. The nature of this blame and guilt being borne by the females who both work and live with physicians is an extension of our religious training. Here the Judeo-Christian ethic dominates the institution of medicine, as it does all of our modern institutions, and does indeed affect the manner in which the indiscretions of physicians and their wives are viewed by others.

The same woman who thought it was safe to be intimate with a doctor at the hospital and ignored other feelings of blame of guilt if one of them was married, suffers greatly as his wife. She may have mistakenly thought she had license to fool around while they were co-workers. Truly he was the only one with the power to "fool around" and not be as demeaned or damned by it. The double standard in the medical profession is not unlike that in political circles in which married presidents, political candidates, or men in high positions have been linked with one sparkling female after another, and extraordinary care is taken to protect and split that extracurricular love life from the image of the family, as well as from his ability to lead the country.

A wife is not accorded the same privilege, nor does she, if she is able, have the luxury of denying her feelings of trust, intimacy, sharing, and love that may and usually do accompany her sensual and sexual involvement with another.

(I have focused here on heterosexual affairs. Lesbian and homosexual extramarital liaisons occur with as much frequency in medical marriages as the general population. That discussion is addressed more fully later.)

For a doctor's wife to have an affair is highly traumatic. She deals with her internal conflicts — silently, isolated, and with reprisals from society when and if she's discovered. No one covers for her. Nor do they secretly or blatantly encourage her activities. She treads the line painfully alone, or she may have an affair to bring her internal discomforts with her marriage to a head. Whereas a man has always been given the blessing of other men to have a casual affair while married, a woman has been told that she is the cause of his philandering. She tempted him, like Eve did Adam, and any sin is usually hers to bear. The world view of the doctor's wife is that of all women: the cause of man's fall from grace. So she may look for an affair to call attention to the unsatisfactory relationship by doing what she has been taught to do, sin, and then rebuild and save the marriage. Add to that the view that a doctor is in a chosen profession of service to mankind. Any question of guilt or blame would fall heavier on his wife as an adulterer.

Women were reluctant to share with me the intimacies and pain of having an affair. Calling it an affair has a different meaning to a woman than to her husband. He does not have to be in love or even contemplate leaving his wife and family if he so chooses, since there is collusion to keep his behavior secret from his family anyway. To a doctor, the woman he sees outside of his marriage, whether for a few weeks or for many years, is considered his mistress.

Since a physician compartmentalizes his life—work, hospital, family, home—he can add lover or mistress to that list and put her into another compartment fairly easily. Recall that he has been trained to keep his inner feelings at bay. Adding another woman is likely done in a clinical, controlled, and distant manner. The availability and even the distance is quite possibly perfect for him.

Felicia, slightly tearful, shares her sadness:

> After we were married six years and Robert was in his residency, I was at home alone with two young children and never saw Robert. I met a man casually in the library. I spent time in the library when the kids were little. Books and reading were my best company. This man was quiet and kind and there whenever I went to pick up or return books. We talked at first, then went for coffee once in a while. I started looking forward to my trips to the library, and soon found myself getting a sitter so I could be alone with him. We ended up in a lovely relationship for a year. But it tore me apart inside. I lived in fear of Robert finding out and at the same time I think I really wanted him to know. We weren't talking. He didn't seem to care any more, and I wanted to feel some warmth and love. The sex was fine, but it was the understanding and talking I loved. Mel and I talked for hours about literature and philosophy, and I ate it up.

Felicia expressed the anguish of taking her commitment to Robert, her husband, very seriously but also taking seriously her relationship to her lover, though in some ways finding it more fulfilling.

The more frustrated I got with my home, the more lonely and unattractive I felt, the faster I wanted to turn to Mel.

Would you have left Robert for Mel?

I don't think so. Although that wasn't an issue since he was moving away, and I wouldn't do that to my kids. Actually that year kept me whole, I think. But what I really wanted was a more loving, more available husband. The loneliness in my marriage was unspeakable.

An intimate relationship with warm communication and connectedness is extremely important to women. Unable to succeed in establishing that with a physician husband and feeling despair over the failure of the marriage, an affair is tempting. The lonely wife doesn't usually look upon an affair as a sordid, purely sexual liaison, but rather sees the arrangement as a person with whom to share intimacies: intellectual, spiritual, emotional, and physical. The affairs may even provide the type of relationship that she would prefer — greater equality, respect for herself as a capable individual. But the complicated and humiliating task of breaking up a marriage to be with a lover is overpowering and most likely will keep her in her dry, distant marriage.

Clearly we need to distinguish between emotional and sexual affairs. For some of us, the touching and closeness that is involved in the act of intercourse is so compelling in itself that it is enough to fulfill our physical needs. It may satisfy needs for closeness without generating other emotional ties or desires for everlasting connection with that person. So the occasional sexual contact feels good and has no strings attached. Traditionally, men are said to more frequently connect in this way.

An emotional bond can include sexual relations or not. Friends have deep ties but don't necessarily have sex. It can be just as intrusive to a couple to have one member of the couple in a deep, emotional bond to a third person. In fact, it is more complicated and consequential to the couple than if that extramarital relationship were only sexual.

For those interviewed, when sex was involved they had an emotional bond with that person. But they also felt that they had attractions to third parties in which no sexual activity had occurred, and they were as potentially powerful and threatening to their marriage. In fact they felt that those relationships were more lasting and could be more important. The bond of emotional closeness and friendship at times had more impact on their marriage if not explored and confronted by them and their husbands.

So having a regular ski buddy or tennis partner or movie friend or conversation person or one with whom to share philosophies, but excluding sexual activities, can be extremely threatening to the primary relationship (marriage). As couples, we are not yet able to bond strongly with more than one person without our spouses feeling some jealousy and insecurity. Without equality, communication, and trust between the married couple, the bond outside the marriage can soon become the primary bond. So we then have a triangle, and what I would call an emotional affair. The affair threatens the marriage. It also serves to arouse the areas of conflict within the marriage and at best enables communication to increase and resolve those conflicts. We can love many people, but without trust and open sharing and a respectful equality with our primary partner, he or she risks becoming secondary. Physicians risk being secondary, as do their wives, throughout their marriage. Unequal relationships preclude trust and open communication, and patriarchal, traditional institutions give only lip service to the family and the marriage having equal priority with the world of work and commerce.

The outside relationship, if important, always contains the element of sexual possibility. That may be what fuels the fire and increases the bond. My point is that the affair may exist even though the people maintain celibacy.

Linda, a nurse presently working part-time, brought her lover to my office for "just one consultation." She had been trying to get her husband into marital counseling for years. There were sexual difficulties and basic troubles with communication. Linda described her husband as "too good to leave, I'd be crazy to give up what I have." But she was very attracted to another man and had been seeing him for eight months. They were in aerobics class together and both were crazy about physical fitness. They started seeing each other for ski trips and hiking, both of which her husband hated. So it was easy for her to go unnoticed and unmissed. Her husband was "completely absorbed in his work anyway and was rarely home."

> One day we just couldn't keep our hands off each other any more. Then we met at motels and went away for weekends when Ray [Linda's husband] was at a meeting or something. Well it's too hot to handle now. We both would have to leave our spouses, and neither of us really wants to. So here we are. You have to help us break up. We get too upset whenever we try being apart for long.

She was distraught by the strength of this relationship, but she eventually confronted her husband, told him about the affair, and insisted that he have counseling with her.

Throughout her affair Linda was very nervous. She lost 15 pounds, couldn't sleep, was irritable and depressed, and yet at other times felt wild with joy. But the pressure of hiding out and sneaking around overwhelmed her. Her feelings were sincere and loving, but the guilt was intolerable. She had told no one of her troubles, not even her best friend.

The liaisons that occur during these marriages fulfill the much needed bonding that does not happen in the marriage. The rare but evident extramarital relationship that went on for years was filled with conflict but resignation.

Eleanor, a teacher married for 21 years and mother of two sons, remains in a relationship with an unmarried co-worker of hers. After struggling with her options, she decided:

> Sure, it's a little crazy I guess. I have a husband and a boy-friend. I can't call him a lover because I consider him my best friend in the world. We're not having an affair either. This has lasted 11 years now.

> *Why not get a divorce and marry Paul?*

> A lot of reasons: religious, moral, my children, economic. I haven't been able to confront it. Actually, at this point I'm sure my husband knows (although it hasn't been openly

voiced), and I think we both like it this way. At times I feel very schizophrenic and say, "What are you doing?" But I've gotten used to my life this way and now I rely on both of these men for different things. Altogether, I guess, I feel like I have a more full existence.

Few women bragged about their sexual prowess or their "conquests" from one liaison to another. Rather, a long contemplated and conflict-ridden decision to be with another man to cope with whatever was sorely missing from her marriage was the rule. In secret or with maybe only one close confidant, meetings were arranged. At no time were they devoid of guilt or remorse. Even those women infuriated at their husbands were usually torn apart by conflict in time.

The irony is that if she chooses to be with another doctor outside of her marriage, a woman may end up with two uncommunicative, distant, restrained, and controlling men. Hoping for greater understanding and fulfillment, she finds herself living with the same feelings of rejection and loneliness, but this time from her lover. Since doctors' wives, especially when not working outside the home, mostly meet other doctors socially, the likelihood of an affair with another doctor is high.

Suzanne, a 48-year-old mother of two girls and a marriage counselor herself, recalls:

> In my 20 years of marriage there have been times when an outside relationship seemed the only way to handle both my inner turmoil and my marital stress. Whether a sexual liaison or an emotionally supportive one, I can look back now on my attractions to other men and pinpoint the motivating factors for acting on them.
>
> A relationship with another physician was the most ironic since he was more distant and stingy of himself than I perceived Craig at the time. I was left feeling helpless, alone, and betrayed. What I realized for myself was that my needs had to be met in my marriage. Either stay in and work on it, or leave and find what's needed with someone else.

Interestingly, being alone and on their own never was an option.

There are so many ways to separate within a marriage. Most women married to physicians try to counteract their loneliness with the separate lives that their husbands lead with some kind of action. Affairs are just one of the actions available to her. However, the success of the action can only be judged by each woman for herself. For some unwilling or unable to leave and unable to get cooperation from a distant husband, the idea of enriching their lives periodically with another man is very appealing. Our society, however, makes that a very costly action for her to take. She bears the burden of guilt for what is seen as a great threat to her husband. In reality it's a greater threat to her husband to work on a shared-equal marriage. The affairs are a weak bandage; keeping her self-esteem at constant risk, she still remains unable to demand her rights within her home.

If we look at what motivates an extramarital relationship for a woman, so many of those forces exist in her marriage to a physician: lack of intimacy, warmth, sharing, attention, self-esteem, confidence, and economic independence; inability to deal with conflict; overpowering inequality in the marriage; poor communication, secrecy, distrust, little shared time and/or interests. All of this is paired with his denial, inability, or unwillingness to see these difficulties. A relationship with another who can provide some of these missing forces is a clear option, if she can survive the social disapproval and consequent isolation.

Chapter 17

Competition:
I'm Running as Fast as I Can

As soon as I started getting good and winning races, Bill took up running. He wasn't very fast. Soon he forbade me to keep racing. — Charlene

A psychiatrist thinks he's being consoling by sharing tidbits from his own experience. He's a physician also, after all; his wife is in my shoes. How can he have the objectivity and genuine understanding of my point of view? Isn't it colored by what he needs to rationalize for his own sanity when he reports how he and his wife have adapted to their lifestyle?

"She has found places in her life where she excels, where she feels no competition with me," he says, "and I encourage her in those endeavors. She is a better golfer than I am and I'm happy about that. I know she needs something in her life to boost her self-esteem. She also has a better rapport with our kids. When they want to have a long talk it's always with their mother. I know and understand that," he says.

Or, "I like to buy my husband's clothes. He has awful taste," she says to me.

"I keep the books in our house."

"I've started running marathons."

These are all statements designed to prove how much power the doctor's wife has, either personal or within the relationship.

"She takes care of our social life."

"My husband says he wishes he had my schedule, all that time on his hands!"

If the truth be known, he is likely not the least bit interested in that which he allows her to be in charge of; in addition, he might also feel frustrated, unimportant, and unfulfilled with all that time on his hands.

Competition underlies a surprising number of social relationships in our society. What's unique about the medical marriage? It includes not only issues of power and control, but also entitlement. In fact, it's difficult to separate self-esteem from the latter.

In my opinion, being married to an MD in the U.S. is like struggling with an older sibling who is competent, revered, and successful at whatever he is involved in. The system (marriage) itself incurs competition, and in fact magnifies it in some instances. We all struggle to be respected, loved, and competent beings who are valued for ourselves. The medical marriage is almost in opposition to that basic need for the woman. Human nature insists that we struggle to create, develop, find ourselves. How is that accomplished when paired with a supposedly equal mate who is indeed unequal in the eyes of the world?

Measuring up becomes our primary motivator, although unconsciously at times. Being as worthy, as smart, as valued, as respected, as loved, as needed keeps us on our toes constantly. Oh, I will admit we are not conscious of these stirrings 100 percent of the time. If we were, life would be unbearable. But think about our actions, the ways in which daily concerns revolve around improving self-esteem. Would this high-performance striving be necessary if we did not have to measure up to the unreachable?

A younger man, even an MD, could probably tolerate the fact that his wife was valuable, respectable, and experienced without any real threat to his position. I must say that I didn't speak to women married to physicians much more than four years younger than themselves.

How do we compete? In small ways, such as who got the last phone call, to large important ways, such as who has the last word or decides the important things between us.

I decided that I wanted to spend the evening with friends not connected with medicine. He then arranges the next four weekends with people of his choice. Where we go on vacations and what we do with our leisure time are issues of competition which include power and control. If I like to watch television to relax, why is it that our TV is down in a dark, dreary section of the house, while he relaxes in the lovely living room, well lit, warm, and cozy?

When I think about competition, winners and losers come to mind. How can a marriage survive in a healthy manner when there is one primary winner and one predictable loser? I know I'll get some disagreement on this point. There are those of us who have figured out ways to feel that we have won several battles.

She says, "He got me a new mink coat this year."

Or, "We're going to Nepal or perhaps the Barrier Reef in Australia next spring."

"My new charge card for Saks just arrived."

All these statements are designed to make us feel as good about ourselves and our worthiness as we perceive our husbands feel about themselves. The "winnings," sending Johnny to private school, using the best housekeeper, ad infinitum, are only superficial, temporary salves to our bruised self-image. They cannot replace the inner strength that comes from our own accomplishments and feedback from the outside world.

In my childhood household, I had two brothers. My father was an attorney. Mother didn't work outside the home. There was always competition between my brothers and myself, probably for my parents' affection. Having competition is supposed to make us work harder, perform more astutely, play the game better. This is not a treatise on competition, so I will forego my in-depth theories about its worth or otherwise. I will say that the notion of winners and losers makes cooperation difficult, if not paradoxical.

In my childhood home, cooperation would have felt better to me. Less threatening. Less anxiety provoking. I would have been more certain of my worthiness. Trust might have been developed more easily. Perhaps the same is true in a marriage. Cooperation sounds more as if the partners have an equal stake and responsibility, and therefore equal worth!

The other aspect of competition that wives experience is among themselves, wife against wife. To win what? The record title of the World's Greatest Doctor's Wife. Would one rather win the title of the Wife of the World's Greatest Doctor? I suspect the latter to be closer to correct.

Examining this issue, we should recognize the negative effects on the individual women. When they attend a meeting of the medical auxiliary dressed and jeweled impeccably, what is the message? What do they feel inside?

Some expressed the wish to me that others lay down their affectations, "be themselves," relax more in the company of other wives, be more open, less threatened, "less competitive." What this image does is put off the other women. There is an insulated shell around each one so that true intimacy is difficult to achieve. We end up being too protective, losing the support of perhaps the only people who can truly know what it is to be in our shoes — other doctors' wives.

Yet the competition forces us to stay at arm's length. What are we afraid will happen? Will it cost us the little self-esteem we have left?

Chapter 18

Homosexuality:
The Not So Gay Truth

I'm not sure I'll ever forgive Brian for using me so that he could pass in the medical community. —Rachel

What happens when a partner in a marriage realizes or finally admits to being homosexual? In Woody Allen's movie, *Manhattan*, with Meryl Streep, the bittersweet statement, "My wife left me for another woman," is meant to be funny. Mr. Allen expects sympathy from the audience. Underneath the superficial snickering is the reality that couples live in this situation.

In the literature on physician marriages, there is again greater attention to the homosexual physician than to his wife's experience. The pain and humiliation of a woman struggling to keep her marriage intact for her and her children's sake even though she now knows of her husband's sexual preference for men is indescribable.

Until most recently, in our country's medical community the knowledge of an MD's homosexuality could ruin his career, and there is still that possibility in some places. It is impossible to estimate the number of homosexual physicians in school or in practice, as public acknowledgement is unlikely if not impossible. As mentioned before, since his career is often based on referrals from other physicians, the knowledge of his being gay could abruptly reduce the flow of potential patients. It is essential that he maintains an image of a healthy, "normal" family life, or his colleagues could single him out for punishment. Being economically or professionally cut off from his peers would be tantamount to ending his career.

Physicians carry the same stereotypes as other people, perhaps more so when it comes to anything related to sexuality and what is considered beyond the normal range of behaviors. A physician is not necessarily more understanding and more educated regarding homosexuality as we would hope or expect. In fact, if we look at the history of homosexuality in our country we could put some of the responsibility for public attitudes on the subject onto the medical profession. It has only been since 1973 that the American Psychiatric Association decided to remove homosexuality as a mental disorder from the *Diagnostic and Statistic Manual*. That was a major step which encouraged greater research and demystification of homosexuality. With homosexuality no longer considered a mental disease, the public and the medical profession could lower the fear threshold. By greater education it is hoped they could embrace homosexuality as another way of relating, not to be feared and ignored but assimilated and accepted within the culture. It is, after all, physicians and then psychiatrists who have encouraged the belief that to be homosexual is to be sick, abnormal, and aberrant. Physicians themselves have greatly influenced our putting the homosexual in the closet in modern history by backing theories with "scientific" proof that to be a homosexual is something you are born with and it is unhealthy, undesirable, and to be condemned. Medicine and religion have married their beliefs and influenced our attitudes. Our present fears and negative stereotypes surrounding homosexuality which we absorbed from religious training were given a scientific stamp of approval.

As stated before, it is understood that male physicians are basically uncomfortable with their sexuality. They are often restrained or obsessive in dealing with sexual issues. Rather than being open and comfortable, they tend to be repressed, shy, and uncomfortable. There are psychiatrists who allude to the possibility that those who obsess in that way are actually dealing with unresolved homosexual tendencies. All this still reinforces how negatively the profession views homosexuality. For a physician to openly admit to being gay is still unlikely, and if he does admit to homosexuality it can be devastating to himself and his family.

A gay physician must hide his sexuality to overcome the common stereotypes. Believed to be more promiscuous, and plagued by short-term, uncommitted relationships, the picture of the sad, lonely homosexual is common, if not born out statistically (Myers, 1988, Kessler, 1983, and Krajeski, 1987). In addition, homosexuals are portrayed as dangerous to children, making both parenting and doctoring children undesirable in the eyes of the public.

Whether in the profession, in schools, or in training, to be gay is still considered undesirable. Students may be denied access to school, training programs, or positions in the hospital hierarchy. Specialties like urology and gynecology are still avoided by homosexuals, because they deal with diseases of male or female sexual organs. Denial and adapting socially acceptable behaviors are still watchwords in this prestigious profession.

It may drive gay pre-med or medical students to marry to prove their acceptability. Or as marriage may be thought of as a cure for the "problem of homosexuality," he may go into marriage hoping his wife will "cure" him.

Homosexuals are often seen in high stress occupations and demanding professions. Perhaps creating this scenario is effective in making it impossible to deal with the reality of an unhappy personal life. Marriage cannot cure problems. A demanding job and extensive social life are used to create greater emotional separation. In the end it is impossible to bridge the problem. It is buried, and at great cost. Even though the underlying reason for becoming time overburdened is different, the result for the couple is emotional isolation and unresolved frustrations.

Since the statistics are showing that at least 10 to 15 percent of married people in the general population are gay and of those, 50 percent have children, there is a reality to be reckoned with. My interviews led me to women married to gay physicians and to lesbians who were married to physicians. I will share some of their perspectives here.

Trudy had been married for six years and had one child before she became aware of strong messages from her husband, Nathan. Generally she said she enjoyed her free time and private world with her son, Timothy. It becomes apparent that in choosing to be with a more emotionally detached person, either unconsciously or consciously, a homosexual, even unadmitted, may be a perfect choice. Sexual-emotional distance is built into the relationship with the addition of the cloak of medicine to justify difficult hours and responsibilities. The combination offers great distance between the couple. As Trudy talked of gradual estrangement and distancing, it was as if she got more than she bargained for when she originally decided to marry a physician.

> I knew Nathan would be busy and responsible. What I didn't know was that he wasn't really sexually interested in me. I thought it was my inability to be arousing, that I must have been doing something wrong. Soon I was picking up signals. He brought home a man, a clerk at the hospital. They planned ski trips together and occasionally went out after work or after Nathan's on-call. In my wildest imagination I never connected a sexual relationship between those two. Then a strange group started coming to our home. I was unfamiliar with gays, so I assumed this group was hospital colleagues even though medical talk was not what was happening. Little nuances and innuendos about men continued to surface. Eventually when we would go to a movie together and I picked up remarks about the movie stars or other people in the theater, it finally dawned on me that I was either crazy or this group was not like the people I was used to. I received lewd sexual statements, embarrassing comments, and continued comments which implied I was wrong or crazy when I confronted Nathan or his friends. "Oh, you're imagining things. Don't be a spoil sport."
>
> Eventually Nathan became obsessed with me being included in sexual activity with this group. "Would you take pictures of Larry and me?" or "Would you please take off my clothes while Larry masturbates." I was afraid. I couldn't say no; Nathan had a history of violence, and I was scared and confused. We had no sexual relationship. I wanted attention. Nathan swore me to secrecy. I had no idea how contemptuous he was of me and my sexuality, but I wanted to be acceptable to him.

Actually, Trudy was cool in her description of painful events. But she was more innocent and naive in her need to be a part of Nathan's life. She respected him, his medicine, and his medical explanations of what she would soon understand as unusual behaviors.

> Don't forget, I had a five-year-old son at this time. I was beginning to fear that Nathan could involve him in their sexual escapades. Confused and frightened most of the time about what Nathan would ask of me next, I finally talked to my best friend. She immediately said she had always known Nathan was probably gay but felt she shouldn't butt into our business. I told her some details and she referred me to a therapist who treats couples in which one person discovers their homosexuality.
>
> I finally divorced Nathan. He swore me to secrecy; he fears he'll lose his job at the hospital. I have Timothy with me and I'm still in treatment.

Five years had passed since the reported events. Trudy continued by saying that she got no support within the medical system or the auxiliary for their problem. It had to be kept secret to keep Nathan's position in the community and profession. Trudy is resentful. Her pain and isolation and her self blame for the situation devastated both her and her son. Confusion throughout six years of marriage, she feels, did influence her relationship with Timmy. She fears mostly for his emotional health and wonders whether he will be straight or gay. The fear expressed by Trudy for her son is common, but research has not borne out the greater incidence of homosexuality among children of gays or lesbians.

Carolyn, who was married for 14 years to Paul before she became aware of his homosexuality, has three children and a business of her own. She decided to remain in the marriage. As she spoke, her lips were strained and her piercing dark brown eyes often tightened, becoming almost closed. Carolyn has short, dark hair, a round face, and a bland appearance.

> Let's be realistic. I had three kids and a pretty solid lifestyle. Whether Paul was gay or not, I wasn't going to change anything. As long as he didn't embarrass me or flaunt his gayness in front of our friends and his colleagues, I would be fine with it. I guess he's really bisexual, because we can still have sex

occasionally and he says he enjoys it. But I know he sees men sometimes.

"Are you concerned about the threat of AIDS?" I asked, wondering how that affects this kind of experience and relationship.

Of course. In fact, Paul has restricted his homosexual liaisons to healthy people. So he says anyway. We have both been tested for AIDS and are negative. Thank heaven. But I am fearful of that. What's really strange is that Paul wouldn't get an AIDS test at his own hospital. We both went anonymously to another city. He was frightened that something would get out in our community. He said he'd be blackballed if his colleagues knew of his sexual preference.

What about your children, do they know anything?

No. We have been careful to guard this secret with our lives. We both agree that they are never to know the truth about Paul. I personally don't want them to know because it would look strange that I have stayed with a homosexual man in a long-term marriage.

It's funny, but in a way we're closer, guarding the secret between us. No one — family, friends, or colleagues — has to know. It's a strain to lie all the time about where Paul is for two or three days at a time, but he's a doctor and they can excuse his schedule and his hours away from home.

It is not uncommon for the gay partner and spouse to develop a facade or a way of dealing with a public mask. The appearance of normalcy is almost extreme to the outsider. Yet both people are rarely able to be authentic. Their true feelings must be denied or at least covered from the world, as they both become adept at playing roles deemed appropriate at the time, losing bits of their real selves little by little.

Melody, an attractive woman in her late forties, described 18 years of a cold marriage to Gregory:

I would have loved kids. I never realized I was a lesbian until my husband came home and told me he was sick of our marriage and had to get a divorce. I had come to believe marriage was cool and not connected. Greg wasn't around much. I enjoyed my work as a librarian, and when I finally realized we couldn't have kids, I'd accepted my life as mostly work and a couple of very close women friends. I had become involved in women's rights but still thought of myself as quite straight. After all, I was married to a physician with a respectable practice in plastic surgery. I was a loner anyway, reading a lot, working on my computer, and waiting for Gregory to come home for occasional company.

If Gregory had not divorced me to move in with his nurse — I know how trite that must sound to you, Esther, but it was for his nurse — I would not have been free to discover my lesbianism and finally be in a supportive atmosphere. Now I am in an all-women's community. We are loving, close, and caring. No men to confuse us or put us down. We try not to compete or compare. I have a good, solid, monogamous relationship with a woman whom I adore. We share intimacies which Gregory could never understand. He always shut me up. Claire hears me and talks to me. Sure I'm guilty for not giving Gregory what he must have needed, but to tell you the truth, he wasn't there for me either.

It appears that for Melody her support system in the lesbian community is greater than Trudy's in the straight community. The partner who is straight experiences lasting scars of inadequacy and isolation since she feels she has to keep the secret of her husband's homosexuality. He may go on to be in a relationship while she is sworn to secrecy. She remains isolated, feeling guilty, unlovable, and a failure.

Pamela carries scars from her coming out of the closet after ten years of marriage. Her husband was an absent cardiologist with great responsibilities in a big city hospital. She tells of his fury when she wanted to leave the marriage.

Pamela, like Melody, belied the stereotype of the masculine looking lesbian. She was petite and had a charming face with deli-

cate features. Her appearance obviously was important to her. Neat
and attractively dressed, she began softly:

> Late in my teens I had some inkling of being more interested
> in being with girls than boys. I ignored the feelings. They were
> horrifying to me. My mother was the epitome of the feminine
> woman — flirtatious, and beautiful, she doted on my dad and
> the men in her life. She never really related well to me, but
> still I knew it was healthy to be like her and "love" men. So I
> was escaping from what my body was telling me and dated all
> sorts of respectable men. My father was a professor, and I
> thought a doctor or lawyer was a perfect choice for me.
>
> Early in my marriage I knew that I was living a lie. The pain
> every day was excruciating. Trying to have a sexual relation-
> ship with Lee was the greatest acting I had to do. I was dead
> inside, and sometimes repulsed by the sight of him. Eventu-
> ally I closed down completely and lived like an automaton. I
> had two daughters and they became my life. That was easy
> because Lee was so busy at work all the time anyway.
>
> Gradually I couldn't stand the guilt and sadness in my life.
> Playing the loving wife was making me sick. But what choices
> did I have? I adored the girls, Beth and Sarah. My greatest
> panic was of losing the girls if I left the marriage.
>
> I joined a women's group, and after two years of listening to
> others, I got up the nerve to share my fears of being a lesbian.
> The reaction was great, and to my great surprise two of the
> group members were lesbians in traditional marriages, trying
> to deal with their problems. They supported me and encour-
> aged me to leave Lee.
>
> Then my nightmares began. Once I told Lee and explained
> my feelings, he exploded. It caught him so off guard and he
> felt such humiliation, I guess he couldn't stand that. His clout
> and power as a doctor started working, and we went through
> two and a half years of legal custody battles. Ugly accusations.
> All the friendships I had with women throughout the years
> were suddenly seen as lesbian sexual trysts, and I was smeared
> publicly over and over. The truth is that I never acted on my
> sexual preference until I was divorced.

Many lesbians wait until they're free of their marriage to be in a sexual relationship with a woman. The threat of losing one's children looms heavily. Plus, the fears and conflicts of their sexual identity stop them from acting on sexual desires.

> Anyway, after guilt and gradual hammering down of my self-esteem, I lost my confidence in being a good mother to Sarah and Beth. They were confused and terrified whenever Lee and I were together. The yelling and anger were almost violent.
>
> Lee had the best lawyers, and homophobia being so rampant, I couldn't get a judge who was unbiased enough to hear our case. Lee was determined to protect his masculinity and to use all his power to keep the girls and ruin my name and my life. He never forgave me for not telling him sooner. He accused me of using him to cure myself, and I guess he was a bit right.
>
> As you can guess, the girls went with their dad and I eventually left the state. I am still unsure if I would be a bad influence on Sarah and Beth. Sometimes I wish I never went to the women's group. This truth has been so painful and I miss my girls to the point of agony sometimes. I just don't really understand it all, I guess.

Pamela was subsequently cut off by her own mother and father, and has had to start an entirely new life as if her past did not exist.

Living a lie and being on guard constantly at work or in social situations is the outcome of accepting one's homosexuality if one is to remain in the medical community. If remaining married, one must lie to a spouse daily to maintain the charade. The dishonesty denies both people the trust and fulfillment of a good marriage. Both partners' self-esteem is questioned. Being regarded as deviant is lonely and emotionally exhausting. Being unable to get emotional support and guidance from fellow professionals adds to feelings of further alienation.

We still have work to do in our culture to accept and integrate those who are not what we consider mainstream. The truth is there is no mainstream. Our institutions dictate what will be socially acceptable. Medicine is a powerful institution and still influences our attitudes on homosexuality, even to the detriment of its own members.

It was the exception during my interviews for a woman to reveal doubt and questions she had about her husband's or her own possible homosexuality. Even the cloak of confidentiality was not considered protection enough. Our prejudices, misinformation, and stereotypes have resurfaced in light of the emergence of AIDS as a life-threatening disease. To be a member of the community that hopes to treat and cure the disease doubly ensures closeting of personal sexual preferences for physicians and their wives. It is imperative that old stereotypes be wiped away with clearer and more accurate information about homosexuality.

Knowing of the pain and perceived threat to their personal lives, I am particularly appreciative and indebted to those who contributed to the material in this chapter.

Chapter 19

Power and Control —
The Money Connection:
Who Decides Where We Go on Vacation?

> We have no problems with money. I make it and my wife spends it. — standard doctor joke

Since in our society the person who earns the most money often has the greatest power in the partnership, the physician continues to be capable of greater earnings and power in the marriage. Even those women who are physicians earn less than male physicians (Bowman and Gross, 1986). Until more women are in higher paid professions, men will be earning more and controlling the medical marriage.

In the discussion on vacations and leisure time I refer to how the greater bread winner controls the choices of how and where leisure time is spent. How do wives of physicians wield power and control in his marriage since the most money is usually earned by the physician? An indicator of power in a marriage is who decides on major purchases and how leisure time and money are spent. The house purchase, the car or cars, the trips or decision not to go, clothing, food, entertainment, education, household help, children's expenses, investment moneys, and insurance expenses all enter the marriage arena.

In most medical families wives have little or no say in how their husband's practice runs or what expenses are involved in their office. Even in these more liberated times the percentage of doctors' wives aware and involved in their husbands' business decisions and expenses is quite low. It still is common for a wife, during a divorce or after the death of her husband, to be oblivious to his bank accounts or to have no information about the extent or whereabouts of his assets. She may have had an allowance to run the house and that's it. No questions asked, or if asked, they often go unanswered.

Many of the women I spoke to never felt comfortable asking their husbands about financial matters. Even as they controlled the household expenses, wives were disconnected with overall or other hidden sources of income.

Janet, married 18 years, was used to being in charge of household finances, always wrote the checks, and felt quite good about her importance and influence in this area of her marriage.

> I'm not sure when this all began, but even in the early years Timothy didn't like paying the bills. He was so busy with school that I felt I could pay the bills and take that load off of his shoulders. So we have had this household account which I write the checks on. Food, kids' clothing, and general household maintenance come out of that account. If the water heater breaks down, the repair money comes from that account. The bill comes for heat, electricity, taxes, mortgage payments — all are paid from there. Timothy puts a certain amount into that every month and I pay the bills. It seemed equitable to me. I also bought personal stuff for myself from that account. I loved it because on the months that I had extra or spent less for the house I could spend more on me and kids personally, like extra sneakers or a pair of skis or anything.

"What about major purchases, vacations, a new car, or moving to a new home? How have you handled that?" I questioned. Janet continued:

> The first house we had we sat down together and figured out what the down payment and monthly fees would be. The money was there, or at least Timothy provided the money for the household account. So that happened comfortably for us both. Vacations are always a hassle. There never seems to be money for that, or redecorating. Cars are purchased as Timothy needs a new one for work. I get the other one that he's finished with. Once I got the new one to cart the kids around,

but usually he pays the down payment on the new car in cash and I pay the payments out of our account.

"Who is making the decision as to which car, which house, etc.?" I asked.

Well I guess it's up to Timothy since he's got to have a nice car for work, and as long as I have a roof over my head and we're all warm, I'm okay. It's true that I feel good knowing the money to cover our expenses is always in the account. So I don't ask too many questions. Whenever an unusual expense comes up, like something special for the kids' school, I let Timothy know that we might go over this month. He's pretty good about covering the expense. I feel good since I pay the checks. I feel like I'm involved and know where the money goes for our daily existence.

"Suppose you decided to go travelling abroad, or go back to school, what would happen?" Janet thinks a minute.

I'm totally dependent financially and I realize that, but since I've never been denied what I need, it hasn't been a problem for me. I'm not extravagant and I think Timothy depends on me not to be. If I suddenly wanted to start a business, like I've thought about before, I'm not sure Timothy would agree. About three years ago I brought up the subject of opening a small antique shop and tried to feel out Timothy's reactions. He flew off the handle then. "You have responsibilities here to me and the children," he said. "Don't I provide for you well enough?" Later he calmed down, but using family re-sources didn't seem a likelihood in the case of my opening a business.

Family resources—what does that mean to a doctor's wife? Generally it seems to mean the expenses required to keep the husband's and children's lives running smoothly, living up to the standards of the particular medical community of those involved. Cars, houses, furnishings, clothing, even vacations and sports are determined most often by the social system to which the family belongs. The wife, though, quickly finds out that her personal endeavors — a new business, education for her profession, a trip to reunite with her family of origin, or just ways to nurture herself that may require financing — are not often thought to be covered from "available family resources." So women in this situation repress their personal desires which cost money. Or they figure out indirect ways of having those needs met under the so-called family resources.

Maria, recently married to a physician, reported,

> I figured that in order to get what I need I have to make it look like it's for the family. If I say I want us to purchase a piece of land and cabin in the country so that I can go and write or just have a place to get some tranquilty, Marty says, "That's ridiculous," and sees no benefit to us or reason for it. If I make it sound as if we all need a getaway place or Marty could use it to do his computer work, he goes for it.
>
> Even my interest in nuclear arms reduction issues and causes have to be made to look like it was Marty's idea, that it will benefit him and his kids to spend money on it. It's crazy really, but indirect is better than nothing. I can't compete with his pocketbook and earnings. He's a gastroenterologist. He probably rakes in the money. [She evidently didn't have any real sense of his earnings.] He's got trust funds for his kids and pays his ex-wife a huge amount from their divorce settlement. I only brought a little money into this marriage. So I know that family resources are available according to what Marty determines they will be.

In my own house, financial management has always been an issue. Either Jerry decides on the way we spend money and then asks whether I'm in agreement, or he probably doesn't spend it at all. Our houses are purchased based on his determination of whether it's affordable. Within that framework I may have input into the decision, but the ultimate yes or no has always been his. Cars and vacations are the same. Generally, how money is spent (whether I pay the checks or not each month) is ultimately decided by Jerry. Since I hate paying the bills, I let him do it, but then I really don't know what we have or what it costs for us to live.

Input gives women a sense of participating, but not a sense of real power, because input can be ultimately overridden, discarded, or ignored. So saying you would love to go to the beach this year and wondering why you're skiing in the mountains can feel confusing. On the one hand you are away on a lovely vacation that is much needed and truly appreciated. On the other hand, if the beach vacation was truly your first choice and to feel powerful and fulfilled only the beach would do, denying this choice leads to repression, frustration, and powerlessness. Telling us that we are involved if we write the checks, but still not giving us the ability to determine where the checks are finally going, creates a dishonest gap in our experience.

We have heard, "But I'm only doing this for you, for the family." "We're going on this trip for all of us." "A new boat is for everyone!" "I can take our son hunting with this new equipment." "This weight room will be great for the kids." We know from experience how much conflict we feel about these statements. If we disagree, we lose. A fight ensues. The breadwinner seems distraught. He really seems to believe his altruism. The fact that we could care less about boating doesn't seem to matter. "What about the course on improving my French so I can converse with people and improve my chances of purchasing antiques for my new business?" says Janet, whom we heard from earlier. "The only way I can have a complete say in how the money is spent is to earn my own money."

How do we equitably account for the years of not having earned "her own" money? Even if earning her own, the greater dollars earner is entitled the greater say. We delude ourselves if we feel we have an equal say over how money is spent when we earn little or less than our partner. Even handing over a paycheck to his wife, a man feels entitled to a greater say in large money decisions if he earns more than she.

Nina, going through a divorce, was finally made aware of various accounts that her husband Miles had kept secret from her. She wrote checks from a household fund which he replenished. She had no idea that he was accumulating a fortune without her knowledge. There are a few ways to avoid those deceptions in a relationship. If a partner is going to be secretive, that's a reality one cannot change.

Physicians do have ways of acceptably but nonetheless secretly covering their financial earnings. In fact, it is probably easier, when there is adequate money coming regularly into the kitty, to close our eyes to other sources and accounts. Why should a trusting wife even question her husband's business manager and other financial counselors if she has enough?

She should if it is a true partnership. She should know what there is to work with so that she can participate in decisions regarding future expenditures. The final and underlying question in the financially unequal marriage, as physicians' marriages most often are, is: To what is the wife entitled? Traditionally, couples decide on their own, in private and personally, and in so doing, have encouraged unequal distribution of the funds, the decisions, and the power in the relationship. The physician earns more, he's highly valued in the society, he thus has greater entitlement to the spoils.

To what extent this greater entitlement affects his wife can only be guessed. There have been numerous times when doctors' wives denied or repressed their own needs which might cost money in favor of the family's needs or her husband's desires. If it is a need, it's easier for a woman to accept it and feel entitled. If it is a desire, it may seem silly or she feels undeserving and unentitled. Her husband works hard, earns the greater money, and is more deserving of the rewards. So first his needs are met and then his desires are attended to. If that happens to be clothing, housing, and leisure time expenditures that make her look and feel good, the doctor's wife wins. She begins to desire those things which she knows he will agree to, still denying her own creative desires. Of course she needs to be warm, fed, and sheltered. The extent to which those needs are met depends on the taste and generosity of the physician to whom she's married. If he has a great need to be perceived as affluent and generous to his wife and family, she makes out well. If he doesn't, she may go without things very basic to her, so accommodating her husband's spending habits is to her advantage. Using the resources without her husband's knowledge to meet her needs is another possibility. Denial or conflict about dishonesty then seem to be the common choices. Either way, Mrs. Doctor doesn't feel like a powerful, entitled, fulfilled adult, but rather like a dependent child.

Entitlement must be addressed. Supporting husband's career and maintaining the household while she rears the children or works outside the home for money, the doctor's wife must be made to feel entitled and powerful. If she waits until she is capable of earning both the money and prestige that he has, she will be disenfranchised for a long time to come.

There are hints that women are breaking through these patterns. We may even know of women married to physicians who hold jobs in political office or responsible and powerful positions in business and industry. Their numbers are gradually increasing. But there is a long way to go, and even these women may struggle with similar issues until equality is commonplace.

THE SACRED MAGIC OF LAW AND MEDICINE

My father, a lawyer, had
in his office the largest
volumes of books known to man.

There was no way a mere girl
could know the meaning of the words
or understand the power in his hands.

Mysterious, magical potions and incantations,
that's what I always thought of the law.
An interpreter and a special education needed
to pass through the portals of justice.

The dark robes, the wigs worn of old
the gavel, the judge at the helm,
nothing more imposing comes to mind

to bring fear into the hearts of men.
"Don't tangle with the law," they say.
"Don't take the law into your own hands."

Fear, mystery, magic, trust and mistrust,
the unknown makes us so needy, so afraid
and so helpless.
Those books distance us
they keep us in awe and yet increase our curiosity
along with our fright, our fascination
and our rage of impotence.

My husband, a doctor,
was also schooled in magic.
His office, too, is filled with volumes of
words and information indecipherable by most.

Instead of black robes and long, grey wigs,
the scalpel, the stethoscope and the white coat
separate his clan from the rest.

He holds the key to the knowledge of medicine.
Only those who go through Hippocrates' doors are
    taught the forbidden secrets of our bodies.

Not a body of law but a body of knowledge
just the same, a body of mysteries, potions,
a hocus pocus that imparts power on the
bestower of knowledge and claims fear,
gratitude and need on its clientele.

I always thought the inner sanctums of
law and medicine were forbidden holy shrines,
territories not meant for little girls.
Girls couldn't possibly understand, nor
could they wield the power of the throne.

I shudder when I walk through the halls
of a justice building, just being there
the ominous shadows of childhood return.

Our institutions of law and medicine are the stars
in a sea of disciplines, but they remain
alone sparkling like diamonds with their
    status.

What gives the gods of medicine their
even higher, more revered image?
The addition of test tubes and chemicals and machines
to their repertoire of books.

The surgical suites, the anesthetics, and the chemicals
and
    x-rays
are even more mysterious
as our bodies and our minds are
pressed, probed and photographed.

Even the lawyers can't offer us that kind
of witchcraft and mystery.
Lawyers have words, a long history of cases.

Doctors have multitudes more to confuse
and keep us in the dark.
In their magic is held
the future of life itself.

Now I understand why people cower
in the presence of a medical man.
It is the childhood belief that within his grasp
is the special magic of the universe,
    that other mere mortals do not
        and cannot rightfully own.

Congratulations to medicine, the teachers,
practitioners and purveyors of all that you guard sacred.
You have convinced a whole world of people
that the secrets of their bodies are only yours to possess.
You have taken away our personal powers of body
    and mind, and convinced us
that without you and your special knowledge
we cannot survive.

Chapter 20

Has He Changed or Have I?

He wasn't God when we said, 'I do.' — Ellen

It's Tuesday noon in mid-October 1988. Six well-groomed, attractive women are setting up for a meeting of doctors' wives. It has taken months to get this particular group going, people dropping in and out over that time, somewhat committed but with feelings of guilt and apprehension about sharing an experience that is supposedly quite respectable and desirable for women — marriage to a physician.

This is a group of young women. Some (about four) are mothers as well as wives. What brings them together is a program for wives of residents at this mid-sized hospital in Santa Fe, New Mexico. With more research materials coming forth from medical researchers, medical schools, and women's auxiliaries, the knowledge is getting out that medical marriages aren't all that perfect. The directors of the residency program suggested that having group sessions for the residents' wives would give them a chance to share difficulties, voice their opinions, and, it is hoped, resolve some of the increasing conflicts within these marriages. The group was to meet weekly with wives or spouses (but no male spouses attended). The doctors were to join the wives for an occasional weekly session also. It is rather interesting that the residents were not having their own meeting once a week, but let's continue.

I had the privilege of attending three of these meetings as an observer during my work for this book. I was intrigued that the training program for the residents would include this type of discussion for wives and couples, and I was delighted to join them. I was not invited to sit in on the couples' sessions, just the sessions for the wives. Had these meetings helped them?

> Yes, I think so. It's so important for us to be able to communicate with other women living in our shoes, so to speak. I don't feel so crazy or so alone any more.

> I've learned better ways to deal with my husband's temper and irritability. Plus, I know if I have a problem I can call any of these women for help.

> The best part of this group is knowing that we don't have perfect existences. When I met these couples at a party for residents, I was sure that my marriage was different, a special case, that it was me who was causing trouble. All the rest of these women seemed assured and confident in their relationships. Until our meetings we were so superficial with each other. I feel accepted by this group no matter what I say.

I sat for many minutes, enjoying the banter between these intelligent, lively, articulate women talking about how they came to be in that program, and their struggles in everyday life. I was touched by the caring and delicate support they gave to each other. They seemed to pick up where they left off in a previous meeting, discussing a very sensitive sexual issue. One of the women whose self-image of her sexuality had deteriorated greatly in recent months feared she was not as appealing to her husband as earlier in their marriage. I suppose the previous meeting's conversation led to some ideas to improve her sexual attractiveness. There were questions and replies as to her success in the matter.

The more I listened, the more I realized that the thing all six women had in common was the confusion about whether they were different since they were first married, and whether changes they were experiencing were their fault or within their control at all.

In the age range of late twenties and one in her early thirties, these women shared their confusion in comments like the following:

Whatever I suggest to Stan, he seems to ignore me or put me down. What am I doing differently?

Charlie used to be so delighted to spend time alone with me. We'd go away for a weekend retreat and tell no one where we were going. Now I can't interest him in anything.

I'm starting to get depressed. We don't laugh and joke much any more.

My mother calls me every other day. She says she's worried about me. Rick actually hit me last week. It was just a slap, but I told my folks about it casually, and they're nervous now.

God, I thought Mark was a quiet, sweet, kind guy who wanted to take care of the world. Now I'm intimidated by him. Plus, I don't think I'd go to him if I were dying. I feel so awful saying that, but it's true.

Regret, confusion, pain, and loss. Those were the feelings expressed or shown on the faces of these attractive young women.

When I decided to marry, while he was in school I thought we would be in this together. Instead we get further and further apart.

I feel like I don't belong here. They're all speaking a language that I can't understand. I don't have the key.

What is the thing troubling you most?

Being left out of my husband's life. Before we were so close. We talked, understood each other, and seemed to relate easily. Now I feel useless. Ignored and useless.

"What has happened since you were married? What's different?"

The consensus among the women was that although they tended to look for negative behavior changes within themselves, they came to realize (as a group, I will add) that their husbands, the doctors, were different from the men they married.

I try too hard to recapture pieces of the old Stan. Going to our former haunts, serving favorite meals, spending time with old friends, not medical people, taking time for relaxation for each of us, together and alone. Nothing works.

It's scary. Until I started talking to this group I thought for sure I was losing it. I was too picky, too critical, expecting too much, maybe I was tired or maybe I just had fallen out of love. Now what I understand is the change that has come over my husband.

Now he's a doctor. A resident, yes, but a doctor nonetheless! So it improved their self-esteem to take the guilt and blame away from themselves compared to what they had done so automatically before their group meetings. But now what hounded them was this undeniable fact that the sweet, loving, interested, innocent, idealistic men they fell in love with were becoming tyrannical, bossy, irritating, irritable, and impatient doctors.

They now had a safe, protected environment in which to ventilate their fears and confusion in their relationships. Whether this would work toward changing the reality, it's too early to say.

Somewhere between deciding to become a doctor, training, and becoming one, the expectations of these men for themselves, their wives, and others around them had changed. At least this was clear to these wives.

I asked, "Do you discuss these things at your couples' counseling sessions?"

Those sessions have been somewhat of a disappointment. I always go with the idea of confronting these issues, but it gets turned around to how we can make life easier for the residents! So I've learned to be quiet and listen in our couples' group.

The groups were led by older couples who had been through this stage of the residency program, and the women's groups are now leaderless, run by the wives themselves.

We're trying to make some headway. It's tough. The older couple [mid-thirties] who led this group was pretty directive. They shared what their experiences in residency training were like, and we talk about ours. Since the men don't have any other group meeting though, I think we [the wives] feel obligated to let them talk more. So we end up helping them figure out how to fix things about what we're doing that they'd like us to change.

I like the women's group, but the couples' group is not too satisfying for me. The men don't talk about the things the way I can understand. To them it's more like, "Can't you just cooperate with us? This is hard work," or "I'm tired all the time. Can't you just understand that and keep the kids quiet?"

There seems to be a long road to bridging the gap of communication. The good news is that this hospital is acknowledging the difficulties inherent in residency training, that the wives have a shared experience. The wives have learned that this business of being a doctor affects those who choose to be their spouses.

What I didn't realize was that a soft spoken, shy, slightly built, caring man would soon think he was God, and expect all of us to treat him that way.

What is still not addressed is the danger of becoming "God," not only to the doctor, but to his future patients and family. The perpetuation of this metamorphosis from human to "godlike" is impossible for his wife. If she believes along with him that he is above us all, then she stands to spend her life in his service. If she is certain that he is indeed human, the ever-present conflicts between the couple may be irreconcilable due to a likely unwillingness on his part to concede that power of godliness so revered by his colleagues. The hope is that he will return to a state of reality and admit that two people living and loving together will succeed only if they are on truly equal footing.

WOULDN'T IT BE STRANGE IF THEY KNEW YOU BETTER THAN I DO?

Wouldn't it be strange
if someone else's child called you Daddy
If someone else's mother called you Son
What if another woman called you Darling

Wouldn't it be strange?
Oh I wish I knew you like they do

Some day I'll take that bus
I'll buy that lunch
I'll read that newspaper

then perhaps I'll get to know you
   Like they do
   Like they do

Wouldn't it be strange
if the woman in the window
knew you better than I?

She sees you every day at lunch
as you go walking by.

Wouldn't it be strange
if the boy at the newsstand
knew you better than I?

He sees you every day at five
as you go walking by.

Do you speak to them?
Do they know your name?

What about the children in the waiting room
Do you laugh with them?
Do you share your love?

Wouldn't it be strange
if the people on the bus
know you better than I?

They see you every day
in the morning and the night
Wouldn't it be strange?

Chapter 21

Accessibility:
Can He Come to the Phone Now?

Sorry, Mrs. Nitzberg, he can't come to the phone now.
— nurse, secretary, receptionist, hospital personnel, etc.

Infuriated, I try for the fourth time to reach my husband to ask
him a simple question — shall we meet for dinner or should I go
ahead and make plans for the evening for myself. The exchange
can't get in touch with him. He's not at the office, he's not at the
hospital. The woman on the exchange (telephone answering service) is confused. I guess he's not wearing his beeper; he hasn't
called in. The charade continues. The hospital telephone director
says, "He's not here and I haven't seen him recently." Both ask me
if I want to leave any message. His office secretary tells me that
he's not working this afternoon; perhaps he had to make nursing
home rounds or was attending a meeting in the next town. Do I
want to leave a message? I recall all the times I have had to track
Jerry down for emergencies for myself, for my children, for his
patients. Thirty years of chasing him and leaving the same message:
"Call home," "Call your wife," "Call Esther, she's trying to get
hold of you. She needs to talk to you."

How many wives deal with the frustration and helplessness of
being unable to reach their partner in life, the father of their children? Many, in many walks of life. Again I'm certain that inaccessibility is the watchword in politics, business, forestry, or career
armed forces, where a man might be out to sea for six months at a
time or on military maneuvers. Wives get used to it; they take it in
their stride for it comes with the territory, or does it?

Repeatedly women married to nonphysicians said, "How do you

do it? The doctor is never home?" I say defensively, "A travelling salesman is never home. A doctor is home sometimes." Perhaps the travelling salesman doesn't have the entourage and the entire society supporting his inaccessibility to his family. Or when he's physically out of town, on the road selling his wares, his wife knows what to expect. She goes on with her life and has a predictable set of circumstances. He's on the road this week. He calls in regularly, or leaves his number at the hotel. True, the reputation of the unavailable salesman and the snide insinuations about what happens on the road are similar to the innuendos about physicians and what happens in the hospital broom closets.

The clear difference is that the hospital nurses, orderlies, technicians, and in the office the nurses, secretaries, and other help join forces to keep the outside world from gaining access to his life and lifestyle at work; unfortunately, the wife falls into that outside world category. The protective guard in medicine is enormous. Even the telephone exchanges inadvertently or openly work with the physician and against his wife and members of his family to keep him guarded and protected at all costs.

Any patient knows how difficult it is to reach through the medical entourage surrounding the physician. Even during a medical emergency there is a barrage of left messages and unanswered questions before a physician directly responds to any individual patient. The days of calling a doctor's office and having the doctor answer have long passed, reflecting a time much earlier in this century when doctors had offices in their homes and either they or their wives answered the phone. Today it is almost a miracle that patients get to the doctor of their choice while the symptoms are still bothering them.

Being married to a physician is by no means a guarantee of access to this overly protected person. Women related over and over again accounts of having personal emergencies at home — children bleeding, the heater exploding, burglars accosting the house, going into labor, aborting babies, even house fires (the list goes on) — and being unable to get through to their husbands.

Brenda, married only five years, remembered her feelings on this subject:

I was beginning to feel truly paranoid. I was married before to a stockbroker. Simple—when I wanted to talk to him while I was at work and he was at work, I called him on the telephone and he answered, or if he had a secretary she put him through to me. Real easy! Or if I came home from my job before he did and I needed something from the store, a simple phone call and the job was done.

Well, for the last five years my life has drastically changed. Eric's office and hospitals where he works require the old type of a CIA agent to get through to him. And after leaving six messages with different operators I begin to feel vulnerable and terribly exposed. The sound of my own voice seems very whiny and helpless after a while. "Tell Dr. P. to please call his wife at home," begins to sound very pesky to me and makes me feel that I'm really disturbing something quite important. The most difficult are the repeated requests of hospital telephone personnel, "Are you certain you want me to pull Dr. P. out of the operating room? He is in surgery I believe, Mrs. P." "Well yes," I say, "I'm in labor and I'm going to deliver his baby soon. Perhaps he should know that," I reply, angry, frustrated and scared to death that I'll have to go through the experience alone.

As far as I can tell there is not the necessity to keep me from having access to Eric. But there is a traditional view or a concerted effort on the part of those working for physicians to protect their time and space—especially from nonsense calls, of which the wife is considered the greatest nonsense!

"Never getting the message that I called," "Never returning my calls," or "Getting back to me when the need to talk or the reason for the call was long past," were commonly reported by women.

The message is clear that marriage to a physician is not considered by his co-professionals reason enough to disturb his sacred work domain. In fact, it is usually the lowest rung on the accessibility scale. When asking nurses or other work personnel in physicians' work places what happens when the doctor's wife calls, the responses ranged from: "My boss has told me not to disturb him if his wife calls—ever!" "Tell my wife I'll call her when I have a free minute,'' which is rare, if ever (not the free minute, but calling her in it!), to actually telling blatant lies to the wife. A nurse who has since married a physician was horrified when she became the wife:

> I knew about the lies and deceit that fill the office to protect the physician and keep him inaccessible to his wife. All the personnel cover for him, tell stories about his cases and emergency calls. When you're on that side you know that protecting the physician from his family is of the utmost importance. I had a co-worker who was fired from her job by her boss—a doctor—who was furious at her because she gave too much information of his whereabouts to his wife!

We see, then, women who need to get the attention they want from the physician pitted against the office women who want to keep their jobs.

Patricia, who has since divorced her physician husband, describes her dilemma:

> It was a vicious circle. I was frustrated by not having a way to get in touch with Peter when I needed him. The red tape was ridiculous. Worse yet, though, was my sense of self—I was made to feel so small, like a little girl trying to reach her daddy. Humiliation was always what I felt after every phone call. I tried having Peter check in with me periodically, but he soon sabotaged that and made me feel as if I was a helpless nut! The system stinks. It puts me in the position of always having to track down Pete. I'm on hold all the time. I never felt like I was important or that I had control of our relationship. Peter always could call the shots! When he wants me, he knows how and where to reach me. Not me—I had to jump through hoops. After 12 years I never really found out what the password or combination was. The humiliation I felt from the nurses and other women he worked with, like they knew so much more about what was going on than I could ever know. I opted to get out of that situation. Secrecy was a big issue in my growing up, so I decided that it made me feel too small and dependent and afraid. I had to get out and find a relationship where there was open access to my husband's life.

Reserve, control, privacy, discomfort with feelings — these traits contribute to a physician's emotional unavailability. His wife experiences this when he is present, together with the physical inaccessibility supported by his colleagues and associates when he is not present. He lives with meetings, phone calls, presentations, work-related activities, and a totally separate life that she learns is impenetrable, for herself and the family. Unspoken is — live an isolated existence, make your own life apart from your husband's. Take the minor role in his life. Balk about it and be ignored, or be completely miserable. I'm calling this invisibility abuse. Not being seen or heard, as in the adage for the children of old. The doctor's wife is to be not seen and not heard, except when convenient and expedient for the doctor and his profession, as an ornament for him, as a manager of his private life, as a comfort when needed, or as a merely convenient protection to an otherwise totally separate life. Thus, swings of anger, guilt, and disappointment are her common companions.

Every time a person is refused access to a close person's life, the message is clear. You are not important enough or valuable enough for me to interrupt what I'm doing. I care about you at my will and bidding — not at yours. I am in control of your value. Physicians' wives must rationalize this information to their self-esteem each and every day. Unable to understand the feelings and disturbed by them, women suffer in silence and feel guilt for their anger and frustrations. "I shouldn't be feeling this way," "They don't mean to humiliate me or force this isolation on me at his office." Then why is it happening time and time again? Why do I feel so awful when it does?

Chapter 22

Coping:
Drugs, Alcohol, Running, TV —
Take Your Pick

I knew I was in trouble when the only thing I ever looked
forward to was "Bill Cosby" and "Night Court." — Greta

It is generally accepted that medication is easily available to physicians' families. Perhaps it begins with something to help his wife
sleep better. He can bring home samples, and no one need ever
know because no prescriptions are written.

For years I took Valium to deal with increased anxieties, whether
it was giving parties which made me extraordinarily nervous, learning to ski, or when I was terrified of heights. I had a supply of
Valium or Tranzene or Zanex whenever I needed it. Oh you can
say, "Anyone has access to these drugs," or "Women are given
these drugs all the time to keep them quiet and in line." True, but
other women must have some physician, even a kindly friend; but
nevertheless he needs to justify prescribing these drugs.

In my house if I needed them I just called Jerry and he would
bring me sample packages from the office. Or if I was extremely
lucky, a Valium salesman may have just stopped at the office and
Jerry could request a large bottle, which he then brought directly
home to our medicine cabinet.

Coping became easier if a pill was available. I didn't have to face
my fears and anxieties, and neither did Jerry. For years he thought I
was super-sensitive to certain situations. He was convinced that he
was helping me to control some outrageous, uncontrollable, and to
him utterly confusing behaviors.

I would experience terrible cramps and diarrhea before entertaining in our home. Alcohol didn't agree with me (probably fortunate, for I might be an alcoholic now). Since I had to entertain at times, I naively took the doctor's orders and used pills to calm myself.

Then we took up skiing. I thought it looked like fun. Jerry was passionately in love with it. Again I began having terrible nervous symptoms before every ski trip, especially if other people were scheduled to be with us. In order to continue skiing, not to spoil anyone else's fun, I endured terror by taking Valium. Every chair lift ride was devastating, but more humiliating was admitting my weakness. Everyone else was heavy into the skiing by then. I didn't want to be left home, a failure, a wimp, so Valium it was. Eventually I became an expert skier, eyes closed on chair lifts, screaming, not talking to Jerry for days, thinking he was responsible for my misery, totally unable to sort out my fears. Jerry, completely mystified by what he saw as irrational behaviors, said, "Take a Valium. You'll feel better. Why suffer like this? You want to ski don't you?" Who knew what I wanted. Despite my crippling anxieties, I was an athlete and could become good at whatever I set my mind to.

Recently my oldest son and his new wife were visiting. He and his dad were on their way to the slopes. He said, "Mom, you never were enjoying skiing all those years, were you?" Then I was shocked and felt guilty, as if I had deceived my own son. He thought I was having the time of my life—what a great mother I was. Other mothers weren't such sports. Now at 29 years old he revealed the truth: I wasn't really having a good time. Once again I was pierced through the heart with remorse and a feeling of failure.

Valium, convenient and available, covered my fears and helped me cope with life. True, skiing is not essential or even important in the scheme of one's existence, yet at the time it was our leisure time activity, our family time together, and our social time with others. For me it was tied to being a successful wife, mother, and person. The fact that heights terrified me and that I denied the importance of my own experience for years is significant now. And the fact that I did not become addicted to the Valium or the tranquilizers is by the grace of some higher being.

I have become a counselor since those days. I have had therapy, and I hope I am successfully touching my fears and finding better ways to cope with life's difficulties. Undoubtedly my work in bio-feedback, stress management, and psychotherapy with others, especially women, has enabled me greater understanding of my own psyche. But for years I lived with the crutch of medications, hearing over and over that, "Those small doses cannot hurt you. You cannot become addicted at those levels. If it helps you, take it." I know better now. If we have problems of mind or body, usually there are explainable and understandable reasons. Although much more complicated to unravel than to take a pill, it's well worth the effort of discovery.

Greta, whom I interviewed at the country club, talked of her life as a doctor's wife. She had been married 28 years. She had a sad expression on her face, was chic in a hat and suit, and had been drinking at the bar when I walked in.

I've been in this business for a long time. Country club, dinners, meetings, parties. Everyone trying to impress everyone else. My husband, Dick, was at the bottom of the totem pole, a family doctor. Everyone else looked down on him, but he referred patients to them, the specialists. So they looked down on me too, I guess. Snotty remarks would fly around: how much busier their husbands were; how much fancier their trips were or their horses and cars were, whatever; which private schools did my kids go to—all that, all the time. I started drinking to get through the evenings, the embarrassment.

Eventually I drank my way through the day. Dick worked all hours, the kids were away at school, and I would drink through a golf game, until even golf was uninteresting to me. Finally the only thing I did was drink and watch T.V. I knew I was in trouble when the only thing I looked forward to was "Bill Cosby" and "Night Court," and liquor, of course.

What does Dick say about your drinking?

Nothing much. He drinks too and doesn't consider it a problem for him. I periodically try to stop, or one of my kids will express concern, and that catches my breath.

I've seen the way others frown at my loud, boisterous behavior at parties. I know my jokes get vulgar and irritating.

But it's still better than reality: no real friends, no work of my own, no kids at home any more. And worst of all, no real relationship with Dick.

Greta's pain was too piercing to witness. She took out large bills to pay for our lunch and said she should probably come to see me at my office. I smiled slightly, but felt I was privy to and intruding on a personal struggle that would take a long time and much support to unravel. I hope that Greta did get support for her difficulties. Many women suffer alone in silence.

Vera described a history of anorexia and running to cope with a cold, unfulfilled marriage:

I started running to reduce my tensions. Soon I was doing marathons and in order to stay slim I would starve myself; the lighter I could become, the faster my times. I loved running because I could leave the house for hours and not worry about what people would think. After years of ignoring my feelings of fear and incompetence, I decided that exercise would make me look and feel better. I was overweight as a girl and always had to watch what I ate. Running helped me clear my head and used calories to do it. I was good and fast. I won races. I began to feel good about myself. People started congratulating Lyle for my running accomplishments. He began seeing me in a new light, as a whole person, I think, not just an appendage to him. Running started as an escape and has become the thing that saved my life and my marriage.

Descriptions of shopping, eating, sleeping, television, gambling, drugs, exercise, affairs, reading, all in excess, were used to cope with life. Recently some mention of support groups of women experiencing similar feelings have been appearing. It is becoming more acceptable to admit to imperfections in our personal lives and share with others.

However willing wives are to get help for troubles, they are still hoping for support from their husbands and the medical profession, yet their husbands are trained to see physical disease, not emotional distress. Many women are still being treated through overuse of drugs and alcohol for things which could be averted through communication and more egalitarian role dispersement in the marriage.

Flo described her infuriation and frustration at her husband's affair with a computer:

> He's in there [his study] all the hours that he's not at the office, working on his computer. We don't talk at all any more. He loves it and can afford the latest stuff. What do I do though? I read and watch TV. I'm going crazy, and if I get really mad Elliot tells me to be quiet, that he's working on stuff for our future, investments. So I don't complain about it. It does feel like I'm the one who complains all the time. Elliot seems fine — sex once in a while, work 60 hours a week, and the computer. I need more, but I'm frightened of going out there on my own again. I was younger then, now I'm not sure. So I read, watch TV, and try to bury my negative thoughts.

It is clear that our lives are complicated. Television tells us how to be and feel. Donahue and Oprah influence many of us, telling us how to feel and what's important today. But to some, staying inside to watch Donahue and Oprah only becomes a coping habit that is hard to break. They too are part of the cycle of distress. The very suggestions they have for our coping become impossible to accomplish, and we sit in front of the television, watching in a stupor, feeling despair.

Chapter 23

Medical Meetings:
Do You Call That a Getaway?

Well it's either go to those meetings or wait till he has a heart
attack and can take some time off. — Phyllis

Where should we go on vacation? This statement seems innocu-
ous enough. Not true! As stated in the chapter on power and control
describing how the money is spent in a medical family, it is a subject of great conflict and underlying distress to many of these couples. But overshadowing the problem of how to spend vacation or
leisure time money is the question of leisure time altogether. The
often-heard statement, "For years the only time we ever got away
was to go attend a medical meeting," seems indicative of the commitment of MDs to incorporate their social life and vacation life
into their professional life.

A typical medical meeting consists of four days away from the
home and office in a luxury hotel at the sea or some resort area. The
purpose of the get-together is to further medical education, see colleagues, catch up on professional contacts and news, and have a
break from the office or hospital grind. I say grind. It is rarely seen
as a grind to the practicing physician, otherwise a medical meeting
would be the last place to spend leisure time!

All time is pre-planned with lectures, meals, cocktail hours,
other meetings. How the physician behaves at the meeting is clearly
an extension of his daily work and interaction with fellow doctors.
The faces are familiar, and the etiquette has been established since
attending medical school. The scene resembles a Boy Scout meeting of grown-up boys practicing medicine. It is clear who is important, what the pecking order is, who makes the most money, who

can be the most intellectually informative, and who will be the most politically influential. The conversation in between lectures has become predictable, from discussion of classes and lectures attended, to continuing in-hospital meetings. As is found among any members of a close clique, physicians desire interaction.

For wives the medical meeting can range from the only time she sees something other than her home to an abomination of four days of separatism, sexism, boredom, and social climbing for her husband's success. Remember, part of the practice of medicine is the time dedication and selfless cure of others (except oneself and family). That's what makes the medical meeting model work so beautifully. The doctor is not even having to rationalize his time out of the office and away from patients if he is indeed away studying and furthering clinical skills. For most, it is the perfect chance to change the physical surroundings, but the commitment goes on. Through hours of medical talk, the dedicated doctor can still behave exactly as he did in Podunk (his home turf), be surrounded by other dedicated professionals, and get credit toward education—without leaving his milieu.

So the issue comes up between husband and wife:

I would be needing a well-earned break from household chores and children. I would see that Jason was tired and drawn and more irritable than usual. I started begging for us to be able to get out of town, away from the responsibilities of our hectic life. Invariably, in fact always, Jason went to the journal listing of the medical meetings published regularly for this very purpose. "Okay," he'd say. "I'll look and see when I can coordinate a meeting with my office schedule." Later, sometimes weeks later, he'd come home with a list of possibilities. Other couples look at travel brochures; we look at lists of medical meetings.

Over and over I suggested a *vacation*, that meant no medical meeting, just a trip or a leisurely suntan on a tropical beach. It wasn't that we couldn't afford it. Even without the tax deduction of a medical meeting we could afford any kind of trip. I did the checks. I know it was not an issue of money. But something in Jason's bones made it impossible for him to think about going anywhere but an organized medical meeting. I felt really lucky if the meeting was going to be at a nice resort or some place I could do sight-seeing at least; otherwise I felt like staying home. It wasn't a vacation for me to be in some convention center while Jason attended lectures all day.

That came from Helen, a sprightly, energetic mother of two daughters.

Madeline shared her experience:

We went every year to Bill's cardiology meeting, and that was our vacation. I did get to know some of the other wives, but even so, the humiliation of having a wives' luncheon while our husbands were meeting and discussing life-saving measures never sat well with me. They'd import someone to talk about table decorations, or how to buy Christmas gifts for people, and this was supposed to be informative and keep us happy. The only encouraging part of these meetings for the spouses is now they are inviting people to talk about stress management or the troubles involved in being married to a doctor. Still, it seems that even those speakers are patronizing us. "How to make your husband's life better. How to keep him happy and healthy longer. How to know if he's burned out on his work. How to guess if he's suffering from depression." That's what wives hear at medical meetings! Sometimes we get invited to our husband's lecture when the powers that be think we can understand the topic, such as business management or the effect malpractice has on your home life.

It makes me sick to my stomach to go to those meetings. It's no vacation for me and if Bill enjoys it — and I'm sure he does or he wouldn't keep going — I've decided he can go alone from now on. I can't go as an appendage any more.

Kay, married over 30 years, rather innocently and matter of factly shared this:

I've always enjoyed our chance to be at Pine Lodge by the Sea
for our medical meetings. If it wasn't for that trip I probably
would not have gotten out of town, ever. I like the shopping
and the tennis, best of all the room service and meals at which
Ellis joins me occasionally. The Lodge is elegant and I feel
luxurious being there. I don't usually go to the lectures provided for the wives because I like to use the time for myself.
I'm a loner anyway, so time on the beach or on the golf course
is great for me. It's the only time we left the kids and got away
by ourselves. Ellis is in a great mood, so our evenings are
great when we go to those things. We even talk more at the
Lodge than we do at home. I guess Ellis is more relaxed. I'm
not sure, but this is his main vacation and I know he looks
forward to the meetings. Learning up-to-date information in
his field makes him feel good, like he's keeping up with medicine. I just love getting away—I sleep late, have wine with
dinner, someone makes my bed for me. It's great!

Here we have the incorporation of professional life with social
and private life epitomized. As brainwashing continues into leisure
time activities, the hold of the medical model and paternalistic medical father marches on, affecting the doctor and his wife in ways
unknown to other wives of professionals.

Suddenly, the phrase from George Orwell's *1984* comes to mind.
"Big Brother is watching you!" How to be in private life and leisure time is dictated to a medical couple and family by the big
brother, or the profession itself, which is taking care of the couple
even on vacation, having an acceptable place for him to go to
"learn" while away "relaxing." The little woman is debriefed
early on to learn her acceptable behaviors at these meetings. Entertainment, comfort, and thoughts will all be provided in exchange
for a tax deduction. No one needs to think, or act for themselves.
Conversations among MDs are predictable, and among wives they
are predictable. The big hand of medicine is powerful and continues
to rule even on vacation, or supposed vacation.

Eliminating the need to think about where to go during one's
leisure time implies there are no other choices to make. To be a
good doctor one takes medical meeting vacations. No planning, no

conflict, no thought required. No choice either. It also implies that women married to physicians are to go along with the program with gratitude. It's either the medical meeting or no vacation at all!

Victoria described her decision to send her husband to his meetings alone:

> Now I go away somewhere else, or back to Montana to my family, while Roger is at his meeting. I always felt self-conscious there. Other women seemed to like it and to know what to do and say. I felt horrible. All I did was sit around and wait for Roger to come get me and take me to dinner. Roger always wanted me to come. "Everyone brings his wife," he said. "I'll be the only one alone." So I'd go and hate it. I'm a freelance writer. Most of the other women put down my work as taking time away from family and Roger. I didn't feel comfortable talking about it. I thought the lectures for the wives were insulting to our intelligence, and the act to impress everyone else made me puke. After five years of this I told Roger I would go home while he went to his meetings, so I would be taken care of and he needn't worry. Gradually he's gotten used to going alone and I've been able to do whatever suits me at that time. If you live differently or feel differently there is no room for you at these types of gatherings. It's like being blackballed in a college fraternity or being shunned from your religious group if you are out of the fold.

The profession of medicine is filled with means to keep members in line. Like a religious affiliation that makes questioning or difference sacrilegious or sinful, so does living with medicine. The medical meeting is still another way of ensuring cooperation and complicity among its practitioners. Wives are a nuisance at the very least, and can be considered trouble makers or dangerous to the profession if they deviate from the appropriate practice of medical wifery. Being ignored by the other wives is quite a powerful influence. Being left out until you cooperate will ensure either cooperation or desperate loneliness.

Chapter 24

Entitlement

I have a vague notion of what it's like to have to sit in the back of the bus. — Esther

In my own therapy the issue of being deserving and entitled keeps looming as a great conflict. It seems that although I married a physician, one of the most entitled and deserving members of our society, I continually doubt my worthiness.

It is striking to me that marrying a doctor only complicates the confusion already existing for women in a world where men are much more highly favored. If the confidence and inner self were not strengthened and nourished when we were children, we are prey to looking for ways to supercede the emptiness as adults.

My family was a troubled one as I was growing up. My brothers, although the favored gender, were somehow a terrible disappointment to my parents. Many causes made it impossible for them to become competent and proud professionals in their adulthood. I can only now imagine how that affected my parents, to whom professionals were everything successful and American. Consequently, my messages, although mixed and confusing, left me feeling inferior as a girl but with the script to fix the disappointments that my brothers wrought upon our household.

My mother never worked outside the home. To her the ultimate accomplishment of a female was in her choice of husband. I think, looking back, that she also struggled with entitlement — what did she deserve? She was a powerful, bright, witty, competent woman who did not succeed as a mother or as a wife in the eyes of the world. Her sons deviated from the norm, one emotionally disturbed, and one less able intellectually than she hoped, and nonmotivated in a home that was materialistically and intellectually striving.

My mother lived through her children. Her entitlement came only through what her husband and children could achieve. She herself was entitled to little or nothing apart from what others could give. What could she teach me then? In a world where men could ask for things and accomplishments for themselves but women could only live through the men, what could she pass on to a girl child?

My legacy was to succeed through the choice of husband, to have children, and through both husband and children define myself! Her definition must have been pathetic. My poor mother—a husband who may have been unfaithful and whose sexual preference was questionable, and two sons who were incompetent to deal with the world, and a daughter who could not really provide vicarious success or entitlement for a mother unless she married well.

I did. I married a Doctor. True, it was not just for my mother, but as I look back, a good part of that choice was to provide my mother with some personal success in this world. She died within months of my marriage.

Why else would marriage to a doctor seem to be the ultimate fulfillment for my generation, an accomplishment which continues to have appeal in the hearts of millions of parents and daughters? Until women are entitled to accomplish and achieve in their own right—intellectually, economically, creatively, and with prestige and respect for their contributions—marriage to a doctor seems to provide the second closest thing.*

---

*A curious thing happened when I was researching this book. I regularly called the research librarian at a local university and asked for assistance. At first she said, "Are you a faculty member? Did you say your name was Dr. Nitzberg?" After saying no twice and getting the cool response, "Our hours are 8:00 to 5:00. Please come in yourself and get what you need," I finally called and said, "This is Dr. Nitzberg. Would you please locate these articles," etc. etc. She was all over herself with accommodation and helpfulness. "Certainly, Dr. Nitzberg. Is there anything else you need? Don't hesitate to let me know how else I can help you with your project. I'll have this information for you as soon as possible." I, needless to say, was both horrified and amused at the power of the "doctor" word, be it a doctor of medicine or doctor of whatever. How unconsciously we suscribe to the belief that a doctor is more distinguished and they and their time are to be treated with utmost respect and consideration. Pity the rest of us.

Herein lies the conflict. Marriage to a doctor does provide special kudos — at times more money than average, respect in the community, a sense of being close to one who provides great service to that community. Why does she still struggle with her own entitlement? Why does she, as I often have, still feel empty and without real value?

For those whose marriages provide fewer societal perks, a wife who earns her way at home or outside has a chance to sort out and ask for that which she is entitled. Not so a poor little rich girl.

I was reminded of Grace Kelly's marriage to Prince Ranier of Monaco. In *Grace: Secret Lives of a Princess*, Spada reports Grace Kelly never felt accepted in her own family (1987). She longed for approval and a solid sense of worth. What better way than to marry a prince and have the entire kingdom of Monaco at her feet? How must she have felt when she gave birth to her first child, a girl, and realized that her job was to provide a son to the throne? It wasn't until her son was born a year later that Monaco rejoiced and celebrated wholeheartedly. Grace had succeeded; only now was she truly entitled to the luxuries of her position. She bore a male child. Sadly, though, neither she nor her daughters Caroline and Stephanie were really valued as whole participating beings with voices to be taken seriously by the entire population. I can only begin to imagine what her tender sense of self, her meager inner core experienced.

It is to that meager sense of self and inner core that I speak. Doctors' wives cannot claim a place of their own in their world, but only in relation to their husbands' lives, or their children's. We struggle with the real question: What rights do I have? Do I have the right to think, to speak my mind, to disagree, to make a mistake?

The current president of a local medical association auxiliary has worked diligently to be heard. She has introduced drug programs into surrounding communities to help relieve the high drug usage and accessibility in schools. She is enormously effective politically. But with her accomplishments she remains Mrs. Dr. _____. Her rewards and audience see her only through her connection to the medical establishment. Her achievements come as an auxiliary achievement, related to the medical profession, and to her husband's achievements, not an individual one belonging to her.

When I feel squeamish about having a typist help me finish a book and my husband questions my need for one altogether, my entitlement button gets pushed. When I assert my will for time uninterrupted by phones or chores for my husband's office practice or chores for our home, my entitlement button is again pushed. I am not entitled to an education, a full-time career. I am not entitled to think. I do not go to law school; rather, I do part-time counseling education to accommodate the family. Again, what are my rights as a wife? A woman? A person?

Since the public thinks I have it all as a doctor's wife, they are less apt to take my conflict seriously. They see no conflict. They see only what they need to see – the doctor who is important, valued, and entitled to all that society can offer him to maintain our health. They see me, his wife, as an appendage, connected at the hip. Others are unwilling and unable to view me as a separate person. And I am in conflict about whether I am entitled to be viewed at all.

Grace Kelly was viewed as beautiful, glamorous, charming, and witty while a starlet in Hollywood and while a princess in Monaco. Still the prince determined that her career would discontinue upon her marriage, and then her townspeople forbade her to return to movies later when she desired that for herself (Spada, 1987). She must have felt an enormous need to be creative and be seen and heard in her own right in the '60s when she was to return to Hollywood. But marriage to the prince and responsibility to her kingdom precluded her career. Those married to physicians experience similar responsibility to the whims of their husbands, his career, and the medical community. Each doctor's wife lives (although not as luxuriously) as though in the municipality of Monaco as the princess, unable to think for herself, limited in her need to truly exert influence for and on her own.

Gradually, after being unentitled to one's own will, the will is broken. As with battered wives or cult members, a doctor's wife loses the ability to make her own decisions and carry them through without an enormous amount of guilt, conflict, and insecurity. How dare I ask for more? We feel anxiety and fear of reprisals or retribution for going against our socialized limitation of rights. The "how dare you" is haunting. The punishment and humiliation awaits as blacks in the front of the bus knew, and still know. Can I disagree at all? Little by little the center of decision making and responsibility is the doctor's. I do not refer here to actual work done to keep the house and care for the children. That his wife does beautifully. I refer rather to the how and when and where things will happen. Who will be included in their lives? What will their lives be involved with? Can she, the wife, be separate at all? I sadly think not. At this point she is unable and therefore unwilling to chance it. And in small and big ways those around her reinforce her unentitlement by ignoring her wishes and opinions, ridiculing and humiliating her, cutting her conversations short, and applauding only that which benefits the household and her husband's career. She cannot stand up for herself and yell "Foul!" Others see this as ungrateful and unworthy of a princess. They may tell her she's crazy.

Over and over I have referred to those of us in the medical marriage as couples who adhere to very traditional values at all cost. In that framework wives have expressed their confusion: Why am I frustrated? I thought it would be different.

How can it be different when the meager or shadowy sense of self denies our entitlement and renders us unable to speak up, act, decide, create, fail, or succeed for ourselves? The profession of medicine expects its auxiliary people — nurses, technicians, secretaries, researchers, and wives — to continue to build the strength of their highest and most revered: the doctor. As a woman, to be married to a physician is to ensure his entitlement through our unentitlement. She can have a little room in the back of the house to start her soon-to-be successful dried flower business. He gets the rest of the house. He is the doctor. The phones are for his use. The cars are used at his discretion. Leisure is his choice. Play is his domain. Money is in his account and he doles it out according to his level of generosity or parsimoniousness. Life in the home is determined by his routine and will.

Sitting in my office across from me is a slightly rounded woman with a delicately soft, expressive face. Her warmth is easily accessible, as are her confusion and sadness. She began:

It's so difficult. All the years I was raising a family, taking care of my husband and three children [two daughters and one son], I wasn't earning any money. I feel so guilty now. That's been such an issue for me since I was a girl. We never had money. My mother raised me alone, working two and three jobs at a time. So for me not to have earned money the whole time my kids were growing up makes me feel unworthy. I haven't put anything into our retirement fund. Ken [husband] is talking about retiring in ten years. How can I retire in ten years when I'm not sure what I want to do with my life yet? I'm 48 years old and I feel like a 20-year-old. I don't know if I can get through college at my age. I feel guilty using money that my husband earned, and absolutely feel unworthy of dipping into savings for a career for me now.

Tears are welling up in her eyes. Occasionally she wipes one off with her fingers and keeps talking.

I don't know what I feel about this money thing. All this time I've been living on my husband's earnings. My head knows I've produced and contributed to the famiy. All those years of parenting, housekeeping, and nurturing everyone. But my gut, it just knots up and gets tight. In my gut I feel little, insecure, and like a failure. How can I be sure I'm entitled to our money for retirement or for anything? I never got a pay check, I didn't earn it.

To what is the doctor's wife entitled? She is called by his name. She lives in his home. She goes to his social or professional functions. Ironically, she even rears his children, as they too are known as Dr. Jones's boys and girls. When I write an article published in our local newspaper, people congratulate Jerry as if he, the doctor, had some influence over it. I get none of the accolades for his business success. The public assumes his competence. They somehow also assume that his competence is responsible for my occasional, lucky, or chance touches with personal accomplishment. "Isn't it wonderful that Dr. Nitzberg's wife writes well? He must be proud." As if I were one of his children and without the privilege and advantage of his attendance in our home my successes would be impossible.

Again, I am only entitled as it relates to my husband the doctor. Whether or not you enter into the medical marriage with a meager sense of self and entitlement and the marriage reinforces these feelings, or the rare self-confident woman loses her sense of entitlement within the marriage, is difficult to fully determine. However, it is apparent that the decision to marry a male physician is a clear choice leading to secondary and dependent status in a highly organized, authoritarian, male-dominated existence.

EQUAL TIME

It occurs to me now
as I look back
that my projects have
never been as important as yours.

When I wanted to go to school
getting a baby-sitter was up to me.
If I needed some advice
I had to wait for your convenience.

When I'm on the phone
I have to get off in case
you get an emergency call.
So I cut my conversation short.

When I'm reading or doing research
if it's dinner time I'd better stop.
Cooking and shopping are priorities
of how my time must be spent.

Maybe I can pursue a career
as long as it's part time
or on my time
and dinner's on time.

My meetings are fit to your schedule
and yet I can be kept waiting
for your last patient to leave
before I can meet on your territory.

All the time I was with the kids
taking care of home and hearth
like Hera and Demeter the goddesses
seeing to the needs of others.

When do I get equal time
Can I begin my career yet
Is it time for school or work
And if so, will you bake the bread?

Is it time for writing my poetry
singing my songs of life
Will you listen when I speak
ask or insist on my due?

Why is my time treated so carelessly
I'll be here only as long as you
Why do I protect you and free you
when my hours are being used up?

Does it seem fair to you
that my job is part time
Writing, counseling, acting
anyone can do.

And parenting—what about that one
Caring for your children and you
Can anyone do that
while trying to develop one's self?

There is something strange about
the system that gives one being
more time than another
though they are both the same age.

It seems as if you will have
lived to be a hundred
while I will get only one-third.

Perhaps the real reason women
live longer
is that the first sixty years
for women is handed over to their men.
In order to be equal they are
owed at least thirty more
to make up for what they gave away.

Chapter 25

Loyal at All Costs

I close my eyes and ears to most of it now. — Tracy

The loneliness is overshadowed by activity and responsibility. After years of secrecy and overprotectiveness we don't even remember that it is painful to keep our real feelings and experiences inside. Before the popularity and accessibility of psychologists we were even more closed, perhaps even shut down completely when things were disturbing on a personal level.

Grace is a 68-year old with a charming, soft, round face and exquisite smile which belie her years. Her eyes twinkled and alternately told of all her happiness and sadness as she spoke:

> When we were first married anything that troubled me was kept within the confines of my small apartment. Duane would tell me about his patients at the general hospital where he was on residency rotation. He'd complain about their inability to give adequate care (it was a city hospital in a large midwestern city) and as an idealist he was torn to pieces. I had to sit and listen to him describe how patients were left in the hallways unattended for long periods. They might be screaming in pain or in situations dangerous to themselves. Once he told me how someone lay unconscious for two hours until someone finally realized and attended to him. He was a 13-year-old boy who had an epileptic fit on the table. He almost died choking on his tongue. It makes me sick to recall those stories now — my stomach tightens in the same knots as in the old days. As Duane's wife I would tell no one of any anguish. I wanted to say, "How could you leave a 13-year-old child unattended on a stretcher in the halls of the hospital! How could you? What if

you were that child's father?'' But instead my job was to comfort Duane — to listen, be quiet. I felt like the receptacle for enormous secrets. The public has no idea of the inhumanities and indignities of medical care in a city hospital. I promised myself that under no circumstances would I or anyone close to me ever get medical treatment in one of those institutions.

I asked Grace how she coped with not telling anyone what was inside all the years of her marriage (over 40 years). Her somewhat rough, low-pitched voice seemed surprised as she continued.

I grew up in a family where no one shared intimate thoughts or feelings. We spoke only about practical issues, things to be done. Not like today where people say what makes them tick. A secret is a secret, at least that's how I was raised. So you take in information and put it somewhere safe where no one else can ever get at it and use it against you. In fact, after some years of listening to Duane's medical stories and his eventual humorous attitude about how people are taken care of, he became blasé and somewhat jaded when the bloom of idealism faded. My sense was that he married me because I was so good at keeping his secrets. He knew they were safe with me and would go with me to my grave.

Grace has loosened up a great deal and is able to share those long guarded secrets now that Duane is dead. He died of heart trouble two years before our interview, and she has spent the last two years in therapy with a woman she admired greatly, unraveling aspects of her life with the doctor. She continues:

Had I been able to talk to Toby (the psychologist) 40 years ago I would have felt much more authentic. I felt tremendous guilt all those years, caught between loyalty to my husband and a struggle for my own integrity. The only way I was able to deal with anger, rage, and sadness through that time was to hide it even from myself. I delved into activities, became a super responsible mother, wife, and volunteer person. Anytime I heard Duane laugh about a patient or hang up the phone and make a snide remark about Mrs. So and So's gall bladder acting up again and how he wished she would wait until morning or get off his back, I cringed inside. When he and his colleagues were having drinks and laughing hysterically about their favorite pesky patients, detailing how they would finally get even with them by sending them to the emergency room in the middle of the night or keeping them waiting in a dressing gown in their office for an unreasonable length of time, or how they would devise rectal exams or tests to humiliate the patients to keep them in line or get them off their backs entirely, I was horrified and numb. Should I laugh or cry? Should I call the patients and let them know of the disrespect and irreverance of their god-like physicians?

I gradually became depressed. I never even talked to other doctors' wives about my feelings. Duane was a good husband. He provided well for me and the children. What could I say to them? Their husbands were the ones laughing and joking together with Duane over drinks on their evenings off. So I assumed that they too thought this was the way doctors all were and I was crazy to worry about it.

I withdrew into myself. Duane never knew that I found his attitude horrifying. How could he take money, prestige, and respect from these unsuspecting people? They trust him and rely on his judgment. I was afraid his attitude would cause some terrible repercussions and even worse, someone's death. As far as I know no real danger was ever caused by Duane's pranks, but I would not have wanted either him or any of those colleagues to administer medical treatment to me!

Anyway, I guess keeping my feelings inside made me sick eventually. I blamed the depression on my chemistry and one of his colleagues eventually prescribed antidepressants, which helped only mildly. But at least I didn't have to deal with my feelings of disloyalty and inadequacy as a wife. As far as Duane knew I was depressed. He could have actually felt disdain toward me at the end just as he felt toward his other patients when they were depressed. I don't know, but my trust and respect for him gradually diminished and I guess I have to admit I lived in a cold, distant marriage for the last ten years.

I've never even talked to my children about some of my

feelings. I always felt that would be disloyal to their father. I wanted them to respect him and the medical profession. After all, I was raised to believe in the sanctity of medicine and doctors.

We as a rule are compelled to keep the secrets of our husbands, their profession and our own personal lives. We feel certain that no one will believe us anyway. We're probably just speaking out because we're upset or angry about something petty, and truly our husband the doctor never said or did anything so inhuman or unkind. The catch-22 is there always. His reputation is invincible, not to be marred by marital discord or his children's misbehaviors.

As self-protection it is almost impossible to break the code of silence. I have tried and have been hushed directly and indirectly by people who need to see my life as perfect. Whenever I write or speak of the negative feelings and doubts of my existence as a doctor's wife, the reaction is the same. Fear, denial, or patronization. Soon we all learn to keep the secrets, as I have.

The medical institution itself capitalizes on the public's need for idealization of medicine. Nurses, staff, and families all overprotect the doctor. Mistakes are covered to the outside world even as they are joked about within the hallowed walls of the hospital or doctor's office or privacy of the bedroom.

It's not always personal or family issues which are covered up and kept quiet, as with a wife who's an alcoholic or a doctor who's been having a long-standing affair with his head nurse. Rather, careless patient care is the big secret kept by wives until they die or are divorced from their doctor husband. The ultimate fear of the lay public (a patronizing description those in the profession call those out of the profession) of being given the wrong medication or the wrong test results, of taking home the wrong baby, of the nurse flirting on the floor and ignoring an emergency in one of the rooms, of the doctor not leaving a golf game or a few minutes of fun with his lover to respond to another emergency — is that those moments of humanity do sometimes cause death or irreparable damage to patients. Those moments occur with great regularity. Witness the New York hospital's questionable treatment of Andy Warhol. We may never know if the true cause of his death was negligence (Stone, 1987; Wallis, 1987).

The secrecy or the cover up is so careful and so unconscious that the perpetrators don't even admit their mistakes to themselves. On some level it is similar to the institution of slavery in which the slave experiences extreme guilt and panic if he or she finds fault with his or her oppressor. The rage of oppression is overpowered by the fear of being helpless and abandoned. So it is with the medical establishment. It's hard, if not impossible, to call our medical care-takers on any mistakes or wrongdoing without experiencing guilt, anguish, and remorse. Recall the times when a medication didn't agree with you or a suggested treatment went awry, but as the duti-ful patient nothing was ever said to your doctor for fear of reprisal. Perhaps your doctor would blame you for not following his instruc-tions. You end up feeling as if it was your fault that you were sick, blinded to the fact that it was his responsibility to correct an error.

Secrets are ultimately destructive and can turn the victim into the persecutor. So nurses keep quiet about hospital and doctor errors, and wives keep quiet about husband's secrets. If the information is clouded with enough guilt, it's almost impossible to track the re-sponsibility to anyone.

And if the revealing secrets and unsightly truths hold the threat of punishment, neither the nurses or wives will make the attempt. Loyalty is defined as "steadfast in allegiance . . . faithful to a per-son . . . feelings of devoted attachment and affection to a person, ideal or custom" (*American Heritage Dictionary of the English Language*). Synonyms include words like idolatry, worship, religi-osity, and devotement (*The New Roget's Thesaurus in Dictionary Form*). Those words describe the essential view of those handmaid-ens of medicine toward their doctors. A wife cannot turn against her husband, regardless of the conflicts she may feel about his behav-iors. Medicine demands ultimate loyalty of its subjects, assistants, technologists, nurses, secretaries, and undoubtedly, wives. Wives are likely to know the least authentic information about cases and professional information, but it is assumed that what we do know we will guard with our lives. It is also assumed that we will stand by our husbands through malpractice cases, affairs, public criticism, and professional and personal crises, even if our values and personal integrity are compromised.

Chapter 26

Vacations and Leisure Time

We schedule our vacation time five years ahead. — Kim

The more I spoke to physicians' wives the more I realized play was not a true part of the vocabulary. Play is probably too spontaneous. There is too much chance for loss of control in play. So we look at how leisure time is used and how wives experience their attempts at play with their physician husbands.

Control and controlling — a central and recurring theme in this book — is alive and well when leisure time is the issue. Often the choice of how leisure time is to be spent is an indicator of who has the power in the marriage. In the chapter on power and control, I indicated that wives of physicians usually are allowed control over certain moneys — household decoration and children's goods like clothes and school supplies. Money for leisure time is usually the domain of the doctor. Even if his wife does the books, since he brings home the bacon he gets to have greater input into how his free time will be spent and how much will be spent on his free time.

Remember, it is difficult for a physician to enjoy "free time." As with any workaholic or compulsive person, a vacation or day off is more likely spent going over unfinished cases, reading journals, or catching up on paper work. Actually, the doctor often goes to the hospital to see patients or to the office to organize unfinished work on his days off. Physicians are unlikely to be comfortable with free time. Even though they desperately need time away, they are most comfortable in the medical environment and feel most useful when doing work in their field (Konner, 1987; Fowlkes, 1980; Myers, 1988; Gerber, 1983).

Women frequently talk of husbands coming home when half the day off was over, or staying at the office all of their day off "to clean up the desk" or "to go over charts" or "to talk to partners about upcoming projects."

The style and requirements of medical practice make it necessary to plan leisure time. Every Wednesday off for golf, every other weekend off, and four to six weeks off a year are not uncommon. Whatever the schedule of the doctor, his wife accommodates and plans her life accordingly (Fowlkes, 1980; Lorch and Crawford, "Role Expectations," 1983). Planning and scheduling are essential to their vocabulary. Unlike other couples, medical wives become accustomed to regimentation and routine, even for their leisure time together. Sometimes as much as two or three years in advance, leisure time, trips, and meetings are organized and anticipated. In fact, most of the family time is allocated so that there is little spontaneous or unexpected play or fun (Fowlkes, 1980; Lorch and Crawford, 1983; Gerber, 1983).

As stated before, the medical meeting is most often utilized as the vacation away from home: a controlled environment where tax deductible meals and room planned at some resort area is the major getaway of the year.

What about the couples who do get involved in activities away from medicine on days off? Judy describes days skiing with Arny:

> I was always nervous. Arny kept criticizing or lecturing me at the ski area. I felt like I was with my father. He would say, "Go faster, face down the hill, don't be so chicken, don't be a pansy." I hated going skiing after a while. I felt so inadequate. We would go and I would be cold and wet and afraid, and Arny would want to get out on the slopes at 8:30 and be first on the lift. Then he'd want to stay out until the last ride down the mountain. I either had to take Valium to go skiing or be a nervous wreck. Toward the end of our marriage I decided to tell Arny I'd just come onto the slopes a little later in the morning after a hot chocolate or some relaxation. I also began going on the easy trails at my own pace. We just couldn't go together without me feeling bossed around and totally incompetent. Instead of having fun, I felt like I was letting Arny down and not living up to how he wanted me to ski. So I, of course, never had fun; in fact, I started getting stomach aches

if I knew we had plans to go skiing for a day or a few days. The strange thing is that I always felt guilty about not wanting to go. I was miserable and scared, but I felt guilty about spoiling Arny's day off from work!

I am reminded of the story of a couple who went on a high country pack trip—horses and donkeys carried them into the high wilderness and there they were to spend 10 or 12 days trekking and riding in the mountains with only a leader and guide as human companions. The country was gorgeous, the trip costly and quite exotic. I listened to the pack guide describe this couple and how the wife of the couple was terrified of heights and had a great deal of trouble on the trip. "She required medication, actually," said the guide. "She totally panicked and became paralyzed with fear of the wide and high open spaces while on horseback." The details were familiar to me. The wife fearful, but going on anyway. The husband ignoring her discomfort. "He said she would be fine, not to worry about her," the guide continued, "but I know how scary these trips can be if you are the slightest bit afraid of horses or heights. It's so hard to get them out of the wilderness. Well, we had to send in a special rescue team for this woman." I couldn't help but say to myself—I bet the husband was a physician. How did I know? He was well-off enough to afford a trip of that kind, and quite inflexible about his wife's discomfort. In fact the denial and seeming disinterest of the husband for his wife's safety in spite of obvious physical and psychological indications cued me to the fact of his profession. "Yes he was a physician," said the pack guide. "What a strange couple, I thought at the time. We had to bring her down by herself. He gave her something to calm her nerves and said goodbye right there. 'She'll be fine when she gets out of this altitude,' he said, and went on with the trip. We brought her down, and sure enough, after a while she drove off to a motel and told me to tell him where she'd be. Crazy huh?" she finished.

The exotic nature of the trip, the stoicism, stubborn holding to plans, and seeming cool attitude of the physician, combined with the wife's compliance and accommodation followed by the strong, "I'll handle this alone" attitude are familiar. He would not have his long-planned vacation spoiled by her weakness and fear, and she, although humiliated, frightened, and totally unsupported emotionally, carried on like the trooper he married.

The control and compulsions follow doctors' wives on vacation and during so-called play time. Dolores talks about how their trips to India, which she so looked forward to, turned out to be working vacations:

> I'd always wanted to travel, so when Allen suggested a trip to Nepal and India I jumped at the opportunity. Before I knew it we were taking an entire surgical team to work on the local people with eye problems there. The first time I went I was sick for three weeks and still had to assist in surgery. Now we take a team every year. I get to do a tiny bit of sight-seeing, but mostly I work. We all work very hard there. Okay, I know it's altruistic and charitable, but what about me and my marriage? We not only didn't get to travel alone and discover wonderful and beautiful sites and cultures, but we don't even get time off. Allen doesn't deal well with time off, but I do and could. I'd love to check out the sites, talk to the people.

Roberta, married "forever" according to her description, talks about bicycle trips to Europe:

> Most people would kill for the opportunity to take some of the trips Phillip and I have taken over the years, in many parts of this country and some European countries as well. Phillip loves to plan and organize trips, and I mean organize. Everything is done from the minute we leave home. So there's hardly time for me to stop at a fruit stand and admire the oranges! Or when I suggest an alternative route or place to stop, Phillip gets very defensive and insulted, like I'm taking away his special toy, his trip-planning toy. Of course, since it's his money that he works so hard for, I don't feel very comfortable insisting on my choice. Actually, I'm so glad he likes to plan these trips that I keep quiet and go where he suggests. Many of my friends married to physicians never go anywhere at all! So I'm very grateful for Phillip's interest in other places. The worst trip was the one to Greece. It could have been great, but I got sick and spoiled the trip. Phillip didn't know what to do.

Every day was pre-planned. We were to ride our bikes 40 miles a day to the next destination. But I was throwing up and had diarrhea, so there was no way I could ride my bike. Luckily we were on this trip with friends of ours, another physician and his wife. She felt sorry for me and was worried about my health. She told Phil not to force me to ride, that she'd stay back and keep me company, so that Phillip and her husband Rod could go sight-seeing that day. They went! I threw up all day and the next while Susan nursed me. What a nightmare, but I shudder to think of what I'd have done without Susan.

In fact, vacation trips were often successful relative to whether a good woman friend was along. Janice, in her second marriage but first time to a physician, spoke:

After two trips to the beach with George, I realized that he used the word vacation when he was working away from home. So I made sure our next trips were with another couple so I could have fun sight-seeing or swimming with someone else. When George plays, he plays at least as hard as he works at the office. He calls the hospital every day and has his nurse call him if anything needs his attention. If he's on the tennis court, he wears a beeper and makes sure a phone is close by at all times. He wears a watch and times everything. I get uncomfortable with his pace and insensitivity. Actually when he's relaxing he's counting the minutes until he can return to work. He's obviously most at home when he's surrounded by patients. I now take real fun trips without him! A girlfriend is much better company and I don't have to feel guilty about laughing or wanting to enjoy myself once in a while, you know—let loose and dance or have a drink occasionally and tell jokes. George thinks all that is irresponsible behavior.

Again, the words responsible, serious, too tense, compulsive, and worrier all are used to describe these men. The wives are left with frustration or a sense of inadequacy. They find other ways to relax without husbands to insist they be serious. Or the wife becomes serious also, thinking that the only good use of leisure time is time for serious reading, meetings, or charitable or medical-related activities.

Gail shares:

> Even as Evan takes more and more days off, he fills them with work. Paper work. Or phone calls. For a while I blamed it on the money. I thought Evan thought vacationing was too expensive. By the third trip I knew it wasn't the money because he was comfortable spending money on his kids or the cars or house or anything else, just not on going on a trip or time off at all. He'd buy equipment to ski or a boat or hunting gear. We'd get all decked out to go camping. As soon as we were away from the office he'd start finding ways to get us back home. It wasn't the money, it was the ability to let go of work and just relax for a while. He can't do it and he makes me miserable if I'm trying to relax while he's there. So I just go without him now. Actually, I'm upset and angry sometimes, but usually I end up feeling sorry for him. When he goes fishing or hunting it's usually with other docs who talk medicine the whole time. I've come to accept this as the style of doctors. Leisure is extended work time either used to build up business, to repay other docs for favors, or doing work. I've decided to go home to the South twice a year for my fun, and I take my kids to the beach sometimes. I've come to realize that lighthearted fun comes too hard to Evan. My family knows that about him and lets him alone on family holidays like Christmas.

So Gail, Roberta, and others, although bewildered and often lonesome for their husband's company and disappointed that they can't laugh more and play even some, have adjusted to a solitary leisure life or none at all.

PART III:
HER INTERACTION WITH SOCIETY

Chapter 27

Dependency Overdose:
The Human Habit — Tough to Break

I have to remind him to call the exchange, to attend his staff meetings, and to get his nurse a birthday gift. He couldn't survive a day without me. — Marilyn

As we look at the doctor's wife and her interaction with the society at large, recall that it is almost impossible for her to be recognized outside of the realm of her role as medicine's wife. She is like the crew of a ship or the gunner's mate, not the captain of the ship, but a supportive yet essential crew member. The ship really does not move without her working involvement. Yet the power, control, and decision making are conducted by the captain. He is and has the final word. She does have to take orders from him and answer to his whims and desires.

What about dependency, then? Isn't he as dependent on her as she is upon him? They each provide essential services for one another that are required by the other. Without these services the job, or relationship, will not survive in a comfortable, familiar, desirable, and efficient manner. Whether the ship continues on course depends on the crew's cooperation with the captain. So it is with the medical household. However, as the gunner's mate is rewarded, valued, and acknowledged, the doctor's wife is not.

As she deals with the world outside of her family, the doctor's wife is led to believe that she is functioning at her best when she serves the physician well so that he can provide his best for the community. Her image and public interaction meets with standards of approval of the traditional medical establishment. She, in other words, comes to feel that her role is to present in her persona the best possible representative of the physician's happy household.

The dependency interchange is ever present. She relies on his economic potential for her bread and butter. Unable to compete with his earning potential and almost always unable to have enough free blocks of time away from her home duties to commit to outside paid employment, she does rely on his ability to support her financially. Soon she also becomes dependent on his decision-making capacity, on his "steering the ship" and guiding their lives. She upholds her end of the bargain, supporting his need for secrecy, confidentiality, problems with malpractice, or whatever their personal trials may be, i.e., drugs, alcohol, depression, sexual incompatibility. She loses her self in his and their lifestyle. She becomes more and more dependent on not just their finances: she also absorbs the identity derived from this role. The cloak of medicine wraps her and surrounds her with a safe set of rules and regulations to follow for supposed security and ease of living. In return, she provides comforts and amenities so that her husband is able to do his job. She sees to it that the entire household works like clockwork, the surroundings are aesthetically pleasing, and she makes it possible for the doctor to entertain when necessary and relax when desired, undisturbed by the details of personal living. When she calls for babysitters, does laundry, picks up shirts for him, does the family's books and records, calls for appointments, keeps up with details so that he can think only about work and let go of it when he's at home, she fulfills her end of the interdependency. She is trading her obedience for his alleged protection. The trouble is that while she is expected to do this, and is socialized for these jobs, she is not valued or rewarded for doing it. As her dependency on this highly respected husband mounts, his dependency on her increases as well, but is ignored. While he is viewed as irreplaceable to society, she feels expendable at the same time she does indispensable work for him. In other words, the performance of her job responsibilities ensures his success.

However, he doesn't feel dependent upon her, per se. He can get anyone to do her job. The traditional view of men toward women implies that one woman is easily replaced by another. Women's work is menial, trivial, and not important in the commercial sense, which is the most important evaluator in the male view. She is made to feel that he's a great catch and she needs him more and more for her survival. Since her skills and jobs aren't valued, her dependency is heightened.

As with a drug dependency, the low self-value eventually grows in the user; guilt for the neediness and confusion caused by the chemical itself drives the person to use more, again and again. A doctor's wife may feel useless unless she is giving to a doctor's lifestyle. She may feel her reward can only come from his success. And she may be unable to see herself any other way or with anyone else or, least probably, alone. My impression is that there is a moderate rate of remarriage to physicians after a divorce from one. Once entrenched in the role and sensing protection and familiarity, she may lack the courage or confidence required to release the identity as medical wife and is paralyzed to stretch to find a wider view of herself. Remember, the physician does represent the strong male protector in our culture.

It is curious to me that she feels dependent, vulnerable, and weak while he, though also dependent, does not feel as vulnerable or weakened by the relationship. Rather, he feels strengthened and healthier in it than out (Vaillant, Sobawale, and McArthur, 1972; Gabbard, Menninger, and Coyne, 1987). Perhaps the social, economic, and psychological power that he holds over her, with the sanction of society, does maintain her weak position and reinforce his strength. The balance of the relationship continues to be in favor of the doctor, yet oppressive to his wife. She deteriorates in her dependent role, suffers emotional and physiological symptoms that occasionally debilitate her, while he thrives until she leaves. Let us not forget that she risks becoming chemically dependent because of the ease and availability of drugs from her husband's practice. This keeps her vulnerable and excruciatingly dependent on the system. In that state she may feel completely at a loss to look outside for help, or be incapable or afraid to do so.

The choice to be married to a physician has hazards and risks not clearly apparent to the unwary. Let's look further at her interaction with the public.

MYTHS EXPLODED

I told you so
you and your black bag
What happened to the boy
Who married the girl
Who wanted a life of fun and joy

the trips we would take
the babies we would make
Oh we were so smug and sure

Perhaps mother was wrong
a Doctor's no prize
I shouldn't have listened at all

Alone all day
Alone all night
Waiting for you to call

What is it with your profession
Why did I have to sacrifice
Why did I have to serve you,
so that you could serve others?

I got no applause
I got no reward
No one even knows my name.

Again and again I ask myself
Was it my fault or yours
Did I expect too much
or did you not expect at all?

Marriage to me meant connection
with a language all its own
instead what I got was silence
Or a word from a telephone

Send me your picture
I'll take it to the next
meeting for fathers and sons
What if your son says who is that — I can't
cover any more

Smart and gay so they say
What do they know of it
One more night, one more pill
It will all be over soon

Doctors should marry each other
It's really what they deserve
Serve the community together
Applaud each other, talk medicaleze
No one else belongs there. No one is really allowed
Not even a wife who helped make it all happen
She's always lost in the crowd.

Sure your patients love you
Your nurses and technicians do too
What do they know of your habits
Your cruel inconsideration and lies
What do they know of life with you?

Of giving up my self to strengthen yours
Of covering your mistakes
Of paying your bills
Of smiling through the tears

The doctor is our hero, our savior or god
But he forgot the woman who knew him
When he couldn't tie his shoes
When his tie was loose
When he answered to his first name
and didn't flinch

I hope you realize what cost it was
to Doctor the rest of the world
I'm on my way now
to find a place to sort this out
Explain the whys and hows

Medicine is your wife, your love, your life
You chose it way back when
I was starry eyed and strong
I thought I could weather anything

How wrong I was
How wrong were you
Medicine won
    Medicine won
        Medicine won

BUT THERE REALLY IS A CHOICE!
BUT THERE IS NO CHOICE, SAYS HE

I can't come home yet
I've miles to go before I sleep
Patients to see
People to heal
Don't you see it's the only thing I can do?

Another meeting at 6 p.m.
Sorry I'm late again
Had to miss Jimmy's game
Couldn't pick up Bill at school
Don't you see I have to follow the rules?

This isn't the time, dear
Mustn't start anything now
The phone can't be off the hook
the hospital might call
Don't you see everyone needs me?

We have to move now
there's a better offer there
I'll be in charge of the ward
It will make me feel great
Don't you see what I'll miss if I stay?

I'm so tired, I'm so bored
the meetings are dry
the work is too hard
But no one else can do it
Don't you see I'm indispensable?

I'm perfect—you have to be too
I'm smart—so everyone says
People want me everywhere
Speeches, and parties, politics, whatever
Don't you see I'm irreplaceable?

Slow down now so there's time for us?
You must be kidding
You are really nuts
I'll retire some day, I'll slow down soon
Don't you see it has to be — there's no other way.

The kids are grown
Are you still there?
The house is bigger
All I have is my stethoscope, my scalpel

Don't you see it's too late now?

Chapter 28

Aura of Medicine:
I Married an Institution

Doctors take care of their own. It's the wives who are forgotten. — Marilyn

In a superb book, *For Her Own Good*, Barbara Erhenreich and Dierdra English included a history of medicine in the United States from the mid 1800s to present. Their focus was on the influence medical experts have had on women's lives to the present, including the direct influence over attitudes and values which spill into our systems of education, family life, laws, communication, work, and even spirituality. I was particularly struck by their piecing together the rise of medical establishment as we know it today, systematically and deliberately eliminating women lay healers and midwives, and women and men of lower socioeconomic classes from being the legal bearers of medical knowledge and practice.

The American medical establishment copied the English and then German influence in which physicians were members of a traditional elite class. They were required to be trained in the new scientific laboratories with studies focused heavily on the biological sciences. Eventually with the help of Rockefeller and Carnegie moneys, physicians in this country were directed to scientific research and elaborate laboratories, while the American Medical Association asserted its growing influence by strict regulation and standardization of medical practice and education throughout the country. Numerous smaller and some larger schools were closed, including schools for women and blacks. Small hospitals were shut down, and any irregular health care practices and practitioners such as homeopaths and midwives were eventually shut out of practicing through legal means. Money was pouring into the "new scientific medicine." Johns Hopkins in Maryland became the model medical school like those in Europe, and soon all schools here would follow that model or be closed. Extensive years of training in biological sciences was required. The expenses, time, and prerequisite requirements would eliminate the lower classes from being accepted. To become a member of the modern profession of medicine would take money, breeding, and influence, meaning those who would be in charge of our health would be predominantly white, Anglo-Saxon Protestants whose families touched the Mayflower somehow. Only a few were women, blacks, or Jews. The aura was thus entrenched, and copied from Europe — stuffy, staid, traditional, and then later cool and scientific, with long training requirements and regimes, dedication to the spirit of that tradition, and of course mostly male-dominated.

From the early 1900s to the present, a limited fortunate few would be able to enter and walk through the hallowed, secret halls of medical science. Only in the past ten years are more women, blacks, minorities, and members of the lower-middle class entering and completing the rigorous training.

The aura includes elitism, classism, scientification, formality, traditional male patriarchal values, separatism, Good Old Boy networking, clubiness, exclusivity, and a capitalistic view of charging what the traffic will bear while limiting the flow of the goods and services. By tightly controlling the supply into the marketplace and convincing a naive public of their essential value, the medical doctor had a monopoly on his services in the marketplace. A true profession with a secret body of special knowledge which would take years to learn would be developed and savored by the special few.

There is a religious fervor in the study and practice of medicine. Historically, those who have opposed its values and tenets were considered heretics, shunned and cast out, and at times sacrificed.

Much remains so today, and with that in mind, when a woman marries a doctor she marries into a long, hard history of fiercely fought and won battles against egalitarianism. She marries a member of a special society with sacred traditions and values which are upheld and adhered to valiantly by the teachers, practitioners, and students of medicine.

Developed through means of paternalism, and sometimes punitive authoritarianism, the medical establishment's great influence over how our culture views women, and our supposed capacities and weaknesses, even its claiming authority over how women think, feel, and act, permeates all areas of our lives. The doctor has been blessed with a long history of control over much of our experience. His wife is presumed to share his beliefs and to retreat under his authority.

Here is my view in poetry:

I MARRIED AN INSTITUTION

On the walls of my kitchen are healthy eating tips
My cupboards are full of brans
The coffee tables have medical journals
We do whatever they say we can.

Years ago we gave up butter
It was margarine or nothing at all
Next, eggs were suspect, then sugar
Or was it not too much salt?

Somehow the black bag is always in sight
The beeper and the telephone too
Become signs and symbols of someone's distress
More often than not it is ours.

The latest views on exercise
Have us all increasing the rates of our hearts
If we overdo and pull a muscle or two
It's to physical therapy we go for repairs.

When others get a cold or flu
They stay in bed so warm and cozy
For us it's a shot every fall
And then an x-ray if we become too queasy.

The children's toys are stethoscopes and Bandaids
of many colors, textures and kinds

They learn to make a tourniquet
and take a blood pressure, height and weight
To them it's fun and games to bring home doctor supplies
   for their friends

The parties and gatherings we attend
Smell of antiseptics and pills
The oath of Hippocrates on at least one wall
The decor, the food, the wine
It's hard to forget who's paying the bills

The people gathered are easily detected
An aura surrounds their forms
Ancient rituals, practices, beliefs, and protocol
Those before them and before them
Held their minds and hearts the same

When I married you all those years ago
I suppose it wasn't as clear
that you would become a representative
of a fraternity, old, established and severe.

The initiation was quick, sharp and distinct
Learn the rules and obey
The way I think now was influenced by your clan
Sickness to me is dry, clinical, harsh, rude

Paintings, architecture and books
Philosophy, religion and sports
Politics, schools and play often
seem to revolve around the persuasion
   and values of those medical men.

I'm not sure we realized it at first
You thought it was just a job
A creative, helping line of work
to provide a secure and rewarding life.

Then as years went by
The influence became more apparent

Health care, health foods, health nuts
Medicine, medical, medicinal
Wherever we look and turn.

It gets into your blood stream
Into your pores
Until you can't see that
Medicine has opened and shut many doors.

Once institutionalized hard and fast
The rules of living become ingrained
But I want to believe that solid or not
We can still be open enough for
   change.

My brush with the power of medicine was close
The institution almost won

The samples from salesman so free
The therapy so prescribed
Separating my body from my mind
Taking the will away from me.

Now as I look back to review and reflect
At times when you come home from the hospital
and wash off the germs from your hands
I wonder what life would have been like for us
If instead of doctoring all those years
You played the French horn in a band.

Chapter 29

Public Image:
You Sleep with My Doctor

If anyone else tells me what a great doctor Frank is, I'll explode! — Sandra

When I knew this interest of mine in the experience of doctors' wives was to be more than a personal diary, I began listening, looking, and asking the general public what they envision, what they think of a doctor's wife. The range of responses has been from no response or rather, "Who cares?" to "My doctor's wife is a wonderful woman," and all sorts of information in between.

For years I hid the fact that my husband was a doctor. It seemed that assumptions were made about me that I refused to accept. The public's stereotype is one of the spoiled, selfish, dependent little woman who has many advantages and doors open for her by virtue of her husband's rank in the world.

To review, in the earlier history of our country—the mid to late 1800s—a doctor's wife was seen as a dowdy, self-sacrificing, extremely charitable woman who usually had a large family and spent any extra hours in her day volunteering to help her husband with his work or help others less fortunate than herself. However, there is little documentation or diary material to draw upon to validate what her personal experience was or to be certain that a doctor's wife in the 1800s or early 1900s lived differently from other women of her time. We know that the physician has had different statuses in society, from being available on a private retainer to those who could afford him, to not being taken very seriously at all due to the lack of technical knowledge of the times. As the doctor has emerged as a more necessary, valued member of society in the last 50 years, he has enjoyed prestige and benefits before unknown to health care providers.

Interestingly, doctors' wives are the one group of women kept locked in a stereotype by the public, even as views and opportunities for women move forward with a closer approximation of equality to men.

Recently I was told that it was understandable that I behave the way I do because I'm a "doctor's wife." Having heard this more times than I care to count, this time I pursued the statement, or rather persisted with a confrontation with the person who shared it. First, I had to work through my hurt and surprise because the woman who made the statement (this time) is one whom I respect greatly. She is an elderly, well-educated, influential woman in the community who is working in academia and also is considered to be a very charitable person. Specifically, the conversation was in regard to my commentaries which appear regularly in our local newspaper. Her feeling was that a newspaper is the wrong place for personal commentary and the only reason they were published was because I'm a "doctor's wife." This is a woman who has done enormous work for the women's movement. I valued her opinion highly. I felt patronized, misjudged as an eccentric, and invalidated once again by the catch-all derogatory reference to being a doctor's wife.

My instincts early on in my marriage were probably correct. The public is rather impatient with a doctor's wife.

I am always struck by the impression of others that doctors' wives have no feelings. We have no capacity for pain, hurt, or insult. Truly my fantasy entails the general public in a vivid conflict of love/hate for their own personal physician. When we're ill, we are helpless and dependent on our doctor. This can be overwhelming. While we may feel unable to express fears or anger directly to the doctor, it is much safer to voice our prejudices and angers toward his wife. Therefore, when someone says, "She's only a doctor's wife," or "What do you expect, she's a doctor's wife," or "Did you hear about Dr. Jones's wife, Eleanor?" or "God, I really feel sorry for Dr. Jones's wife," they are probably expressing more sentiment for the doctor than for his wife.

Over and over women talked of their discomfort associating with women not married to doctors. Repeatedly they concurred that others either put them on a pedestal or view them with jealousy and disdain that made it practically impossible to remain socially intimate.

"You don't have my experiences. You're a doctor's wife," should be emblazoned on the hospital auxiliary door. "How would you know, you're married to a doctor?" was said over and over until our ears screech. The daily life of a doctor's wife includes variations on the theme of all women, but — and the but is enormous — we are human, women with thoughts, feelings, and spirits. As Shylock says in *Merchant of Venice*, "If you prick me, will I not bleed?"

When will the cloak be removed so the woman underneath can be seen, heard, and understood?

I feel it essential to address an unconscious conflict operating here. The love/hate which people feel toward their doctor operates when referring to his wife. She is, after all, sleeping in his bed. It is remarkably like our parents when we are growing up. We are dependent on both for our survival. Clearly as adults and perhaps as children, we are aware that our fathers provide for our security. They are out in the mysterious world doing magical jobs to bring us money to keep us alive. Our mothers provide comfort to us, but without food provided by father, we go hungry and mother's comfort is not too helpful. (That he could not be free to provide food if she were not caring for the young is ignored.)

So it is with our doctors. In very mysterious ways they bring magic to heal us and keep us alive, akin to our fathers. Their wives exist only in that they sleep with our doctor (to keep him happy, presumably), but offer us even less than our mothers did in terms of our survival.

How should we (the public) feel toward these women who sleep with our doctors? For some there may be jealousy, thinking, "I would like to sleep with my doctor; perhaps that would ensure my physical safety indefinitely. It would also make me privy to the magic that he has at his fingertips." For others there may be a need to deny the wife's existence altogether, thinking only of the doctor's existence. He is omnipotent, needing nothing or no one for his strength and succor. For still others, the animosity and rage of being dependent can only be expressed toward her. "My doctor is necessary, he's wonderful, I need him. His wife is insignificant. She's unnecessary, just a leech on society." It's as if some members of the public are saying, "I hate you, Mom. Leave Dad alone. Get off his back [literally and figuratively] so he can take care of me, pay attention to my needs, keep me alive and well!!" We then all become dependent siblings in rivalry for the doctor's affection and protection, i.e., public and wives (See Part IV, "Metaphorical Relationships: Wife-Husband, Patient-Doctor").

It is unreasonable—the fear that she, the doctor's wife, knows something or has something of the doctor's magic that those not intimately tied to the doctor aren't privy to. Should we be nice to her, provide her with comfort, be loving, or should we be hateful and quietly outraged by her and driven with jealousy?

The unreasonableness of the conflict is apparent to the doctor's wife on some level. We realize we're people. We're human beings. *There is no magic!* Our husbands are human. *There is no magic!* Leave us alone to be like all women, all people.

At another, more insidious level, the doctor's wife can't understand. Why the unreasonable rage toward her? What has she done to deserve people's scorn? The scorn of strangers? She's denied jobs and then is criticized for not working. She's offered special services and then is criticized for taking the offers. She is invited to social functions and then is criticized for her appearance there. She is asked to volunteer her time and then is criticized for being a volunteer. She keeps to herself and is criticized for being so private. She is publicly visible and is criticized for being too public. If her children fail, she is criticized for their failure. If her husband fails, she is criticized for his failures.

It would seem that the only chance the wife of a doctor has to maintain her self-esteem is to deny that she is the wife of a doctor, to live as an individual, severing connections to the public view of her husband.

Punished by the public for sleeping with the doctor, punished by his co-workers, including nurses who are the other women who care for his welfare, the doctor's wife learns to live with distrust, hurt, anger, and confusion toward the general public. When and if she is liked or loved, is it for herself or for her husband the doctor?

Julia, a client in her late fifties who had been treated for depression originally but who more recently was working on self-esteem and marital issues, related her interpretation. Julia is a woman of imposing stature, dark hair, deep-set, expressive eyes, and an unusually engaging smile. Her ongoing frustration in therapy has been her weight, which while on antidepressants had been quite reluctant to leave her rather large frame. In addition to her wonderful smile, I greatly admired Julia's spirit. She had always been a feisty woman who easily spoke her mind, and although it was somewhat blurred by depression, her feistiness was not easily stifled, which, incidentally, always delighted me in our sessions.

Julia is quite reluctant to tell anyone she'd married a doctor.

> In our community when we were first moving in we were told to live on the right side of town. All the doctors live on the northeast side and we were assured that to live anywhere else would be unheard of. That was many years ago. I'm not sure if it's still that way.
>
> People would expect me to drive a certain car and buy my clothes in the right clothing stores once they knew who my husband was. I got so I went incognito into the neighborhood stores.
>
> My favorite story is the car shopping one. "What does your husband do?" the salesman asks. If I say he's a doctor, then his eyes light up and he immediately wants to show me a more expensive, sleeker car. He might even say of them, "You can't drive this car. It's too plain." Imagine being told what car to drive!
>
> Even my daughter hides the fact that her father's a doctor. After being asked, "What does your father do?" she's already been told by her boss in the store where she works, "Oh, you're one of those spoiled, rich bitches." She was horrified. In college she's quite careful to keep her father's profession a secret. She feels she's prejudiced quite negatively because of it.

When Julia describes her anecdotes, her story is tinged with resentment, anger, and confusion. The question seems to be, "Why judge me or my children by my husband's job title? I'm probably more like everyone else than you think I am.'' In our sessions she is able at times to see the irony of the situation, but only after many moments recalling what she considers unfair prejudgment and treatment by an unfamiliar and often hostile public.

> Some of the same people who are often very flip or short with me in a store or on a committee are the same people who have been seen by my husband in his office for medical treatment. What do they want from me?

I'm still not certain whether Julia, if given another chance, would choose to live her life unmarried, or with a partner who is not a physician.

LAMENT OF WOMANHOOD:
VISIBILITY PLEASE

Can't you see me standing there?
Open your eyes —
wider, wider please.
I've been here all along.

Don't you hear me speaking to you?
Prick up your ears —
more, more please.
I've been speaking for years.

What do I have to do to get your attention?
Stand upside down
Shout, scream, cry, holler,
    or be silent?
What is the matter with you all?

Is it my voice?
Is it my words?
Is it what I mean?
Or is it my face,
is it my hair,
is it my costume?

Somehow since I was a girl
I feel I have offended you
by my very presence.
My voice was too coarse,
    too harsh, too strident.
My humor was too self deprecating.
My thoughts were too different from your own,
    somehow unacceptable or misunderstood.

I have made myself
    smaller.
I have tried being quieter.
I have stopped thinking
    and feeling.

I am slowly, ever so
  slowly disappearing
  from view.

Is that what you wanted
  for me all along,
to be just an apparition,
  to be summoned at your will?

I'm holding on as
  tightly as I can.
But, you're winning,
  you're overpowering, you're
  dominating.

I am now nearly invisible.
I am now alone.
I am now truly lost.
  I am no longer.

Where am I?

Chapter 30

Friendships:
Woman to Woman

My women friends are the foundation upon which my daily
life thrives. Without them the isolation would be unbearable.
— Pat

Women have counted on their friendships with one another
throughout history. They support and educate each other, pass cultural traditions from one generation to another, assist in childbirth,
sickness, loss of children, and death of one another. Much has been
written on the importance of friendship between women. Unfortunately, until this latest surge of feminism in the last 20 years, indus-
trialization had caused a diminishment in the accessibility of
women to one another. Friendships among women were on the de-
cline due to isolation of the nuclear family, role changes, and probably most of all to the reduced status of women in the society. No
longer would we value women's advice, or women's support and
guidance in time of need. Women became more reliant on male
institutions and males to provide the support, education, and health
care formerly provided by women themselves. With feminism and
the modern women's movement, the value of sisterhood, friendships of women, and female bonding have been rediscovered and
encouraged. We are freer to enjoy our women friends and can gain
the nurturance and understanding from women that may not be
available in our male-female relationships.

What of the doctor's wife? How do female friendships fit into her
life?

When Alyson talked about friends, her eyes lit up at first, like
candles, and then they glistened with tears.

I had been close to Sandy since we were girls together in Vermont. We went to school together and decided we would go to college together too. We went to the University of Vermont. I was studying language and Sandy was a history major. We roomed together for three years. Then at the end of that year I met Marty and we fell in love. I tried to include Sandy whenever we did things, but she felt awkward. We graduated and Sandy went to graduate school. I married Marty. He was a med student on his way to Pittsburgh for a residency in internal medicine. Sandy and I wrote to each other and saw each other that first Christmas. Gradually we saw each other less and less. Marty and I started socializing with medical people. I had two kids and Sandy went to work at a university in the South. It's so hard to keep up with friendships, no matter how close. When Marty finished his residency we moved out West for his post-residency training. He got a fellowship and we went where he had to study. I didn't dig my heels in to friendships the third time we moved. I couldn't stand the pain of separation from people who became very close friends. In residency, since the guys are always at the hospital, every two or three nights, I think, the wives come to really rely on each other for help, moral support with kids, and just company. I made two great women friends there in Pittsburgh. But when we moved out West I couldn't keep up with them either. Moving day is so horrible. More goodbyes and you know you may not see each other again.

Was it hard to start up friendships after moving into a new area?

Not really. The medical community always reaches out to its own. Someone always calls on you to invite you to a coffee for new members. The trouble is that after a while I stopped trusting the length of time we would stay put. So I'd be moderately sociable, but not totally. Just surface. You know, talked about general stuff, acceptable chatter, but not what I'm really thinking about. The other thing I came to realize is that it's hard to have friends who aren't in the medical community. In some ways, since there's only so much time to socialize and since we all live in the same area of town, we are limited in our range of contacts. Plus being here to entertain the staff members at the hospital, to impress them, I guess, for Marty's professional advancement.

Well, I'm not too comfortable with the older doctors' wives. They're too conservative for me, but I spend a lot of time with them at the dinners and cocktail parties that we can't refuse. Doesn't leave time for down to earth friendships for me. I haven't really been able to replace Sandy in my life. I'll always miss her. She got married to a sociology professor and they live in South Carolina now. I keep planning a trip back East to see her, but you know how that is — other things always seem to come first. I can hardly get back home to see my family, let alone my old friend.

It is true that in today's world, with its inordinately fast pace and time commitments, friendships between women are difficult to nurture. Due to our role expectations, the pool of women we see will most often be other doctors' wives. For those whose interests deviate from the norm or who find things other than their husband's medical practice important, finding friends is a time consuming proposition.

Hilary, who has been a doctor's wife 32 years, had her own way of solving the dilemma:

I wasn't the type to join Junior League or League of Women Voters or Women's Auxiliary. Nor did I want to spend all my social time talking about hospital-related issues. Chuck's friends were married to nurses who all worked at the hospital. When they got together I always felt like an odd woman out. The names they tossed around meant nothing to me, nor did the medical conversation. I quickly discovered that to feel alive and interested I would have to seek out my own social group. I went to school and then worked part-time in real estate. My specialty became farms and ranches. I am doing quite well and have made a few fairly close friends in the business. Sometimes Chuck comes to parties of realtors and I go to his medical parties. But basically I socialize with my close friends

on my own time so as not to interfere with our free time together. At first my acquaintances were strange about me being
married to a doctor. They'd imply I didn't have to work and
they assumed I wasn't a serious person. But as with everyone,
once you get to spend time with each other the prejudices are
broken down and all that doctor's wife stuff faded away.
"You're okay," they'd admit, and we soon built fairly solid,
dependable relationships.

In fact, not being in medicine, it's easier for me to complain
about my personal problems. There's no chance of Chuck losing referrals from other doctors if I'm not speaking badly to
their wives. I know the docs' wives must think I'm a maver-
ick, but you do what works best, I suppose.

Shirley talks of her lifelong friends:

We met when we moved to town. Our husbands work together
and we golf and tennis together. They understand what it's like
being in an MD marriage—weird hours, hysterical patients
calling at all hours, stepping in for our husbands when they
can't come to dinners and occasions. Only a medical wife will
accept not showing up at the last minute or our leaving
abruptly in the middle of a card game. We've nursed each
other's wounds from medical school on, some of us. There are
no secrets here.

True there seemed to be similar styles, acceptable rules of
the friendships. For example, if there was a choice between a
commitment to a friend or a husband's emergency, the emergency won and everyone seemed accepting of that.

The conflicts recur when professional demands override personal
confidences. Friendships seem to be deeply prescribed in restrictions: cheerful, pat conversation to make the doctor look competent
and successful at his profession, talk of children or of ourselves, but
never anything to shed aspersions on the character or dedication of
the physician. When not working, there is great pressure to do the
same things, buy the same things, so that the conversation remains
within the prescribed framework.

The competition for referrals is always operating. She may be torn between loyalty to him and her own need for personal intimacy with women friends. However, it is a rare wife who shares with another doctor's wife the intimate details of an affair of hers or her husband's, or fears of any abusive situation at home, or marital instability. The gossip quotient is known to be higher and the trust level therefore drops accordingly.

Georgia described the gossip network succinctly:

> I told one "friend" that I was worried about my husband seeing someone else, and in three days it got back to me — that he indeed was, who he was with, and for how long.

The grapevine serves to keep our behaviors rigid and appropriate to the needs of the medical culture. The existence of a gossip network also reinforces careful observance of superficial verbal interactions among its participants. Enough is said to keep the gossip alive, but not enough to damage its members, especially the medical practitioners.

If the postulate that women married to doctors tend to be comfortable with more distance in their relationships is true, then the social life even among other women supports the superficiality. On the other hand, it could be that warm, friendly women able to bond normally are deprived of these close attachments by the medical sociocultural system.

I can recall being extremely busy with my children in the early years of my marriage. I kept to my home and family. My children were my closest friends at that time. The demands of husband's needs, home, and children left little time for personal friendships. Those important to me were gradually forgotten as I struggled with priorities and loyalties. Soon my ability to be close with other women was like an atrophied muscle. Unused, it became more and more uncomfortable. Jealousies, envies, unresolved angers, social climbing, making best friends of those who can refer the most patients, or merely having friends who feel secure that they befriended a doctor gradually eroded my confidence in intimate interactions. Did they want me or Jerry? Were the women encouraging my friendship to improve their husband's professional chances? Uncomfortable with the games, I withdrew into a smaller and smaller circle. Superficiality was loathsome. Instead, I opted for loneliness, or one or two trusted friends who were not connected to the medical profession. This was an unconscious process in which Jerry and his profession colluded. The result reinforced either playing by the rules within the system or living in relative isolation. Eventually I too believed that I had no choice but to befriend people from Jerry's pool of colleagues, or to befriend none at all.

TO MIMI AND LU

We met when our children were small
our husbands were merely boys
Each of us in our own way
was sorting out all the toys.

At first I had no idea
how important you would be
in the scheme of my life to come
or the day-to-day frame of just me.

What joy in all the hours of talk
sharing whatever we felt
our thoughts hardly needed be aloud
the others knew the meaning instantly or before.

The games we played together
as our children ran and jumped
meals watched over, husbands soothed
laughter and tears over the years
almost never being stumped.

I marveled at how strong you both were
you came through any hardship with grace
How do they do it? I often thought
they manage their homes, their families, their
husband's careers
taking on more than most
without complaint.

One father fights with his son, his son fights back
you center yourself and calm them both
One's parent gets sick and eventually dies
you soften the blow and wipe everyone's eyes.

I watched you and learned
Not quite understanding, always admiring
your patience, your energy but mostly
your humor — the laughter that elevated us all.

Our children have grown
Have lives of their own
Mimi moved first—far away from us both
I had no idea the effect that would have.

Next I would move—we go where our
husbands need to be
What I never realized
when Lu brought me here and returned to her home
was how important you both were
to the very essence of my life.

Our phone calls diminished
over the years
Even though we can pick up right away
from where we left off.

I'm as much at fault as any
Life is so busy and the distance so far
But to both of you—Mimi and Lu
You are always in my heart
Guiding my hand as I write.

I had no sisters as you well know
and my mother died when I was quite young
You both have been my female light
My truth in a world of men.

Without your friendship and love
Without your example and support
My life would be barren and lonely
For none could ever measure up
to the sisterhood you provide.

You both have kept me going
Just knowing you're out there somewhere
Whenever I need understanding without judgment
support without criticism
Whenever I need a true and valued friend.

Chapter 31

Women's Medical Auxiliary:
A Rare Institution

I'm no longer welcome at the meetings. Once I gave up being Mrs. Doctor, I gave up rights to the Auxiliary, I guess.
— Barbara

Picture an extremely well turned out, socially knowledgeable group of women at a luncheon meeting, picking at light fruit salads, sherbet, and tea. There is an agenda, officers up at the head table, and even a podium and gavel. The meeting comes to order. There's a treasurer's report. The secretary takes notes. The topic might be: the location of the next meeting, flower arrangements, getting more members, or fund raising for charity. What do these women have in common? That they are all married to physicians forms the basis for their gathering and whatever activity follows.

The Women's Medical Auxiliary (the name before feminism; "women's" is now deleted) is a special phenomenon for physicians' wives. It is a highly organized support and service group which meets monthly. The system, county-based at the local level but linked state and nationwide, is the primary source of interaction between women married to doctors. At present it is one of the few groups that bases its existence solely on the spouses' profession.

The first group of women in this country to formally organize a state medical auxiliary met in Hot Springs, South Dakota, September 29, 1910.* At that time there were fewer doctors in any given area, and the practice of medicine was much less specialized. Any-

---

*From "Historical Highlights" of the American Medical Association Auxiliary, Inc.

one could practice in the healing arts in the late 1800s and early 1900s. Few formal requirements were yet established.

We recall the tradition of the old time doctor: house calls, horse and buggy, trudging through the snow, sleet, and hail to help patients and their families. At that time women often assisted at home births and were called upon to use family remedies to heal the sick. Physicians were called upon to care for the well-off.

In the 1920s and 1930s physicians became more organized and elite by refining their qualifications and requirements for licensure. They enlisted the help of their wives in their fight to keep homeopaths, naturopaths, chiropractors, and osteopaths off hospital staffs.

In May 1922 the American Medical Association House of Delegates approved the organization of a national auxiliary. At that time 24 women from 11 states attended their first national meeting in St. Louis. At their husbands' suggestion, wives formed the auxiliary as an educational and political counterpart of the men's medical society.*

In the auxiliary, women discovered they enjoyed the idea of getting together with others who shared their experience. The auxiliary worked as a support group, and an organizing forum for community activities. It soon became the social assemblage that reinforced the separation of the doctor's wife from the rest of the female world.

It is noteworthy that the national auxiliary membership grew from 4,000 members recorded in 1926 to as high as 80,000 in 1959, and has since dropped down into the 70,000s and has remained at that level.+ One could speculate that the '50s were the height of auxiliarydom, just as it was the time of "the feminine mystique" of women staying at home and supporting one's husband's profession. The leveling off and then steadiness of the membership since then might imply a strong core and philosophy of traditionalism in the medical marriage.

As time went on, medicine changed. Doctors were caught in the scientific revolution. Specialization evolved and our worship of sci-

---

*From "Historical Highlights" of American Medical Association Auxiliary, Inc.

+Telephone communication with American Medical Association, Inc., Historical offices.

ence as a religion changed our interaction with medicine. Doctors and their wives felt the repercussions. The auxiliary became a place for meeting other wives and sharing fashions, recipes, hairdressers, and conversation. It was used less for formal political action and more for planning community work. She lost the little esteem received as the doctor's right-hand woman, and her rewards from social work continually diminished. Wives couldn't compete with the organized medical associations as a political force.

Paid work was not a choice for these women. Volunteering became an art. The auxiliary worked to combine social needs and creative involvement as a doer of good works. Few other groups met and organized purely on the basis of their husbands' occupation. Only military wives and faculty wives at the university level readily come to mind. Just because he was a physician of any kind, his wife was and is automatically a member of the Women's Medical Auxiliary of his county.

I am aware of the positive accomplishments of local and state auxiliaries. Through fund raising auctions, benefit dinners, and volunteer work, members contribute to the needy. In fact, in the Physicians Health Program of the Medical Society of New Jersey, moneys raised by auxiliary members are earmarked for the impaired physicians program. Other funds might benefit children's hospitals or any number of charitable causes. The wives volunteer; the physicians gain community appreciation; and when the system is working at its best, an addicted physician, or his wife or child, may receive support and care from these fund raising efforts. Still, in New Jersey 5 percent of the treatment available in the program is given to wives and children, while 95 percent goes to impaired physicians. Indirectly, she works to see that her physician husband keeps functioning at the office.

Networking, that effective technique of combining business and social interaction used for years in the male world of business and professions to gain and renew a cross-section of professional contacts, hence gaining access to increased business and opportunities, has long been utilized by wives in the auxiliaries and at their husbands' professional meetings. Once again, however, being adept at networking enhances their husbands' professional reputation, patient referrals, and ultimate professional success. I believe doctors' wives unwittingly became the first collective group to develop and perfect networking skills among women. Its ultimate economic value was quickly recognized by their husbands and has been encouraged and supported.

My early experiences with the medical auxiliary 25 years ago were disappointing. I have a vivid recollection of myself as a young woman with the very recently attained status of doctor's wife. It was terrifying to be surrounded by those experienced in doctor's wifehood. My clothes were wrong. I was too shy. The two most commonly asked questions were, "Where did your husband go to school?" and "What is his specialty?" That rankled. What dues would I have to pay to belong to this established society?

This was an exclusive organization whose members sported clothes befitting *Vogue* magazine, complete with matching attitude. Welcoming committees graciously engaged the new wives into the community — the medical community. I was told where to buy the right clothes, get my hair done, buy food, and enroll my children in school.

I had great difficulty being comfortable because here was a place where my status as a doctor's wife was also examined and judged. Was he a surgeon? Then other wives showed reverence and expected that your clothes and jewels would be more expensive. As a general practitioner, Jerry was low in the pecking order and I, consequently, was also. It was humiliating for me to feel like an outsider; membership was rightfully mine. Had I desired election to an office, the likelihood was slim — only through displaying hard work at telephone calls, envelope stuffing, meal organizing, and other mundane accomplishments would I be considered. Perhaps then even a GP's wife might be considered for treasurer or secretary. Because of the competition and insecurity, intimacy fails.

I recall Eileen, a 48-year-old mother of two, during a nine hour interview in her gracious home:

> It was incredible. I played cards with the same women three times a week for 11 years. One day in the newspaper I saw the name of Ruth's son! He'd been arrested on some horrible drug charge. . . . Ruth had never, in all those years across the card tables, let on that there was a problem at home. I felt awful,

terribly hurt, and powerless to be of any help. It was infuriating to think that she didn't trust us enough to share that!

She described the disappointment and loneliness she became aware of after that incident:

> It was as if the card games were on automatic—like going through motions with no real meaning behind them. I felt more distant and apart from those women than I ever felt possible.

I knew her disillusionment and emptiness, and hated the blank expression in her eyes.

Certainly there are acceptable points to share among the wives: pleasantries, generalities, superficialities. Nothing that smacks of negativity at home. The image of the doctor is always at stake, as is the related image of his wife.

Secrecy and competition join forces to separate these women. Overwhelmed with the expectation of loyalty, devotion and undying faith keeps her from revealing private and personal needs and feelings. Often this silence is accomplished without conscious discussion on the part of her husband. It is a learned or assumed response in all medical families.

Broken marital bonds result in broken ties to the auxiliary. It's rare when a new wife is cheerfully accepted without proving herself first.

Being replaced in the medical auxiliary by your ex-husband's new wife is a painful experience. Women, who put years of their lives into the organization, having a social life, friends and perhaps a system of volunteer work and activities fostered by the auxiliary, are mercilessly shunned and deemed outcasts. They lose their prestige, social system, identification with a support group and club membership. I can think of little else about marriage to a physician that so poignantly highlights the status of these women. Replaceability, disrespect, insult, and profound humiliation occur over and over again. Age is no longer an indicator of this problem. Whereas formerly a new wife was likely to have taken the place of one who died, now a woman is likely to be remarried through divorce. Then, still alive, the ex-Mrs. Doctor loses friends and suffers the sting of total exclusion from the club.

I ultimately realized that this group was used to further the men's practices more than the women's self-esteem. In early years the auxiliary published and nationally distributed *MD's Wife*, renamed *Facets* in 1977. It is sent to all members of the organization. Other publications, including *Hygeia* and *Today's Health* magazines, are seriously promoted by the auxiliary to increase public awareness in medicine and related issues. The local and state auxiliaries publish newsletters. Beneath the guise of professionalizing the organization (for example, a complete biography of the newest president) are the articles suggesting ways to advance the public view of medicine and methods to improve the doctor's practice — increase efficiency, avoid malpractice, etc., once again as if the wives were physicians. More confusing for one's identity.

Recently, when invited to speak at our local meeting held on the same night as the physicians' general meeting, my talk was entitled, "The Empty Nest Syndrome." The men met downstairs in the country club and were served roast beef in a lavish, large, comfortable dining room. The women met upstairs in a tiny, windowless, attic-like room, and their menu was a small salad bar. This gross inequity had been a monthly occurrence in this country for years. Some people weren't aware of the effrontery and indignity of that situation. I was infuriated and voiced my dismay at the beginning of my presentation.

Today there are auxiliaries that allow male spouses of female physicians to join, although I've never seen a man attend a meeting. The club is a backlash organization. Women have been excluded from their husbands' meetings and organizations for so long that the men's groups have enjoyed exclusivity, and only now are reluctantly accepting the attendance of female physicians. The clubby atmosphere, separatism and competitiveness of the auxiliary promotes the men's business, narrows the women's focus, and discourages them from spreading their wings. The amount of work and time spent on club activities is enormous and exhausting, and the rewards are few.

Women are ostracized within the group when displaying enthusiasm about leaving the fold and going back to school or work, even part time, at anything which suggests a focus other than medicine. Nursing is acceptable and is encouraged today as in the past.

To their credit, there are local auxiliary groups around the country who are informally offering group support to spouses. Mercer County, New Jersey has such a group, which has been meeting since 1987. Groups in Oregon, Florida and other states have been springing up to attend to the special needs of medical spouses, hoping to break through stereotyping and eliminating isolation of wives from each other. Being attended by spouses of all ages, these groups are apt to begin as complaint sessions against the husband, the doctor. Soon and with commitment on the part of those attending, the topics move on to personal issues not unlike those covered in this book. It is heartening to see wives increasingly supporting one another, often having to go against the threats and fears of their husbands if they attend.

Louise, a therapist group leader and psychologist married to a physician, shared:

> Our group is attended by auxilians [affectionate name used for those in auxiliary] and non-auxilians. My biggest shock from working at the hospital and seeing the doctors there is their ignorance of each other's marital problems. In the group, their wives are becoming more intimately aware of each other's problems. Yet the doctors remain aloof and cool. At first this made it difficult for their wives to attend the meetings. The husbands have said things like, "What's going on at your coffee klatches?" or "You don't need to meet with those people." The doctors are in therapy, their wives are in therapy, and so many couples, especially the younger ones, are in marital therapy. Yet, the doctors don't seem to be aware of this fact. They behave as if everything is fine in their lives and in the lives of their colleagues. Amazing.

Though encouraged by the support offered by these groups, it disturbs me that they meet under the auspices of and as an adjunct to their husbands' profession. Perhaps women, meeting with other doctors' wives and nondoctors' wives to share and exchange human problems and eventually encouraging men and women in dialogue, would increase our knowledge and information base even more.

Generally, the auxiliary got mixed reviews among the women I interviewed. Some were delighted to have a group with which to identify, and found it a valuable outlet for their commitment, time, and energy.

Jean, a soft-spoken, charming mother of six, married 42 years, said:

> I don't know how I would have survived without them. To move around a lot and automatically have a group who speaks the same language and shares the same life has been a lifesaver for me! I've been active in it all my married life. I'm sort of the mother of our group here. The young wives look up to me for advice and inspiration. I guess I get a lot of strokes at those meetings.

She was quite careful, proper, and gracious while I was in her home. She showed me her husband's works in sculpture, of which she was obviously quite proud. She had trouble focusing on herself.

Lila, married to Tom for 12 years, recently moved to the area and joined the auxiliary to meet people. (In the auxiliary directory, the doctor's wife is listed alphabetically by last name and husband's specialty.) Lila describes:

> It's the only group I can interact with which doesn't turn their noses up at me for loving clothes and jewelry. Anywhere else, I feel reverse snobbery. It's as though I have to act like I don't have any money at all or the other women will be jealous of me because my husband's a doctor!

Some actively involved women saw the aura as often too stiff and formal. "Uptight" was frequently repeated. While we all enjoy letting our hair down, the protocol and tradition of the auxiliary precludes this. Others violently opposed the auxiliary. Annette, the newly married second wife of Hal, readily agreed to an interview. I can't forget her red hair, carefully tended but fashionably outrageous. Even though the phone was constantly interrupting our interview, she was anxious to share this:

I was horrified at the attitudes when I went to my first auxiliary meeting. People all wanted to talk about Hal's first wife [she was very active in the auxiliary] and they hoped I would follow in her footsteps and wasn't it a shame that Ellen [another wife] had to take over as treasurer because of Joan's divorce? I felt as if everyone knew everyone else's business, and was terribly intimidated!

Through the years, I have occasionally had reason for guarded optimism. Recently, this article appeared in my auxiliary newsletter:

The Medical Society president is asking that one member of the Auxiliary be sent as a representative to the next meeting of the County Board of Directors. Please call this number if you're interested.

What did this mean? Why after all these years was the medical society including one of the wives of its members to their board meeting? At first glance it could mean removing the cloak of secrecy of their meeting, allowing a spouse to be privy to the inner sanctum. My second reaction was that it was a bone being thrown to the auxiliary, a ploy to keep them interested in spending their time and energy on their husbands' careers; include a token wife and give all the wives a false sense of participation, knowledge, and communication. Or it could be seen as a bridge between the groups, as an honest attempt to accept female input into the organization. Why did that seem so hard for me to believe? Or could the female physician members have suggested to their male colleagues the wisdom of including an auxiliary member?

As it turned out, the auxiliary had printed the news prematurely. The county medical association had voted *not* to include an auxiliary member onto its board of directors after all, to the great dismay of the auxiliary members. My speculations on the subject became moot.

Some women feel a strong negative identification with the "auxiliary woman." She's the consummate doctor's wife, seen as the perennial helper, perfect in all aspects of social grace and charm but not to be trusted. She's too sugar coated, an opportunist, working only to further her husband's career. Many purposely shun the auxiliary to avoid the image, a denial of being seen only as Mrs. Doctor. A female seeking her own identity has a difficult enough time without coping with an auxiliary group based only on the job her husband holds!

Chapter 32

The Women's Movement:
Effects on Me and My Marriage

It hasn't affected my personal life in any way that I'm aware of. — Nora

The most traditional women married to doctors were insulated for a long time from the rumblings of feminism. The concept of equal work for equal pay would not directly affect women who were not working outside the home. The fact of their not receiving payment for their services as essential partners in the medical profession had not occurred to them. The fact of their prestige counting only as a silent partner to their husbands did not bother them. The setting aside of self for the support and success of the men they married was part of their early training as women in our society. Medicine would turn out to be one of the last professions where a woman was still essential to the success of her husband's career — as long as she fulfilled the role traditionally. In fact, without her (or someone else like her), he could not pursue and achieve his career goals at all (Fowlkes, 1980; Lorch and Crawford, "Marriage to a Physician," 1983).

Interestingly, an overall percentage of those I interviewed complained that the women's movement did not belong to them. They were not working anyway and they did not want to shake up the security of their economic position. The more I spoke to these women, the louder the words of Betty Friedan's *Feminine Mystique* seemed. Here was her '50s woman in all her glory in the late 1980s, and absolutely confused as to what all the shouting was about.

"Feminism has escaped me, I guess," begins a 46-year-old wife of 23 years. Diana is an attractive, small, well-built woman. She has warm brown eyes, and curly, well-coifed dark brown hair with two sturdy combs in it. Her posture defies her 47 years. She studied dance for years and her athleticism shows. She is a consummate host, serving me tea and small, buttery iced cakes and chocolate drop cookies. The striking difference between her home and the others I have visited is the abundance of dolls of many sizes from all over the world. Many sit on the furniture and line the walls on shelves. She explains they are from her collection which she started as a girl in Iowa.

> My mother loved beautiful things and she encouraged me to be a collector. She brought me dolls from wherever she went. She and my father traveled in their mid to later years. When I became an adult I held on to my doll collection as if it were my very self. In fact, when we started moving around for Barry's [her husband] training in medicine, he always told me to get rid of my dolls. It's probably the one time in our lives when I stuck to my guns — or my dolls, if you will — and refused to go along with him.
>
> Later as we started taking trips of our own, I got very excited about expanding my collection. Now I've even loaned these to local museums as part of certain exhibits. I guess they really feel like mine. They represent me and my past to some extent.

Diana did sparkle when showing me each doll, meticulously describing the origin and details of how it was made. It was difficult to bring her back to the effects of the women's movement.

> I can't see that it has entered my life. Oh, a few years ago I got excited about some of the books. I read *The Women's Room* and *The New Assertive Woman*, but generally I have not been a politically active person. Whenever I get excited about a cause, Barry gets nervous and gives me all sorts of projects at home or at his office to get involved in. My very latest interest was Students and Mothers Against Drunk Drivers. I volunteered to get a program going at our local high school. The more involved I got, the more Barry and I started getting irritable with each other. If I had night meetings, he would explode

and stay at work later and later. I had to hand over my responsibilities to other women. Barry has depended on me for years to be here for meal preparation and generally when he comes home from the office. I can't stand the fighting, so I give in to his wishes.

He's never minded projects for the kids [they have two sons]. Being involved with their care and school activities, or anything that I can do at home doesn't seem to phase him. But throughout our marriage, even my taking a class in doll making or pottery seems to get him upset.

It took me years to realize that Barry's moodiness and irritability with me and the kids was directly related to me doing something strictly for myself. I guess perhaps the women's movement does relate to me and my situation. Barry usually does call the shots around here. But in the early and mid '70s when I was reading that stuff, I thought—this isn't about me. I'm not oppressed. I have everything and I don't even have to go out and work if I don't want to.

I do remember getting angry once in a while when I tried to assert myself with Barry. He seemed to overreact so that I'd be overwhelmed and crawl back to my more quiet self. He'd point out that I was being unreasonable, that women's lib was for lesbians or women who had to work and weren't getting paid enough. He'd say, "All you women are alike—never satisfied. We work our fingers to the bone to provide for you and what do you want?" I've never dealt well with his anger. My parents raged at each other all the time. My father threw things when I was little. So I guess it was easier to retreat to the status quo. . . . Anyway, my life was and still is fine. Nice house, great kids, we go away twice a year on a big trip somewhere. I know Barry is loyal to me and as my mother always said, "He doesn't drink or beat you, so what more do you need?"

The increasing rates of physicians' divorce, instrumented by either the physicians or their wives, shows a clear impact of the women's movement (Myers, 1988). Since a successful medical marriage appears to require a strong role definition with the doctor as authoritarian bread winner and his wife as deferential and subservient handmaiden, and as women have been questioning their range of choices and are looking at more fulfillment of themselves, the medical marriages, as with many traditional marriages, are breaking down. Obviously we are and will continue to be in a period of great restructuring of roles for men and women in the family institution.

The medical marriage and the medical profession are intertwined, interdependent; one cannot stand without the other working smoothly. As I review my interviews of those marriages in trouble, it seems that the wife influences the course of the marriage directly or indirectly in proportion to her assertion of a clear, strong self.

> It's like dangling a carrot out there for me. I stopped working when we had young children. I raised the kids essentially alone, and now that they're going out on their own, that's what I want for myself. It's an uphill fight. In the early years of the women's movement I was thrilled to get Louis to help me with the dishes once or twice a week. If he called a babysitter on his own, you could have knocked me over with a feather.

Mary Kay has been married to Louis for 18 years. She continues:

> I guess I have been a latent feminist since we got married. But hard as I try I'm still the one who manages the household and the kids and the social life and Louis's personal stuff. He gets called out in the middle of bathing our little girl. His meetings take precedence over my project with the HELP Line, so I have to get the babysitters. When I decided to go back to work [Mary Kay is a medical illustrator] there was no option about moving to where I could get a better job—a bigger city. In fact, I was offered a job in Chicago with a big publishing firm, but Louis's position here is solid. Or so I always thought. He'd say, "It's taken years for me to get on the staff of this hospital and to get everyone's respect. I may even get to be the chief of staff in a couple of years. How can we move to Chicago?" So women's lib or not, I've taken free-lance work where I can get it. My job will never be taken as seriously as his. If I stay married to Louis, and believe me it's been touch and go ever since I've tried to become my own person more, I'll have to accept the fact that my own work life is second to

his career, and if something comes up where I have to represent him as chief of staff or something, that will always be first.

The range is enormous. The younger women do appreciate the ability to at least work in a part-time job. They still do most house-related tasks for their husbands and family.

A career requires more time and energy, full-time commitment. I can't move up the ladder in banking like John can in medicine,

says Jacqueline, married only three years.

My one-year-old requires full-time care. Think about it — how many full-time careers can one woman have? Even if I'm a nontraditional doctor's wife (which I consider myself), I'm not a volunteer woman and I do want to have my own separate career for pay. Who will take care of the baby? Try to get a doctor to refuse to take call if an emergency arises. Try to get a doctor to cancel his schedule of appointments to come home to a sick child! Ask a doctor who's been in surgery all day and part of the night to wake up with a sick baby at three a.m. the next night or three nights in a row. Let's face it. Someone has to take charge of the kids, and since banking is eight to five p.m., I'm the one who tries to run home for lunch and check the baby, or I'm the one who gets up with the runny nose stuff at three a.m. It's an ongoing conflict! It takes great stamina and fortitude to be true to feminism and live with a doctor!

I loved Jacqueline's forthright attitude and enthusiasm. She's 25, fiery, determined, and enlightened, not at all someone who sees her role as one of adjunct or support system to another. She, like Mary Kay the medical illustrator, is trying to find a way to be both an individual and have an equitable partnership to a man of medicine. Not an easy task.

I have observed at close hand a couple I consider to be quite liberal minded and who strive for equality in their relationship. They work together in an ophthamology office — he is an MD and she a nurse practitioner. She uses her maiden name to retain her professional identity separate from his. They have three young daughters. Occasionally when I enter their place of business the children will be on the premises, with the office help watching over them as both of their parents are seeing patients in their respective offices. At times the office assistants look harried and at times the patients register complaints that the children are disruptive. The parents take turns getting the children to and from school and to and from various after-school activities. The children have on occasion accompanied their parents to office staff meetings if it was absolutely necessary.

Here is a true combining of family and profession. When asked, however, Natalie, the wife of Mason, said:

It takes planning and perseverance. I do all the cooking at home because I love to cook. Also my work schedule is much more part-time. I come in two to three days per week to Mason's full-time. But that's okay. I worked full-time before we had children and I married so late in life I wanted to be a mother for a while. So Mason's is the primary career, and although I take my work seriously when I'm doing it, my patients are the ones who are rescheduled if there's a snow day and I can't get a babysitter. It's weird. I've had it both ways. As a single career woman I could make my decisions, come and go as I pleased. I made a great living and was respected and published in my field. When we married Mason was already a prominent eye surgeon. He was married before and divorced. I had seen doctors, worked with them, taught them, but still, being married to one requires giving in and giving up one's feminist principles at times. Mason considers himself a feminist. He's against competition and definitely tries to promote equality, antiracism, antiprejudice, peaceful co-existence, and so forth. However, the practice of his career doesn't make it possible for him to periodically cancel eye surgeries if his kids are having a special show at school. He does a large share at home, more than any other doctor I know. I try to remain grateful for that.

From older, more traditional women I heard,

> I don't care about women's liberation. I've done all the work around here for decades. What can women's lib do for me?

or

> My life has been fine, just the way I wanted it to be. I had enough money to come and go as I pleased, to take care of my family the way I wanted to. What other husband or profession could have offered me that?

or

> If women like getting more heart attacks and strokes like men get them, let them go out and be the doctors. As for me, I'm happy at home, watching the kids and the dogs.

and

> I think everyone has gone crazy. Women have babies, they nurse them. Marriage to a doctor is the most extraordinary way for a woman to fulfill herself as a woman. There are elegant dinners, wonderful clothes, and beautiful household furnishings. Doctors lead an exciting life which she is privy to at parties and meetings. All she has to do is hold up her end of the bargain. Be a good wife, entertain, be gracious, invite the right people over, take impeccable care of the house and kids, be there when her husband comes home from a hard day at the hospital and be willing to make his life a little easier so that he can go out in the world again and do this thing. It seems an equitable arrangement. No wonder the doctors leave for younger women — they need someone to fuss over them, to protect them like their mothers did from the big, bad outside world. I see it bright as day. A young woman wants to do her own thing; even the young doctors are joining group practices to get out of working so hard. What is going on? Where are the old-fashioned values of hard work and helping people? Everyone is into helping himself more. I see it all the time. No one wants to give in to the other, so divorce, divorce, divorce. Then

what? A bunch of kids floating around with no adult supervision. I never minded motherhood. Now no one wants to do it. Well, if you marry a doctor, either don't have kids or prepare to be a mother to them.

The latter was spoken by a 72-year-old retired doctor's wife of 50 years. She reflects, quite astutely I think, the dilemma of women married to physicians in the '80s and early '90s.

Where is it all going? There is a backlash of traditionalism. Whenever doctors' wives try to fight for a more equitable arrangement, they come up against the proverbial brick wall. Fowlkes talks about medicine as the male-dominated, traditional hierarchical authoritarian institution which attracts traditional men who need to receive a great deal of personal deference and must be able to be in a superior position over co-workers and wives (1980). If he doesn't find the traditional wife, he will make her into one or the profession will require it of her. And if that still fails, she will be replaced with a more traditional model who will support, nurture, and revere him.

I think the women's movement forgot that until our mothers stop fussing over their boys and making them need constant attention and adulation from the public and the women they marry, failure will dominate the realm of the doctor and his wife. Until their girls are fussed over as much, they (the girls) won't ever be able to demand the same care and treatment from their husbands, the doctors, as he can and does demand and receive from her, wife number one, number two, or number six. She will always be out there. Until she is paid a salary for her essential task at home, she will not feel truly productive, or as if she has achieved something of value in our society.

Even Fowlkes' wonderful sociological study comparing twenty MD's wives to 20 academician's wives could not quell the bias that what the doctors' wives were doing was somehow empty and shallow (1980). Perhaps the medical profession should include spouses on their payroll for providing essential tools to the physician so that he can achieve his success. She is indeed an associate, a co-partner, in the profession of medicine. The institution keeps her that way. Perhaps equitable pay and prestige for her skills, acknowledgement of her value, and contribution to the continued successful practice of her marital partner would allow for her increased self-esteem. She can then freely choose, with dignity, the job of physician's wife-associate. If not, the traditional physician marriage is going to continue to disintegrate through serial divorce.

The high percentage of volunteer work provided by doctors' wives in hospitals, auxiliaries, and in the community leaves them vulnerable to nonsympathy or even attack from feminists. They end up doing purely women's work and are unpaid for it!

It saddens me when these women feel they don't fit into the ideals of the women's movement because they have privileges provided by their husbands' income. Other women may feel that feminism does not apply to the doctor's wife. How wrong! Why women who work at home or volunteer their time should feel disenfranchised from the women's movement, or why those in academia or in the board room should feel unsympathetic toward those at home, is distressing and confusing. It's clear that we need the support of the most ardent feminists. We need the most help in discovering how to attain more equitable arrangements in our home lives and freedom to work outside the home so that our choices are broader and more satisfying. We need the women's movement to help us to find ourselves!

As for me, when my husband comes into my room on his day off and sees me writing and asks—if I'm not doing anything would I please arrange to pick up a birthday gift for our son because he's not sure but he might want to be available to go skiing on his day off—I want the women's movement to march one-million fold behind me with banners saying, "I am working. I am writing. I am serious. You use your day off to buy the gift. You take care of it for a change!"

THE LAMENT OF A WOMEN'S MOVEMENT WOMAN

I tried and tried
God only knows how hard
I went back to school
I went back to work

The more I did
The harder it became
I joined a group
I asserted myself more
I embraced other women

I tried being more open
I stood up for ERA
I stood up for the right to choose

I took off my make-up
I shake hands with a firm grip
I bring my child to his father's work place
and say you get the babysitter
my job is calling me

I give speeches
I carry banners
I confront the issues all the time
Equal pay for equal work
Free choices — the same as them

Don't ask me if I'm married
Or how many kids I have
Not my age, or home situation
If I'm going to get pregnant
Or what if my kids get sick

Don't ask me who my husband is
Ask me how I'll do the job
Where I went to school — not when

What if I have a different color
Or a body that doesn't work like yours
Women's lib promised to open up the doors

Why then are there so many doors still shut
Tighter than before
All those figures statistics and percentages
Don't mean much any more

I come home from work and bake the cookies
I see the dishes still in the sink
I take the baby to the dentist
Why must I be the one to think

Where's my wife and savior
My mother's helper and cook
I've done everything they said to
And still my work's not done

Women's lib you've deserted me
You've sold me a bill of goods
Till home and hearth is valued
And men take care of kids
What's the point in me doing double duty

There's more to do
More to fight about
More to remember
And more to regret

What price this so-called equality
This greater freedom of choice
I can't tell if I've won or lost

If I'm the one who struggles
If I'm the one who slaves
To make it work for others
And still never get repaid.

THE GIRLS IN THE BAND

This is for the girls in the band
marching along
tapping out a time

Aren't you wondering who hears you
Doesn't it seem as if your flutes are mute
Are the drums resounding
Are the tubas really hollow?

They say you should march to a
                    different drummer
Speak a different time
What you play is not to be said
What you say is not understood.

Where will you go this time
Up to the park or down to the avenue
the buildings are bare
No one is there to hear your song

Why not play for each other
hold each other's hands
March together side by side
Embrace your sisters loud and strong
the melody and tune rejoices
What you have to say is clear
the girls in the band are here to stay
the girls in the band are free
No one need applaud them
For they understand one another
they hear each other play
the harmony comes easily
when each one sings her way

He says how sad and lonely
to be outside and alone
She says her music is the universal song
shared throughout the world

She understands that to be truly free
The band must be heard
the band must be understood
the band must not only be
          inside of me . . .

The girls gather to rehearse again
One more time — we'll see
Another note another refrain
Louder here, then soft, and louder still

They are cheering
They begin to tap their feet
Strum Strum the beat picks up
the girls smile, then they turn to
          one another and nod
It was worth it after all
We are great musicians
We'll take our song along the road
Let the other girls know — let's lighten their load.

Another place, another time
          another song

Strum, Strum along
Here's to the girls in the band
Play for each other, play for yourselves
the music will soothe you and bond
          you together
Hold hands, bring your daughters
teach them the song — they'll need to know

Remember you are the girls in the band
From you comes the music of tomorrow
I'm proud to be playing your song

Your sounds echo in my ears
and brings me hope and joy
Stand tall, be quiet for now
Remember the band must always play on!

Chapter 33

Trouble at Home:
Who's the Patient Anyway?

For years I thought it was normal to go to sleep drunk. No one
ever tried to stop me. — Elaine

Reviewing the available literature, though scarce, had me convinced that physical and mental illness was rampant among doctors'
wives. Medical research done by physicians themselves, especially
psychiatrists, has pointed out the high rate of depression, suicide,
and alcohol and drug abuse reported for physicians' wives.

It is my impression from my review of the literature that statistics
regarding impairment of the physician or members of his family are
not available in reliable numbers. The American Medical Association Information Services was unable to provide any information on
this.* I was told by the Impaired Physician Division of the AMA
that several states have allocated moneys for research and care programs for impaired physicians and their families.

There is an increase in these programs and in group support treatment for these problems. Otherwise, there has been no attempt to
compile data on the national level or to track trends and changes in
the area of problems in medical households. It could be surmised
that there is not enough interest in a broad overview of the data. I
was told also that each county or state study done defines abuse and

---

*Center for Health Policy Research, the National Center for Health Statistics,
the American Women's Medical Association, the Bureau of Health Professions
Statistics, and the Alcohol and Drug Abuse-Mental Health Administration also
were unable to provide these numbers.

impairment differently, and this hampers the comprehensive compilations of data on a national basis.

Having surveyed many reports by those who treat physicians' wives, physicians, and their families, it appears there is an increase in reported complaints. Marital stress, drug and alcohol abuse, and depression apparently are rising in medical families. As of this writing, there are no hard numbers available to compare to those not in medical families. It would seem that, for reasons of privacy, reporting impairments and personal problems is discomforting and unlikely, as is true in the general population. In fact, the public's expectations and demands of greater personal and interpersonal success of physicians and their families hampers the reporting of difficulties outside of the medical profession, which does not desire further public exposure.

Florida and New Jersey presently have the longest standing programs funded by their state medical associations for physicians. Oregon, Ohio, Iowa, and others increasingly have offered volunteer help programs for impaired physician treatment. The threat of loss of medical license brings MDs into treatment. Some programs encourage the involvement of spouses and families in the treatment. A few programs have assistance for the addictive nonphysician spouse, and unfortunately, there are reports that co-addiction between physician and spouse is increasingly prevalent, as is the growing use of alcohol coincident with other drugs (Getz, 1989).

A landmark study done in 1963 by James Evans, MD, reported in the *American Journal of Psychiatry*, entitled "Psychiatric Illness in the Physician's Wife," was and is still cited as the last word on the subject. Evans made a detailed study of 50 women admitted for psychiatric care to a private hospital. He never actually spoke to these women, but used records of their treating psychiatrists. Thirty-one of these women had a history of mental illness in their family. Nineteen were college graduates, nine had partial college, 12 were nursing school graduates, two had partial nursing training, and eight were high school graduates. Reported symptoms included: "anxiety, muscle spasms, depression, excessive drinking, attempted suicide, chronic pain, excessive hostility, withdrawal, mania and feelings of rejection" (p. 160). Also, 75 percent reported sexual incompatibility, with no further explanation on that subject.

Drug abuse was considered in 22 of the women. Some of the drug use was treatment for chronic pain, low back, migraine headache, abdominal, and menstrual pain.

To quote:

> The contrast between the reportedly good pre-morbid adjustment of the patients as a group and the severity and tenacity of their illnesses is striking [after repeated readmissions]. Nevertheless, prior to illness they had been quite successful. They were well educated and pursued a variety of intellectual and cultural activities in their leisure moments. They were able to marry men with high socio-cultural standing. As a group they had successfully weathered the difficult years of their husbands' training and the early years of practice. Only after an average of almost thirteen years of marriage was an overt illness manifested. (p. 161)

Evans continues in these often-quoted remarks/findings:

> Illness developed when the equilibrium of the adjustment was disrupted by such reality factors as the increasing involvement of the doctor in his work, or a conflict between his personality characteristics and the idealized expectations of his wife. (p. 162)

Depression, drug addiction, and "somatization" are the themes found repeatedly when describing the doctor's wife. Evans uses the word hysteria throughout the article, implying that her distress and physical complaints (somatization) are overdramatized and exaggerated. She supposedly is someone who was overly close to her father and had a father-daughter relationship in her marriage. She is said to be narcissistic (emotionally immature and self-preoccupied), overly needy, overly dependent on her husband, and her physical complaints are a supposed reflection of "hostile dependent" aspects of her relationship. She is trying to frustrate her husband, the doctor, through an illness he cannot diagnose. Evans also suggests that the husbands' lack of attention to their wives and the accessibility of drugs increases the potential for drug dependency and the depression. He implied that the doctors may be in collusion to keep their wives ill by ignoring or medicating so as not to face their own impotence (p. 163).

Others point out "hysterical" personality traits which are revealed by depression, excessive concern about aches and pains, and overly dramatic behavior, implying that these troubled women are imagining their discomforts and discontent. Reference is made to her anger, resentment, and depression, which increase with the length of the marriage. Also common are the words, "husband's responding to his wife's dependency needs" by giving her medication, leading to an addiction. Women were said to be more affective (expressive of feelings), while husbands used more intellectual defenses (Derdeyn, 1979). Or she has an inordinate need for affection, while her husband is detached. She is also said to have a passive-aggressive personality (Evans, 1963). She is called "a dependent histrionic wife" married to "an emotionally detached husband" (Miles, Krell, and Lin, 1972, p. 481).

Newer studies convey puzzlement as to why so many doctors' wives end up in a psychiatrist's office. She's angry or depressed, and neither she nor her husband understands why. She's uncomfortable with her anger since she's living a model, enviable lifestyle, and her husband is "baffled by the turn of events which finds him with a depressed and suicidal wife and problem children" (Miles, Krell, and Lin, 1972, p. 482). The words "needy," "narcissistic," and "dependent" are used to excess when describing a troubled doctor's wife.

Recent literature seems rife with blaming women and mothering for their daughters' troubles. In *Perfect Woman*, Collette Dowling devotes much of her thesis on narcissism of women created and passed on from mother to daughter. The ineffective rearing of girls, needy and unfulfilled in childhood, is blamed for the preoccupation with self, perfectionism, and general low self-esteem. Mothers living through their girls set them up for severe dependency, obsession with others' opinion of them, and a great lifetime need to be special.

Being a doctor's wife would seem to fulfill those "narcissistic needs" to be grander than others. If our mothers passed on narcissism because they lacked a healthy inner sense of self, perhaps it behooves us to look at a society which perpetuates a myth of female narcissism. How can a girl or her mother be totally self-confident and self-respecting in a world where females are denied value from birth? Let us not perpetuate the myth of mother's fault — and female narcissism. It is obvious that mothers and daughters will gain self-respect as society values women and femaleness. The doctor's wife exemplifies the bind of a caretaker with little self-esteem. Her husband the doctor is praised for his qualities of self love and grandiosity, for which his wife is given only reproof and then medication.

Traditionally if there is trouble at home, whether small irritations or large incompatibilities, women have somehow sought to repair the problems. So when a woman has tried talking, sharing feelings, creating romantic interludes, cooking favorite dishes, offering intellectual stimulation, having an affair, etc., if she is not getting any satisfaction and improving the way she feels and the way she and her husband are relating, more drastic measures are necessary. Divorce proceedings are a clear option, but they're not always desirable or possible. While frustrated and misunderstood, she may not have coping skills useful to meet the crises in her life. Unable to understand her own discomfort, she goes for outside help. Women tend to presume that they are the ones to fix a relationship; in fact, since society reinforces this fear, women come to believe that they are the only cause of the crisis.

My clinical practice has highlighted women and children as barometers of family life. If a child is upset and stirs up trouble, often he or she is shedding light on a marital difficulty. Well so does a woman. Unfortunately, when the doctor's wife, or any woman, comes to seek help, she is labeled by the medical community through the psychiatrist as crazy, dependent, narcissistic, hysterical, a fake, overreacting, depressed, and suicidal. In addition, there's an implication, the ominous "overlay," that she has consciously manipulated these symptoms to her advantage, or that she is inherently weak and inferior, and — independent of the relationship with her husband — is showing symptoms and signs of her inferiority. She is made to feel incompetent, and rather than look at the relationship or the entire system of medical care for women, her dependence and reaching out for help is looked upon with disdain and condescension. Then, she is humored along as if she is a weakling who could not be expected to be otherwise.

Somehow distress as enacted by the wife is not the same as that of a distressed physician. She, after all, was already weak and especially needy. Her symptoms are almost expected. If he's depressed or suicidal, it is probably his overwork or case load that's causing the symptoms. If she's sad, lonely, frustrated, and angry she's an hysterical woman. No cause for her rage, just inexplicable rage! Her inherent inferiority, weakness, and tendency toward overexaggeration are to blame for her display of aches, pains, and sadness. Her husband's angry; he's had a tough day. She's angry and it's a problem of her inner make-up. We must medicate the anger and rage away. If she's sick (inherently) we'll fix her with our best potions for inferior, depressed, unpowerful people. The anger is especially frightening to the doctor and his wife. Since anger is powerful and is sometimes a precursor to rage, a more vengeful emotion, they are both fearful of it; she because it's unladylike, unacceptable, and uncomfortable; he because it's threatening to his position in the marriage. Medicate the anger or repress the anger, and show depression instead. Depression is the more tolerable and acceptable emotion, especially for females. She, consequently, is the "identified patient."

Tamara, a woman in her thirties with three children, had just lost one baby to premature abortion. She reacted with a combination of rage and sadness:

> We had just moved from my home town and I was trying to get used to a new place. Then the next thing I knew was I was pregnant. I've had trouble with depression after each one of my other deliveries, and I've expected a lot of help from Ryan [husband]. I guess a part of me has always hoped I'd be protected by Ryan in my life. After I lost this pregnancy, I flipped. Not just depression this time, but great anger.
>
> Ryan was flabbergasted. He could deal with tears and me quietly keeping to myself, but when I got really angry he reacted in a way I'd never seen before. Ryan's pretty sweet usually. Soft spoken. Everyone loves him. In our church he's very active and respected. My family loves him. He's always been steady and dependable. When I got angry and started shouting and hollering somewhat out of control, Ryan turned

on me. He picked up a broom and chased me with it. Then we had pandemonium. The kids got scared and tried to stop our fighting. Ryan was now in a rage and I was then getting terrified. He hit me across the face a few times and threatened to put me in the hospital if I ever yelled like that again. I was shaking.

Next thing I knew I was in a shrink's office. One of Ryan's colleagues. Ryan and he sat and talked about my situation. I was the patient. I had the problem. And they would fix me together. In the middle of that session I got infuriated again and ran out the door of the office. Ryan came into the hallway and brought me back inside. Both he and the other doctor agreed I needed medicine to calm me down. I couldn't get a word in to the other doctor about Ryan's behavior or that I was now afraid for me and my kids. I was trapped, and I knew it.

Tamara went on to describe a few more visits with this psychiatrist. She felt that she was especially vulnerable to depression and subsequent psychiatric care after childbirth.

No one would consider that I was not the only problem in the family. They assumed it was me, my problem. I was a troublemaker, and I felt that no one was listening. In fact they were trying to shut me up. I also had to consider my children. If I didn't cooperate I was afraid of what could happen to my kids. Ryan had never gone crazy before. I was terrified. I know it's weird, but if I took the pills and kept quiet Ryan was fine to us. So I followed the plan. I guess I sort of gave up. No one even mentioned the loss of the baby. The only thing everyone was preoccupied with was my impending outburst of anger.

Others may speculate as to what triggered Ryan's response to Tamara's angry outbursts. My point is the system: doctor/husband diagnoses his wife and perhaps refers her to a male colleague. Both doctors are afraid and confused by her anger; both have an unconscious stake in keeping her as "the patient" and "under control." And both have been taught that she alone has inherent potential for mental aberrations and weakness. If she's not making enough noise to be causing trouble, she will never get to a psychiatrist. She may then deal with her situation on her own or only with her husband's prescriptions.

When a Ryan is distressed, it's not likely that he will be seen or helped by anyone. He's most likely to doctor himself or deny his disturbing behavior or problems. He may provoke his wife to act out his own unhappiness, or he seeks help for them both under the guise of "fixing" her problem. Or she takes too many drinks or sleeps too long when her sexual life is unfulfilling or nonexistent. Or their child fails at school or gets involved with a troublesome group or takes drugs or cuts school or threatens suicide. The family interaction is the problem; the rigorous roles and cool communication, the overachievement orientation, the lack of visible imperfection, all put tremendous pressure on the family unit. The worst part is the unconscious blocking and/or the conscious inability to see trouble and feel safe about getting assistance.

About 20 percent of the women I interviewed admitted to a childhood in which they experienced some form of abuse. The behaviors ranged from neglect of one or both parents to alcoholic abuse, physical violence, and sexual abuse within the family. It is no wonder, then, that a woman with that childhood experience, living in fear of violent outbursts and perhaps personal assault, would be attracted to someone she presumes will be stable and preoccupied with his career. To say that her desire for safety and solitude is a reaction to negative childhood experiences is to state a likely and predictable outcome from our present knowledge of the effects of childhood abuse on its victims (Bass and Davis, 1988).

To choose a distant, orderly man who is pursuing a socially desirable career might be seen as protection to an abuse survivor. To her, her husband's inaccessibility is a welcome relief from her intrusive childhood. In fact, she also appreciates not being sexually active unless she initiates it in a very safe environment. Having a relationship which is intimate only on a limited basis is appreciated. The economic stability, the emotional and perhaps sexual distance, and the predictable order of marriage to a physician are quite comfortable, if not desirable, to her.

It is presumptuous to judge her choice of husband and lifestyle as a reflection of her inferior or unhealthy mental history. On the contrary, a woman who survives this kind of abuse in childhood (and the statistics based on open admissions are likely quite low) instead shows great strength, health, self protection — in other words, excellent survival skills — in choosing a physician husband. He is less likely to stir up her emotional ghosts from her past. It is only as she resolves her past fears that she may find her distant, cool, detached physician husband less appealing. When she is more comfortable with closeness and intimacy, he may be unable or unwilling to satisfy her needs.

If it is acknowledged that the doctor is troubled or "impaired" when he is ill (rather than being labeled crazy or sick as his wife would be), then the wife is called in to sessions to help in the process of fixing him. However, when they are in marital therapy there is a "poverty of communication" between the couple (Miles, Krell, and Lin, 1972, p. 483). There are increasingly more programs for "impaired" physicians, usually kept hidden from the public so as not to tarnish the image. I am told there is a high success rate in the programs designed to reduce his drug and/or alcohol use, or depression (Smith, 1987; Myers, 1988). Impairment means loss of a great deal to a physician. He stands to lose his license to practice medicine, and there is presently increased support for his immediate return to functioning.

Even with drug and alcohol treatment interventions increasing, the more involved the spouse is in her husband's office practice, the more fearful she may be to report her husband's drug or alcohol abuse. She stands to lose not only her husband's income, but also her personal identity in his practice as her work may be lost. In this case, she not only maintains the home, but the workplace as well. Any intervention threatens to crush her entire world. With greater available information regarding co-dependency, these programs are trying to get both partners involved in treatment. She is pressured to report him through threat of loss of available funding for his treatment. She is also made to take part in his treatment as a co-dependent in his problem. My impression is, however, that the funding to date is directed primarily toward the physician. The spouse's treatment comes as a secondary benefit, as it will improve the physician's chances for recovery and return to his practice.

When his wife is impaired, or rather sick or sickly, those very people who work quickly to repair her husband move just as quickly to maintain her illness. They keep her on medication, whereas they remove his. They keep her in long-term therapy, whereas he's out as soon as possible. She is to remain dependent, and he is to return to independent functioning.

Remember, in the last 150 years middle- and upper-class women at various times were either confined to their beds, operated upon, leeched, or otherwise medicated for their supposed innate ovarian or mentally caused illnesses (Ehrenreich and English, 1974). The doctor's wife as a member of the middle-upper-class was viewed as the very epitome of womanhood: problematic and weak and correctable. The doctor took on the role of expert where women were concerned in the mid to late 1800s, first as a gynecologist or surgeon, and later in this century as the psychiatrist, all from the traditional school of thought and perceptions that women required fixing, and the doctors were the only ones who could fix them. How, then, does the modern doctor's wife escape the long-accepted view that her husband and his profession are the ultimate authorities over her body and mind? She must believe the word of medicine. She is either an hysteric or a malingerer; her female organs need fixing; or her brain should be retrained, oppressed, or tyrannized. She is a middle-class housewife, married to our symbol of expertise. She either believes in his diagnosis and treatment of her "illnesses" or is threatened with rejection, alienation, or economic and emotional deprivation. Of course, the lifestyle in which she is engaged may contribute to her "illnesses." Yes, isolation, sensory deprivation, gradual denial, destruction of her intellectual and creative capacities, and relative lack of freedom of thoughts and expression do make her "sick."

Ultimately, whatever she believes, she is the identified patient, the crazy one, the one responsible and therefore the one to be fixed; then our household (or our society) will be well. Pretty unreasonable and unrealistic, this double standard is difficult if not impossible for her to overcome as the present system stands. It's not working to assume that the wife of a physician is a dependent, weak, overly narcissistic, needing more affection than normal, and/ or incompetent, and then to punish her if she does exhibit any of the above in her time of frustration. The stereotypes of weakness, inferiority, and overemotionalism come to haunt her over and over again. Perhaps we look in the wrong place for the so-called patient. Society must take responsibility for such an unjust system and try to deal with greater compassion toward any of us who are in trouble.

In his 1980 article "Suicide in Doctors and Wives of Doctors," Safinofsky reported that the suicide rate of doctors' wives was higher than suicides among women married to men in any other professional group. He attributed this to her unmet dependency needs, perhaps because of her husband's unavailability. There is no reason to believe that the trend toward high suicide in doctors' wives has reduced to date. I suggest that if she is depressed and despairing enough to contemplate and commit suicide, she and/or her relationship to her husband is not all that may be troubled. She may be the victim of unreported distress, poor medical treatment, or worse, her symptoms may be overlooked by herself, her husband, and the medical profession, which does not take her seriously. This is a frightening and dangerous set of circumstances. (See Chapter 12 "When I Am Ill.") Her available choices appear to be: no treatment for fear of being ignored or misunderstood, thus bearing the burden of her depression alone, or collusion between her husband and his colleagues with the threat of ultimately receiving inadvertent mistreatment. We can only guess what the consequences of her committing suicide are for her husband, their children, and the community.

In the medical marriage, if the suicide rates are higher than the general population, and the drug and alcohol abuse rates are higher, and the rates of depression and marital dissatisfaction are higher, and the rates of physical and sexual abuse distressing, then misplaced blame and oppression are not going to fix it. Rather, acknowledgment, awareness, and then some creative solutions are a better place to start.

DIPLOMAS ON THE WALL

(Written while waiting for my physician [female] to examine me for
my regular yearly check-up.)

Here I sit sick and afraid
Wearing only a sheet
With an open back.

My feet are cold, so are my hands
Yet as I try to warm myself
I see the walls in front of me
Framed pictures of writing, seals and signatures.

The words are unclear
Latin I think, or some inexplicable signs
Your name appears in Old English script
Above the names of others who went before.

The walls full of these pictures
In the waiting room
In the examination room
In the halls and in your special office.

As I sit patiently, chilled and worried
I wonder about the messages
In those frames.

Gold, silver and delicate script
Camouflage the meaning for me
But still I know I'm to be impressed.

All that glitter and calligraphy
Takes my breath away
Did you go to all those schools
And study all those years?

Did all those people bestow all those honors
Because of who you are or what you've done?
I'm overwhelmed by your accomplishments.

Honorary this, licensed that,
Phi Beta Kappa, Universitas Pennsylvaniensis
Do those words bestow a blessing upon you?

Or will I feel better
Just knowing a person of such stature
Such special skills and training
Who joins the halls of Hippocrates?

Will that save me from my pain
My anguish, will it subside
Just knowing your history and intentions?

I put my trust in you
My respect and gratitude
Those diplomas on your walls
Help heal me most of all.

Chapter 34

Malpractice and Other Strains: The Individuation Process

We've watched our friends drop out like flies—one by one.
—Priscilla

One of the areas of great concern to medical families is the great increase in cases of malpractice brought against physicians. Doctors live in fear that they will be judged harshly, or make a mistake that will be taken to court. Some cases actually do result in the physician's losing his ability to practice medicine. The costs of insurance have become so prohibitive as to prevent physicians from practicing their specialty, i.e., the state of Florida's obstetric malpractice insurance has caused many physicians to alter or discontinue their obstetrical practices altogether.

Ironically the threat of malpractice has caused changes in medical practice—more paper work, less spontaneous communications with patients, more scrupulous testings, and greater detailed record keeping for the physician for each case. The public demands for overseeing medical care has opened the way for doctors to police their own profession and for the public to gain greater access to their care. The trend seems to be to give greater control of the patient's health back to the patient.

How does malpractice affect the doctor's wife? Insofar as she is primary caretaker of her husband, the doctor, malpractice affects her enormously. Recall, she is empathetic and understanding. In some ways the experience of a malpractice case draws the wife closer to her husband. For the first time in their married lives there is a real threat to the stability of his career. Never before has the MD's word been questioned and threatened as it is today. As technology and overprofessionalization of health care continue to evolve, malpractice is a natural consequence. The more sophisticated the technology and specialized the practice, the more room for judgments and human techniques to fail. Perhaps they are only human, the public is beginning to say.

The pendulum swings from total loyalty, reverence, and admiration to distrust and unreasonable monetary demands for human errors made by doctors. Multimillion-dollar malpractice cases have been tried and settled all over the country and loom over the heads of practicing physicians everywhere. Although it has helped to return physicians back to the realm of humans rather than gods who could do no wrong, the threat of malpractice affects medical practice (which I will not elaborate on here) and also the doctor's wife.

Women described their experiences with great empathy. Some rage at the public, and express a sense of overprotectiveness for the welfare of their husbands. Perhaps for the first time in their married lives their husband the doctor is seen as extremely vulnerable. The threat to his competence, judgment, and self-esteem is greater than at any other time in their marriage. If she is extremely fortunate, her husband will open up to her and share his feelings of isolation, depression, and the terror that he may never again be able to use his skills and practice his craft.

Both are aware that they can't talk to anyone about an impending malpractice case. Loretta, a woman in her late forties, married for 26 years, said she and her husband had gone through a series of malpractice cases. The latest case, which had been hanging over their heads for three years, was finally coming to trial.

> What saved us is that Don was not being sued alone. He was part of a team of physicians in this case. If I had to keep quiet about the case any more it would drive me crazy. At least the other doctors' wives could talk to me a little about what they were going through. Donald became very sullen and moody, and for a long time I had no idea what was happening. I agonized at the thought that perhaps I was doing something to upset him.

Women were relieved to find that their husband's sudden behavior changes, i.e., depression, reserve, irritability, or poor sleep, had a real cause. Usually we blame ourselves for our husband's moods and feelings, looking for ways to fix them. What a great relief to find that a malpractice case is the reason, rather than ourselves or our marriage. During a malpractice saga, wives can feel useful; sometimes this is the only time they feel completely involved and connected to their husband's world of work!

Loretta continued:

Headaches became Don's regular visitor. He stopped sleeping, in fact, began having terrible dreams. I suggested he get checked. He was losing weight and seemed terribly preoccupied. He spent hours going over records. I was feeling left out and helpless for months. He never told me why. Finally one of his partners' wives at a party blurted out, "How is Don handling the _____ malpractice case?" I was floored. He hadn't said a word to me, but had been carrying this horrible thing around alone. Actually, Don seemed greatly relieved once I talked to him about it. It was a case in which a woman's child died soon after birth. Not knowing of the baby's death, the mother agreed to have her tubes tied while still on the table. The baby was healthy up until the last minute. Now she will have no more children. I don't know all the details, but Don started talking about it incessantly once I let on that I knew about it. I became his therapist—hours of constant talk about details, going over and over what else could he have done, and what would happen if he lost the case?

Eventually I had to get away from it. I went from not knowing anything to becoming the receptacle for it all. What could I do, really? I went to court every day when it went to trial. Every night, to calm down, Don and his partners went out drinking after the court appearances. They went over detail after detail. Now I'm not sure if I did enough. Sometimes I wished that he would lose and we could go on to a normal life, like everybody else, away from medicine altogether.

Here Loretta was obviously struggling with conflicts of her own. The malpractice case brought she and Don closer than ever in their marriage. Nothing, not even her three children, had linked them like this. She went on to describe her vacillation from sympathy with the defendant (a woman who had lost the only child she would ever have) to her loyalty to her husband in support of his ability and judgment as a professional.

> I went to court every day. People asked me how it was going all the time. I began to think about the case as if I were the one on trial. I had great fears about my future if Don couldn't practice medicine. Perhaps it would be great to be a regular couple in the world — no demanding patients spoiling our private life. How could those people think Don was an awful man? Don was feeling so disappointed that all his time and effort with people could end like this. "Ungrateful," he would say of his patients. I got so nervous by the end of the trial I flew home to Missouri to be with my sisters and mother. I needed time to talk about things other than Don's malpractice case.

It is not surprising that women feel torn between the guilt or innocence of their husbands and the plight of the suing patients.

Others expressed resentment about the hours away from the office — away from family. "For what?" a woman said. "My husband works hard. He put his life into medicine and look, now he can't even practice. Some lawyer advised his client to sue, and now my life and my husband's are changed forever."

Loretta said Don eventually had to stop practicing in the area. No insurance company would insure him. He's working out of state now, and trying to get hired on the staff of a hospital somewhere. Loretta:

> Otherwise he'll go into the automobile business. I've had it. I'm left to pick up the pieces. The nightmares are coming true. Doesn't the public realize the cost of malpractice on everyone? No one will want to practice medicine. There will be no one to care for the sick!

Loretta's rage was felt by other women, as if they were personally insulted, as if they had treated the patient, as if their professional integrity was being judged. The wives sang uniformly of disappointment, despair, depression, and confusion. "Now where do we go? My husband is nothing without the practice of medicine." What of her? What is she if he doesn't practice medicine? She feels she is left to pick up the pieces, if she stays at all, or if he stays with her after all this. He may leave her, unable to face his failure. Then she is left to deal with her rage and confusion alone.

Chapter 35

Relocation:
Disorientation Anxiety

I grew up in rural South Dakota. Somehow living in Boston was like living on another planet. — Gwen

Part of becoming successful in a career is dependent on the ability to relocate according to the demands of the profession. One of the determining factors in hiring women for certain jobs is their ease of mobility. In studying the pursuit of a professional career, Holmstrom has suggested that it is "advantageous for career advancement if a person can decide where to live without taking into account the interests of the other members of the family" (1973, p. 30). We know that traditionally women went wherever their husband's job required. Usually women are told of their husband's great, exciting, not-to-be-passed-up opportunity for career advancement in Podunk, U.S.A., and although she is being asked how she feels about it, the implication is clear: either we move there to Podunk or my (his) career is down the tubes, and you live with *that* one.

How many of today's husbands are relocating to improve the wife's chances for her career? A few, maybe even some. Still, if there are children or if his profession is one in which that move would be overwhelmingly costly to his job, chances are she'll move alone or she'll refuse the opportunity. How many women refuse to go along with their husband's career move because of the demands of their career or otherwise? Fewer still.

Yet why is it more traumatic for a woman to relocate than a man? If moving is based on a decision made freely for the benefit of the decision maker, there is a chance that the move, though difficult and disruptive, will still be positive. When a move is for the benefit of one's sense of achievement and the other is going along to provide solace and comfort only, that will be traumatic for the comforter.

Like other accommodations required of her, a doctor's wife must move a few times in the course of her husband's training and career. He feels he has no choice but to take the internship or residency or fellowship or practice opportunity best suited to his career goals. He will move, start work soon, become entangled in the rigors of his new professional environment, and essentially remain in the same daily routine. Whether a different house or town, life is the same otherwise: she is still at home to comfort him, care for personal needs, and make the transition as easy as possible for the family.

But the uprooting can be very disruptive for her. Her life, dependent on the familiarity of her environment and social contacts, is barren for a time. No outside work helps her focus and concentrate her feelings of dislocation; she may be bored, anxious, and distressed in addition to feeling homesick and lonely. While the doctor is out doing his job and meeting new people, his wife is isolated in strange surroundings.

Rhoda was reminded of her four moves in the previous eight years:

> Every time I get settled we have to move again. First it was the army. There I felt like such a sissy. The army wives talk about moving like it's water off a duck's back. Some of them move every year or every two years. They said they learn to like it. They become proficient in making friends and feeling at home. Some of them talk about never really unpacking their boxes. They leave things in storage permanently! Can you imagine? Anyway, first it was North Carolina, then Georgia, then out of the army and into a residency program in Ohio for three years. At least it was three years. By then I had three children to attend to. I was home alone, me and my four, three, and six-month-old babies. Alex would go to the hospital and I would be home with kids. We lived in a complex with other residents, but I'm a quiet, reserved person. My privacy is important to me. So I'm uncomfortable reaching out to

strangers. The others would sit out at the playground with their kids and chat, and I'd feel so out of place. It made me feel incompetent. I did finally make a good friend, also a quiet person. She had one five-year-old and we hit it off.

The trouble came when it was time to find a place for post-residency fellowship. Of course, Ohio wasn't the place for that. Now we would have to move again, this time for two years. By this time I was too tired to be involved in the decision. We ended up in Chicago at a big medical center. Ugh. Three small kids in a Chicago suburb, and me from a small New England town. What an adjustment. What a sad moment when we said goodbye to our friends in Ohio. Me and the kids stood outside of our apartment. My girlfriend and I bawled, and my kids and a few of their close buddies also were teary. Alex had already gone on to Chicago. I felt so alone and forlorn.

Because the demand for doctors is higher than the supply, his wife may end up living in a desirable area. Like other entrepreneurs providing a service in chronically short supply, a doctor is almost guaranteed a good income and the related status wherever he goes (Fowlkes, 1980). That guarantees greater choice and flexibility than is available to someone whose company sends him to a branch office — they either must take that location, get fired, or be demoted at least. However, choice options or not, during the training stages of his career, his wife is subject to moving a few times, and she may have only a small impact on the decision about where she lives.

In an article written by sociologists Skipper and Gliebe (1977), "Forgotten Persons: Physicians' Wives and their Influence on Medical Career Decisions," the authors suggest that where he will practice is a decision in which she has the most impact while her husband is a medical student. "The wives' influence appeared to be greatest on the decision about the geographical location of practice" (*Journal of Medical Education*, p. 764).

Her career aspirations and the children's educational opportunities both affected where he would set up his office. In fact, the idea of a group practice in a mid-sized town (over 25,000 and under 500,000 people) was preferred by wives who were hoping for a better family life if her husband had partners to share his call hours. Skipper and Gliebe pointed out that the areas in which doctors are in short supply — small rural communities in more remote areas of the country — will have to entice the wives somehow with the help of medical schools, government, and medical associations if they are to find doctors to fill their needs.

After looking at this study more closely, it became apparent that the information was gleaned mostly from the medical students themselves. The husbands reported that their wives were interested in good schools for their children, possible career opportunities for themselves, and group practice so they might have more time as a family. Out of 45 men interviewed, only 21 were married and only 17 of the wives were interviewed.

Although I am slightly heartened that these women were remembered at all by the researchers, I am doubtful as to the value of the findings. Again, it is patronizing to suggest that wives strongly influence their husbands' career decisions. He has already been severely programmed by his medical school and the long traditions of medicine, and it is considered insulting to presume that she may have influence upon the decision making. While thinking she's involved in the decision to relocate, she actually has little or no real impact regarding her husband's professional moves. She may write the checks, but he has the ultimate veto. So it is with relocation. Being taken into consideration is not the same as being able to say an unqualified, "I will not move again. Even if it means leaving your medical practice altogether and looking into other work possibilities, I will not be able to make this next move." This requires clear thinking based on individual needs with equal rights in the marriage.

The doctor's wife experiences only an illusion of partnership or influence over the course of her life with the doctor, but she ends up with a great many rationalizations about why this move was all right.

Sharon, married 14 years and mother to three school-aged children, is immersed in a social services career of her own while trying to also branch out into a career in business. Her husband was quite successful in his practice for eight years, but some misfortunes in business ventures made remaining in that area intolerable to him.

I loved the area where we lived. The kids were quite settled, friendships, social life, everything. And I finally had the nerve to go to school and stretch my interests a little. I'd been wanting to try stock and bond investments and get out of psychology for a while. I've had success in investments before and felt that now would be a great time to shift interests. But Jim has been depressed in his practice. Too much responsibility on him I guess. Solo practice never did agree with him. We've already tried this once before, but being the one responsible for such a heavy practice doesn't work for Jim. When we moved here he was determined to work a lighter schedule so he could spend more time at his sculpting and other art projects. At first he did. He even started a studio, but some foolish decisions landed his studies almost belly-up financially. He picked some poor artists to work with and just had a partnership arrangement. You know, they say doctors stink at business. Well, he got more depressed and felt like he couldn't face the medical community and his patients any more. So we had to look for another place to move.

How did you handle that?

Not well this time. Uprooting the kids gets harder as they get older. Plus my own interests are just blossoming. When we made this move I thought it would be at least long enough to get all the kids through school. I don't shift gears as well as Jim. He feels if he's not getting what he wants from his work time, he can get up and move again. That's one reason he chose medicine, so that he could work almost anywhere he wanted, be his own boss, make his own hours. But every time I get used to a place, make good friends, and start to really settle in with good career prospects, Jim's looking for a new practice opportunity. He's thinking about teaching in a med school next. So now I'll have to get used to the rules of academic medicine if that comes through.

I am supportive, maybe too much so. If I had the guts I'd just tell him to adjust to my career changes this time. I've always deferred to his job, I guess. Being an MD, he seems to be capable of doing more important work than I do. Plus I can't stand his depressions. If he's not happy, I'm miserable myself. So if he'll be happy teaching, maybe I'll get to select the next move. I hope so. But truthfully, it's hard to imagine that happening.

What seems innocent and caring is costly for women.

When I moved the last time I went into a five-year depression. After counseling, drugs, and time, I finally worked my way out of it. But it was such a shock to move from a small town to a suburban big city in the Midwest. No friends, two small children, never seeing adults, having to learn a whole new area. The pace of living was so fast and confusing for me. No one said hello or looked me in the eye on the streets. I felt so lonely and displaced. I'd never have agreed to that move had I any idea of the effects on me. For a while I wouldn't leave the house. We had to hire someone to take care of my youngest son. The psychiatrist I saw for help wasn't much help either. He gave me drugs and told me I'd adjust. In fact, he told me to try to "buck up" so that I wouldn't cause Bob any worry. I remember so clearly. He said, "Carol, Bob is in a new hospital, new job. He needs your support. Don't let him see how unhappy you are or he'll be distracted from his duties, and his patients might be the one's who'll suffer." Yuk! When I left him [the psychiatrist] and went to another counselor, a woman, she addressed the issue of loss and grief from the move. She helped me to regain my self-esteem a bit. I eventually improved enough to work part-time on a political campaign. I'm a journalist and I did press releases and PR for the local congressman. Without that work I'd still be depressed.

Relocation and its ramifications would require a book in itself. The psychological effects may be enormous. My concern is with the damaging effects moving has on women when there is little or no choice or input regarding the move. Or, if involved in the decision to relocate, is the doctor's wife emotionally prepared to be uprooted for her husband's career? Presently we are all more mobile. We live in a busy, moving society. But while the physician moves from one city or town to another, the daily routine and even the physical surroundings of his job remain frighteningly similar.

The walls and furnishings of the hospitals are alike. The equipment in the offices is similar. Even the placement of staff offices and patient waiting rooms can be alarmingly familiar regardless of the city in which the buildings reside. So the greater part of the doctor's day at work is familiar. Protocol is the same. The work decisions are the same. Even the uniform is the same — white jacket and white uniforms for him and his staff. The names vary, but the procedures in hospitals, offices, and colleges are so alike as to make him almost immediately comfortable with the familiarity. A physician can move into what is called locum tenens and take over temporarily for another doctor while he goes on vacation. It's that easy to use the skills and move them about.

His wife predictably makes the home familiar and comfortable for him. She hangs the same paintings and arranges the same furnishings as pleasantly as possible. He comes home to her and the children and his study, which probably is furnished in a style reminiscent of their last home. He reads the journals, takes calls, and goes on with his life. Social life is built into his professional life.

What of her? So few of the familiar trappings are there for her — she has her children, perhaps her home furnishings, and occasional time with her husband — but usually at this time he is more immersed in work, and therefore he's even less available to the family. To her the physical surroundings make up much of what's comfortable and familiar. The people she knew in her last location are vital to her emotional state and well-being. Close friends are what keep her connected to the world outside. Without them she may wither and feel lost. If she was working outside the home, her job or career must be painfully re-established anew. Contacts are not built in. Women are relaters; people interaction is so essential to our well-being. Once removed from familiar people, it can be years before the new people are as trusted and comfortable. A longing for home and trusted, familiar places and faces is almost always experienced as a great loss.

My move with my husband and then nine-year-old son is as vivid to me today as it was more than ten years ago when it happened. We lived in the same house and reared our four sons there in suburban

New Jersey, 40 minutes outside of New York City by car. For years we talked about crowding and pollution of the suburbs and wouldn't it be nice to relocate. But could Jerry pick up and leave a lucrative group practice and start over somewhere else? Meanwhile I had been going to school as my children grew, and was on my way to becoming a counseling psychologist. I had a year of internship and training in family therapy and biofeedback under my belt. My career was beginning to fall into place. Contacts were being made, and after years of motherhood and isolation, close colleagues in psychology were appearing on the horizon.

Now Jerry would agree to move to the West Coast. "Let's go look and find a place we like," he said. I had talked about it; in fact, it had been my idea years before, so I couldn't disagree now. We searched, researched, and being of an accommodating nature, without strong will and determination, I agreed not only to relocate but to move to another world — a town of 15,000 people on the West Coast! What did I know? Plus, I felt that since it was my impetus to move, the fact that I was just starting to spread my career wings didn't matter.

What a trauma for me! I was totally unprepared for the culture shock from Woody Allen's northeastern intellectual lifestyle of ethnic variety to the colorless lack of differences of a small town. Blond hair and blue eyes looked so uncommon to me, as were the tanned bodies, vegetables, sprouts, and people concerned only with exercise, fitness, and stamina. The worst experience was the unfamiliar business of people calling me by my first name. "Esther, may we help you?" or "How are you doing, Esther?" God, I thought, I've never even met these people before and they act like they were at the hospital when I was born!

I've had to get used to instant recognition, as well as everyone knowing my business and my family's. No privacy. No anonymity. People not laughing at the same things that tickle my fancy. Young, beautiful people out running as soon as the sun comes out in January.

I was truly disoriented, dislocated, and depressed for years after the move. Making new friends and starting up a counseling practice under the influence of relocation anxiety proved to be tricky at best.

I blame my not knowing myself well enough at the time of the decision to move, plus not having the courage of my convictions to say, "No, this move is not timed well for me. We stay or you go alone." I was socialized to go along. Jerry said, "I can't change my mind. I've already told my partners I'm leaving." This after we came to the West to purchase a house, and I had a major personality change. I became distraught, hysterical, and didn't know if I could handle the outdoor, health-conscious, everyone-knows-everyone's-business environment.

The biggest surprise was to come. For the first time in our married life I was to be seen truly as the doctor's wife—the doctor's wife in a strange and unfamiliar environment. There wasn't even a synagogue. Religious services (which I didn't attend anyway) were held in an old church, one of the many filling every corner of the town. What a nightmare to a Philadelphia girl raised in the city and on the subway! The reality of being recognized and treated as the doctor's wife for what felt like the first time in over 20 years of marriage was to be the impetus for this book.

Disorientation, strange faces, different colors of skin, styles of relating, ways of being, and varied values forced me to come to know myself. But it is only hindsight that speaks. People who move biannually or more often experience a haziness, a semi-alertness of consciousness from unfamiliarity. Men go to work, children go to school, but the doctor's wife unemployed outside the home discovers the disorientation and unrecognizable sensations all on her own at home.

I heard over and over: "The move was much harder than I expected," and "It seemed much easier for my husband to adjust to the move than me." If that is true, I wonder why and what should be done to correct the situation.

I am fearful that her self-esteem is delicate enough. Doesn't it seem possible that relocation actually diminishes an already lowered sense of self-confidence? To uproot a cactus and ask it to grow in a marsh is unfair and unrealistic. But once adapted to the marsh, to then remove it to the arctic constitutes cruel and unusual punishment.

Chapter 36

Confidentiality:
Who's Being Protected?

I always act like I never knew Phil was their physician.
— Anne

Picture a round table, a blue linen cloth, a small centerpiece of
dry purple and white flowers, lovely flowered pottery plates, and
purple napkins in rings of green and white. The glassware is sturdy
yet delicate, and the smells from the kitchen are heavenly — seafood
of some sort in a cream sauce with orange cakes for dessert.

There are several women waiting to be called into the breakfast
room and seated at the table. Sunlight shines in from the picture
window overlooking the table, and the coffee is brewing on the
sideboard close by. This is a brunch meeting of doctors' wives who
have known each other for anywhere from two to 12 years. There
are eight of them. They meet every other Wednesday to share one
another's company and catch up on details of their lives. One of the
women, Charlotte, I think, suggested they meet like this. She felt
they could gain something from being with women whose lives had
so much in common.

Brunch is ready now. Deborah, the hostess this time, casually
coaxes the women from the study into the breakfast room. Somehow the subject of husbands not talking about their patients to their
wives had already begun in the study and it seemed as if this one
would hold the attention for a while.

I hate it when Victor tells me about a case at the hospital and
then adds, "Remember, this is just between you and me. I

don't want you to repeat this to anyone." He never mentioned any names, and if he did this city's so big there's no way I could possibly know who he was talking about.

Yes, I know what you mean. When we get into one of those discussions, Herb usually prefaces it by something like, "Can I ask you something, Char? It's about one of my patients. I'm not sure I did the right thing by telling them to get a second opinion." Or, "I wonder if I was too abrupt with Mr._____ today. Sometimes he gets on my nerves." Or he'll go into great detail about an operation, what almost happened and how great it turned out or didn't turn out. And then he says, "You remember not to say any of this to anyone else," like I can't wait to pick up the phone and report to all of you the gory details of the latest case.

When I go to Wally's office to meet him for lunch he's always edgy that I'll see his patients there. He's paranoid about this confidentiality stuff when I'm there. But at home he doesn't realize how much information he gives me. The truth is, though, that I never really connect what he says with specific people. So someone getting a terrible case of the flu or having to have a special set of x-rays of their stomach for ulcers means nothing to me. In fact, I've met some of Wally's patients socially. I know because they tell me that he's their doctor and how great he is. But they seem to think that I know all about their medical history.

I don't know about you, but I resent being kept in the dark all the time. When I worked on the same floor with Mike we could talk about people and their treatments. I knew them. I worked on the cases too. So Mike and I could understand and I wouldn't have this feeling that he was keeping big, dark secrets. Now if I say, "How was your day?" he says, "The usual," and he refers to people as if they're medical names only. You know, "Oh, I did two EKGs, three liver biopsies, lost two, recommended that one have another CAT scan, expect we'll do the new monoclonal antibody treatment on one woman if she meets the requirements," and so forth. Before I knew the people that went with these descriptions; they were real, honest to goodness flesh and blood, breathing, feeling people with complicated illnesses, some very sick. And somehow I felt closer to Mike knowing that we were both out there trying to help these people if not to be cured at least to feel better for a while. Now he keeps them from me. Even from himself, I think. If I say, "Whatever happened to Mrs. _____? Do you see her in follow up?" he shuts me up politely by something like, "I'd rather not say, dear. Please don't use names. It makes me concerned about confidentiality." Why does he assume that I'll use the information in some terribly destructive way?

Lunch is served. Steaming hot crab in a wonderful sauce, an experiment from the cook, who is a caterer by profession. The oohs and aahs go on for a while with questions about the recipes for the crab and the special glazed artichoke and carrots. The cook revels in the response of her guests and continues the previous conversation.

I'm always being reminded of a faux pas where I repeated some statement about one of Russ's patients. Russ had talked for weeks about the treatment of this young boy who had an unusual kidney disease. He fretted about it every night when he came home from work. Should he refer him out or get a colleague to consult with him? Whatever. The boy was 11 at the time, and once when I went to meet Russ for dinner after work I noticed a woman in the waiting room. She introduced herself to me and I recognized her name immediately. Innocently, I told her I was so glad that her son was doing better now and hoped his treatment wasn't too uncomfortable. Well, she told Russ what I said and he blew up at me when we met for dinner. "How could you? Do you know how compromised I am now? What if that boy dies? Do you know what kind of trouble you could have gotten me into?" He raved all night like that—what right did I have to speak to Mrs. _____ out of turn and about her son's treatment, how stupid of me, on and on. I felt horrible. I was being compassionate as one mother to another. I know how I would feel if Tim or John [her children] had that illness. I would be terrified, and I think I'd appreciate the fact that the doctor was involved enough to share the information with his wife.

What happened to the boy?

I guess he was all right. But I was so intimidated that I never opened my mouth about him or any other of Russ's patients again. Only if Russ brings it up himself. Otherwise, it's off limits for me.

Does anyone understand the purpose of the confidentiality, at least regarding wives?

Not completely. It's just always been an unspoken code in our house. When Ed talks about stuff at school or the clinic, we don't impose or ask for details. It's always been a one-way thing; he gives only as much information as he wants to and the kids and I keep our noses out of the rest. I always thought it had to do with being legally bound to protect the privacy of the patients. But what I don't get is why sometimes I get all the details of an entire family for months, or years even, from Ed so long as he's comfortable talking about it. If I bring it up he gets tense and lets me know that's not kosher for me to know the names and histories of his patients and students. We've had fights about it in the past. I get defensive, and question why the inconsistency. Doesn't he trust that blabbing about his work life is not the most important thing on my mind? We've gone back and forth on it in the early part of our marriage. He just would get unreasonable and put his foot down. No real explanation, just, "That's how it is. I'm not supposed to talk to you about my cases," he'd say. "If I do you're definitely not to dare repeat it." I've heard him say that to the kids also, "If you overheard what Mom and I were talking about, don't repeat it, whatever you do!" So we all learned that we would hear things that were not to be let out of our house.

I don't know about you, but sometimes I feel used, like a receptacle or a shredder of top secret material. I feel in a bind.

I'm supposed to be there and listen and be helpful when Frank needs to talk, but then I worry about how he is and how his patients are, but I feel bound to keep quiet. It drives me crazy. In my work I am free to discuss everything, and there are no restrictions. [She owns a book store.] I'm not afraid to mention names and recall incidents that occurred in the shop. In fact it makes me happy to have Frank to talk to when I get home. When my political work gets active I still share everything with Frank. [This woman eventually became a city councilperson.] It's always been a mystery to me. He could inquire as to my goings on and I was free with sharing. Somehow the reverse was never true.

Doesn't anyone understand who's being protected by this code of confidentiality?

I never thought about it that way before. My father was a doctor. I grew up in a medical household. In those days, long ago, his office was in our house and we all knew the patients and their families. My mom helped him as receptionist, girl Friday I guess you'd call her. I remember keeping other kids company or playing with the young patients all the time. No one ever thought anything about it. When you came to see my father you got a family of six at times. In my marriage, work and home are very separate. I really am not aware of who Kyle sees and what he does at work. But I never thought about it as a code of confidentiality. You make it sound like everyone has sworn to keep the work life away from the home.

Don't be ridiculous. I know everything about Carl's work. He never shuts up about his cases and his activities. He even tells me about what's happening between his office personnel. I know when they're fighting, having babies, building new houses, if one of their kids is having trouble in school, or someone had a nervous breakdown. Maybe Carl's a gossip or something. Or maybe I just push him to get all the new information. I've never felt excluded from his work life. He talks technically to me because I'm in the field [a medical technician], so we can converse about the details. He's research oriented, and so am I. So we love exploring those kinds of details of a particular patient's problem. He even asks me for advice all the time. I think he knows that I won't misuse the private information or get him into trouble.

What trouble?

If a legal case comes up, that information is considered private between doctor and patient, I guess. It's weird, though. If you work in a hospital you have access to charts, so nothing is totally confidential anyway.

Yes, I've worked in mental health before, and I'm aware that office personnel and counselors and clinicians all have access to charts, and the personnel do talk about clients occasionally. So I'm not sure what the issue is here.

The dessert was brought out, and it was an exquisite banana flambé, flaming right at the table. It broke the timing and momentum of the discussion. In fact it didn't seem as if any of the women really understood the mixed messages surrounding confidentiality between their husband's work and themselves. Their experiences were different depending on whether their husbands adhered more or less strongly to the professional injunction that wives are not to be privy to work details. Obviously the wives were privy to a great deal of information, at times in total detail and at other times just bare bones with no names attached. The reasoning seems confusing. Is it the patient being protected? The doctor? His wife and family? Who is not supposed to know and who is supposed to keep quiet about what they do know? Everyone ends up playing a game of hide and seek. When I go to a party and see a patient I know has been treated by my husband, I don't refer to his or her illness. I play by their rules. They seem to want to think that either I know all about them, inside and out, or they hope that I don't know anything of them at all. My husband wants to be able to tell me when something's bothering him. If he slips up and does mention any names, he needs reassurance that I'll be mum about who he's discussing. Most of the time he feels he's protecting the patients' privacy by trying not to tell me their names. I'm busy protecting Jerry and his patients for the sake of his reputation and integrity. I'm not sure who protects me.

"I'm bound by my profession not to tell you patient-specific information. I hope you won't take that personally. I can tell you anecdotal information, but I have to keep the names out of it. I know that's bothered you sometimes. It's not that I don't trust you, but over time you may forget that something I said was to remain confidential, and you might let it slip out." My husband's words on the subject to me: "I pride myself on holding to that professional ethic. Even though I consider you my closest confidant, I can't divulge explicit information on people I see professionally."

When asked why, he said, "Because I don't want you to feel uncomfortable with personal material about others you may run into." He held this view even when we lived in areas in which I'd be extremely unlikely to run into any of his patients; the population was too large. He continued, "And I have to protect myself and my reputation."

Somehow there is a presumption that this information about Mrs. M's gallbladder on Mr. P's hernia is too hot for me to handle. I'll be incapable of using the proper human discretion that adults normally utilize when hearing of another's illness or other privacies. Or is it necessary to keep the information privileged as if that's part of the magic of healing? It keeps the physician himself as the one who is in control of the flow of information, and he feels more in charge of the entire process of care.

More often than not when his patients come up to me and talk about their personal stories, I'm in the position of not knowing what they're talking about. Or if I did know, I rarely connect them with their diseases or maladies. In order to protect professional ethics we lose personal intimacy. We also are made to feel untrustworthy, immature, and incompetent by the restrictions and guarded process of medical confidentiality. As the last to know, the wife assumes she lacks the intelligence and perception to have the equal ethical and moral judgments of her husband. There is still within us the belief that a woman cannot be trusted with man's "important" secrets. At the same time she is used for succor and nurturing as needed.

Chapter 37

Me Working:
In His Office or Out

The worst time in my life was trying to work in his office. I'd never do it again. — Cheryl

Today there are over 60 percent of women with children under five in the work force, and the numbers are rising steadily for those working outside the home. The choice of jobs are ever increasing and widening in spectrum, albeit slowly.

Apparently, the majority of doctors' wives who work outside the home are working in the health care system. There are exceptions: the governor of Rhode Island is a doctor's wife. There are state representatives, mayors, perhaps a state senator presently in office, and probably numerous ex-doctors' wives in politically powerful jobs or in executive industrial jobs today.*

The average doctor's wife in 1988 is a homemaker who works part-time in nursing, a health care-related field, office management (in husband's office), or home interior design. Many dabble in fine art or do work that is time flexible and adaptable to her husband's schedule.

The voices I heard the loudest were women railing in frustration that their husbands did not want them to work outside the home. With much conflict and persuasion, some eventually consented to

---

*I have been unable to track this information. Changing statistics in each state make it difficult to keep current. Recall also, as noted previously, the lack of response from the American Medical Association Political Action Committee to my inquiries on these statistics.

their returning to nursing. Another smaller number felt that their wives could provide useful work in their offices.

I heard, "People resent me taking a job from someone who really needs it," in almost all the interviews. "When we were struggling in medical school [notice the return reference to 'we' in medical school] it was completely acceptable for me to work. As soon as my husband became successful it was strongly frowned upon for me to work outside," according to a woman married 42 years. She was free to work outside in the early '40s when women worked much less frequently outside the home. In the late '80s she is told overtly or covertly that marriage to a doctor closes doors of work opportunity for her.

College educated, experienced in volunteerism, and usually terrifically competent and organized, this powerful source of executive material is relegated to the household because either her husband finds it abominable for her to work, or his profession feels that her employment signifies that he's not as successful as he'd like us to think. Finally, if neither of the latter is operating, the work world shuts the door, prejudiced against her husband's earning power, and again she hears, "You don't need this job. We'll give it to someone who does, no matter how qualified you are. You can continue to volunteer your time if you like, but don't consider yourself seriously contributing to the work force!" Again I hear the resounding sounds of the women's plight in the '50s. Now, however, instead of competing only with men who need jobs, Mrs. Doctor is competing with her sisters, other women who need jobs.

I have given group seminars to women married to other professionals, i.e., dentists' wives, lawyers' wives. The subject of working outside the home comes up readily. Women married to dentists traditionally work in their husbands' offices. It is more acceptable within the profession. Lawyers' wives seem to escape what health care professionals experience. They can choose their career or place of work more freely. Within the legal profession there isn't the pressure for wives to stay home or work only in their husbands' offices. Attorneys — even when there were fewer female attorneys — have been less constricting on the personal choices of the families in their profession (Lorch and Crawford, "Role Expectations," 1983).

Dentists' families, probably modeling after medical families, are in between. While a dentist's wife can work outside the home, she is often restricted to working in her husband's office. In fact, by having the dentist's wife on the scene as overseer of the office, she is encouraged to keep the employees in line. Even if she has young children, it is not unusual to see the dentist's wife in the reception room or in the back office doing his accounts.

One woman, 48 years of age, married to a dental specialist for 26 years, mother of two daughters—has worked in her husband's office for 17 years, and explained:

> I've worked with him since we moved here 17 years ago. I did take some time off when Katy [younger daughter] was small, but have kept involved in the office books and management all these years. I think it's important that women know the workings of their husband's office. What if something happens to him? Women are at a distinct disadvantage if they hide in the sand and don't get involved. I'm afraid of not knowing. I stand to lose too much if we divorce or Sam dies before I do. This way I know where to look for figures, I know what they all mean and what is rightfully mine. In fact, even while Sam's alive I feel it's to my advantage to know about the financial interactions going on in this office. It is half mine by law.

She agreed that there is reinforcement from the dentists and their wives to work in the office. There appears to be a greater willingness to perceive the office as a partnership between the dentist and his wife than among physicians and their wives. I leave other researchers to explore this subject in depth.

I bring up other professionals' wives as a point of comparison. Once again, the doctor's wife has more restraints on her choices (Lorch and Crawford, "Role Expectations . . .," 1983; Fowlkes, 1980). Rebecca, 36, worked some before she married a medical student.

While Jay was in school I worked as a technician in a local lab. We thought I should keep working until he finished his residency. As it turned out I got pregnant right at the end of the residency, so that was perfect. Now that Jillian is eight I'm feeling antsy, and all my friends are out working, even with young children. Jay is against me leaving the house. He's making plenty of money as an ophthalmologist. He'll never have to worry about financial security for us, he says. But for me it's a matter of being bored and lonely. I only see Jillian, and she's in school until three in the afternoon. I can't be expected to entertain myself all day long until it's time to prepare dinner. I'm an active person. I bore easily. I've even asked Jay if he needs help in his office, would I be able to work for him, even three days a week? He's adamant about MDs' wives being home raising the kids and keeping the house. It's ridiculous. I have a housekeeper. What is there for me to do? I've tried volunteer work, the auxiliary, for a while. I helped at Jillian's school. For me it's not my own work, my own serious business, where there are people to talk to about what interests me.

Those who have accepted the "doctors' wives don't work" edict may work in his office; however, this has special problems for a wife.

I've struggled with the other employees for years, so they don't feel that I'm getting special treatment as the boss's wife. Realistically I vacillate from feeling like a partner in Rod's practice to a mere regular employee.

Sonya goes on to describe how she and Rod worked together "hard and long hours to make his office and hospital practice successful." Sonya is a nurse practitioner who has worked along with Rod since he completed his training. They have been married 22 years. Along with her office work Sonya managed to parent their three children.

Working in partnership with Rod has distinct advantages. I have the same vacation schedule and the same work day as Rod. Although he usually likes me to go home early and start the household chores — dinner, helping the kids with their lives, school work, social life problems. Now that's much easier because only the youngest is at home. If I worked for anyone else I wouldn't have the flexibility of time off I do with Rod. But the other side of the coin turns up when some other office help are sick or away. I end up doing double time and filling in for them, even if I wasn't scheduled to work.

What about your salary or wages for working — how does that work for you? Sonya smiles a little sheepishly and then responds:

That's always been tricky. For tax purposes I'm on the payroll and have been for years, ten or so since Rod's office was opened. But to tell you the truth I never see any of that money. At least not directly. At first I said, "Okay, keep the money in the till." We really couldn't afford to have anyone else do the work when he was starting. So I actually worked for free in those days. You rationalize, saying, "We're saving all that money by not hiring anyone else." So in other words, I'm contributing my wages back into the office. Rod said he was essentially doing the same thing in those days. . . . Well now I'm on the payroll. But again, we use what we need for household or office expenses. But I don't have or never had the sense of bringing home a paycheck for my work. But I don't see Rod as doing that either. We decide together how we'll spend the profits from the practice, so I feel okay about it.

How do the other employees relate to you?

I've struggled to figure out a comfortable role in this office for me and the other employees. Rod's the boss, he's always been and I treat him that way at work. It hasn't worked for me to get any special privileges. The other employees are looking for that. I go overboard, in fact, to be another hard worker. Women who work for their husbands probably work three times harder than if they worked elsewhere.

Why?

So as not to feel special or privileged. There is a tendency for the others to resent my presence anyway. If I took advantage by going home too early or shirking my responsibilities, the tension would rise.

The other special problem that comes to my mind is the sexual tension or competition for Rod's attention that arises once in a while, where people didn't know we were married. That was interesting for a while. I kept it quiet. The girls would flirt with Rod and make passes all the time. In fact, people over the years have spoken to Rod about firing me, that they can't work with me working there. After one big scene a few years ago where Rod finally had to fire the woman, he made me office manager. And I'm up front with the fact that we're married and no hanky-panky is tolerated.

What happened with that employee?

That incident was devastating to me. A technician was really sneaking behind my back and trying to set me up. She'd tell Rod about mistakes I made, or she lied about what I was doing. She even told Rod I was seen with someone else, stirring up trouble for us both. The payoff was when she called him back to the office after plotting to get me to go home to be with a so-called emergency at home. She was after Rod, and even the knowledge that we were married didn't stop her. Looking back on it, I let myself in for it, I guess. It was a time when I wanted more recognition and responsibility for my work, and Rod had kept resisting making me manager. So we were strained, and this young technician thought she could move in. Rod was flattered, no doubt, and didn't put a stop to it. In fact, he didn't even see it happening the way I did. He thought I was crazy, until she really came on to him that night that I was called home. We found out she set the whole rendezvous up and lied about other things for months. So out she went! And I became manager and Mrs. _____ at work. There's always an adjustment for the other employees. But when they appreciate the rules, we have no trouble.

There's a family business feel to Sonya's description. Their money goes into the same pot and she seems comfortable with her responsibility and status in her job at Rod's office.

In the early days when I was not sure about a personal career and wanted to do work outside of the home, I briefly entertained the thought of working for Jerry. But he had a hard and fast rule with his partners — no wives working in the office. Why? It was thought to be potentially too explosive, creating jealousies between wives and other wives who were not working there and between the employees and those potential wife-employees. What Jerry didn't say was that he and his partners refused to be put in the position of having to resolve conflicts between themselves due to employee friction where favoritism might be construed. He was fearful of repercussions if the wife-employee failed to do her job well. "How can you fire your wife? Or someone else's wife? How can the other workers complain about my wife to me?" That could be touchy between the husband and wife. Unsaid — it could create a rift between him and his partners. Also unsaid but implied — we can have a freer ruling hand over employees if they are not our wives; we risk dealing with equality issues if wives are there. Fear of loss of face between partners seems to be there somewhere. "Can you control your wife?" or "Keep her out of our business!" It's much simpler to have a hard rule — no wives allowed. Keep the mystery alive. Have no women checking up on our business lives!

I took it in my stride then, not realizing the double bind — the potential special treatment given to family members working in an office and the potential mistreatment of those same people. I always thought it seemed like a perfect thing for me. I would work part-time, get the same time off as Jerry, and feel more involved in his work.

The trouble was and is that Jerry and his partners were fearful of a spouse really having inside information about the workings of the office. Keep work and home separate! What she doesn't know won't hurt her! He always told me how his partners hated it when one of the wives came in and looked at the books or checked on the schedule to see how busy her husband was. I was afraid to be compared to her. So the message — stay out of my work life — was loud and clear to me.

Messages are confusing. "Work in my office if I need help and I can't afford anyone else." "Work in my office, because you'll have the same schedule as I need you to have." "You'll be available when I need you." "Don't work in my office, the office 'girls' resent your presence." "Do the books at home, you won't make any waves that way." "Don't work anywhere else. We're partners, but your paycheck can wait." "We're partners, but I'm the boss while you're at work." "We won't ever be able to have free time together." "Sure I want you to work; just remember to have all your other jobs at home and related to my life done first." "Whatever you want to do is fine, but I'm too busy to help."

The question of time priorities is big. For years I put off my school and my work. I really had no time, raising four children (and a husband), to devote to studies and career. "Working part-time" is the cry of many a doctor's wife. "I can't commit myself to any more than that," say many of us. Why not? Our husbands have. They have been free to devote as much time to personal career development as necessary for success. Our time is their time, and that's it.

A pharmacist married to a physician told me that it's been so hard for her to dovetail her work schedule to her husband's.

> I'm just getting back to work now that the kids are growing up. But Clayton always wants his schedule to come first. If he's got next weekend off, I'm supposed to take it off too. He's getting ready to slow down his practice, and I'm just beginning to get serious about mine. Now he's talking about traveling. So it's traveling with Clayton or keeping up with my career. The choice is lousy.

And finally, a poignant point is made by a colleague and friend. She practices counseling in partnership with her husband, who does psychiatry. Her biggest complaint was that although she was making hospital evaluations on clients, the referring physicians always directed their communications to her husband. She said:

The letters would come to Ellison, to Dr. _____, regarding my client, and they ignored me altogether. I may have been treating that person for a year and knew the case like the back of my hand and still the referring docs wouldn't report directly to me. I always had to call them immediately and correct the situation. But I was humiliated every time and felt that the relationships between me and my clients were jeopardized and demeaned.

Working outside the home, while a realistic choice for more women, has a long way to move for those married to full-time physicians.

Rare indeed are the cases of the doctor parenting three young children while his wife goes 500 miles away to finish a master's degree, or of him going along to assist her in her studies and child care so she can complete her education. It's rarer yet when he picks up and relocates his practice because her career advancement depends on it. It still takes exceptional people to accomplish the latter.

The increasing but still rare marriages of two physicians have unique problems of their own. Risking extreme oversimplification, I will state that it is the female physician who works fewer hours, more part-time, is the parent most involved with the children, and who takes on the greater responsibility of the household. In an ironic article, "Never Marry a Doctor," written in 1988 by Michael A. LaCombe, a male physician complained that his physician wife was rarely available, her beeper was taking precedence over their love life and causing a host of other inconveniences formerly reserved for females in his shoes. But in spite of the difficulties encountered, he ultimately wins out:

> He has in the end had his flirt with glory though, his moment of togetherness with his bride. He obligingly cooperated when the bank insisted he countersign her loans. He was for them a doctor, after all, and *she, merely a woman*. [Italics mine.] (*Journal of the American Medical Association*, Sept. 1988, p. 1292)

This was published in a well-respected medical journal. No doubt the irony above was enjoyed by the traditional male readers of that periodical. Those women, however, striving to become professionals equal to their male counterparts, do have a long way to go.

Clearly, the wife of a physician is forced to remain in the dark ages when it comes to working in his office or her own. If she helps in his office at times, she may be unpaid, unrewarded, and unappreciated in her own right, or she is ever reminded that the doctor is the boss and clearly the person to be taken seriously. Her job is secondary and on demand. Even if she is essential to the running of his office, it is ultimately his profession and his office. Outside work requires time juggling and restraints of commitment, determination, and self-confidence, and usually is accomplished with lip service but no active, concrete support from the doctor.

Chapter 38

My Short Career as Host of "The New World of Medicine"

Those doctors definitely could use a new image, but are they daring enough to hire either one of us? — Ursula

Here was my big chance. I was already bitten by the television bug. That is, I liked the work I had done in television and radio to date, and hoped to continue working in the media. Suddenly, and quite fortunately I thought, an opportunity presented itself. The Medical Society was looking for someone to host their biweekly medical show: two half-hour interview shows weekly on pertinent medical issues. I saw the chance to do news pieces live or taped on location, and to interview local health professionals on topics of my choosing. Perfect. I had done two years of programming, organizing, writing and interviewing for a weekly radio show and had regular exposure to television interviews and call-in type shows. Being a ham at heart, bright and articulate, I knew I was the woman for the job. What I failed to see at the time was the Society was looking for a woman (no men applied for the job) to represent the traditional, staid values of the medical community. I, being of wild red hair and sometimes wilder clothing and demeanor, would not do. But I didn't realize that. I thought writing skills, creativity, experience, and enthusiasm would count, and I truly felt the program needed some enlivening to increase the viewership.

Part of the grueling interviewing and final selection process included on-camera testing and a lengthy proposal for new shows for "New World of Medicine." I spent hours preparing, planning, organizing, writing, and actually rehearsing before video cameras. Leaving no stone unturned, I got professional advice and tutoring so that I would be presenting myself most effectively. For days and weeks this was my preoccupation. Could I measure up and be the next Miss "New World of Medicine"? The first part of the selection process was a hot seat interview set in an imposing boardroom before six physicians, the director and assistant director of the television station, and the director of the Medical Society. Looking back on their personal questions about my attitudes, how I utilized my time, and information pertaining to my children, I realize that these questions would be illegal today in most states, or found to be sexist and discriminatory. Then I submitted a written presentation equivalent to a thesis proposal, and finally completed two taped, simulated, televised 30-minute programs.

Actually, of the seven applicants (all women) who went through these rigorous interviews, two of us were married to physicians. Neither she nor I was chosen. My fantasy was that both Ursula and I were much too outgoing, exciting, and aggressive for the job. The pay was almost nonexistent for the amount of work required, and the doctors did want someone who would be passive and compliant to their direction. Not only was it hoped that a woman would be hired, but a woman willing to give her service practically free, and who would be comfortable with doing the bidding of the Medical Society as well. Actually, the person who did get the job was quiet, soft spoken, and proper. Perfect for the requirements. I probably had a sour grape feeling when rejected, but time and insight have shown me that they were correct not to hire me; I would not have represented them well and would have made trouble every step of the way. They really didn't want an exciting show informing the public in creative new ways. They wanted to keep the status quo as they saw fit: reserved, proper, orderly, and predictable. At the time I was also unaware that to hire one doctor's wife and not the other was to make trouble for the doctors. The competition could have created dissension among the ranks, and for what? One of their wives. Any woman would do, after all.

Chapter 39

Divorce:
Where Does That Leave Me?

Don't think for a minute that divorcing a doctor is sedate and civilized. Grant hunted me and my son down with a rifle.
—Sharon

HE'S LEAVING NOW

I put you through school
I took care of your needs
The house was perfect
The kids were fine

How could you do this
Now's not the time

I dressed for your parties
I said the right things
I waited till later
And followed your strings

How could you do this
Now's not the time

The children are grown up
My job's been on hold
Your nurse looks so lovely
I look so old

How could you do this
Now's not the time

Our furniture's paid for
My sister will go
Next time I'll listen
When your nurse tells me no
Next time I'll be better
I'll be sweeter and kind
Then you will stay with me
You're much too refined

How could you do this
Now's not the time

The time would be never
Our bond was forever
Not just through med school
Not just for kids

This was for always
That's what Missus Doctor is.

Historically, medical marriages were less likely to end in divorce
than those of the general population (Rose and Rosow, 1972; Garvey and Tucson, 1979). There is disagreement regarding the divorce rates of male physician marriages. Researchers postulated a
range of theories: doctors have better marriages because they're
happier; doctors are too busy to divorce; they're too traditional; or
doctors don't need to divorce because they can have a loving wife
and a girlfriend if they choose.

It was always idealistic for the public to feel that those in charge
of their health and well-being, the stalwart keepers of the keys to
the black bag, were paragons of virtue. Donna Reed, married to her
doctor-husband of the famous TV show, was what the public
wanted as the doctor's wife. Together their marriage was a giving,
altruistic one of self-sacrifice and care for the community. Together
their marriage needed to be stable so that the doctor would be free to
heal the sick. A divorce would be devastating to the image of the

healer, and in fact there was a danger that a divorce would ruin the medical practice of the doctor.

Well into the times when divorce rates were racing ahead in the country, in the medical establishment they were thought to be poison to a medical career. Whether in academia, hospital, or private practice, a divorce could stain a doctor's reputation almost irreparably.

A carry-over from seeing the doctor as perfect is, or was, the public's demand that his home life be perfect also—quiet, invulnerable, but stable and dependable. With that visage in the background the doctor could then go forth to his more exciting work life of ambulance sirens, litters of bloody bodies, heart attacks, babies born, and continuous close calls with death. This man needed a retiring, dependable wife to succor and nurture him, to keep the hearth warm and the hot chocolate ready for his unpredictable but eventual arrival home. His wife was in the background, ever loving, admiring, and supportive—rearing his "must be perfect" children in their "must be perfect" home. None of the players in the scenario ever complained or thought of changing this picture.

Then the picture did begin to vary. The medical community was the first to hear of Dr. So and So running off with his medical assistant when he was 43 or so and she was 30. He must have gone crazy. Everyone in the hospital, or at the university, knew of their romance, but that was fairly usual among doctors. No one thought much of that. The word was that when Mrs. So and So calls, cover up for the doctor, say he's in surgery or with an emergency, or just finished delivering a baby. Say whatever you have to. No harm done. All docs do it, but they all go home to their wives. And after all, she's the one with the mink coat and diamond tiara and their kids are the ones in private schools. So don't worry—hush. I'll cover for you now; you never know when I'll need the favor returned.

That was before. This time Dr. So and So has gone over the edge. He's actually gone and left his wife! Everyone is in an uproar. The colleagues even think seriously about blackballing him. The other wives are sympathetic with his pitiful wife, who was perfect in every way, and the doctor is definitely the heavy. His practice may drop off. He and his young wife may have to leave town, without the children, and start a new life somewhere else.

The scenario of the middle-aged male physician dumping his also middle-aged wife—you remember, the one who put him through school and gave up the best years of her life for him—is still prevalent today. In fact, it's quite common with all the divorces among medical couples. Eventually, however, the divorced doctor is supported by his colleagues and it is his abandoned wife who is shunned and ostracized while his new, younger wife is soon embraced by the medical community. She will just move right into the same house, same role, sometimes even same shoes of the former wife.

It is not clear why doctors divorced with greater reluctance than the general population in the past, but now are quite comfortable changing partners when their personal discomfort level becomes too high at home. First it was conjectured that finances are what kept medical marriages together—the woman not suing for divorce because she depended upon the doctor's income for her and her children's financial security; he not suing for divorce because his financial reputation was at stake, or he would lose too much money in a divorce settlement to go through with the legalities.

It has been said that medical couples would remain in poor marriages or in deadly marriages rather than risk rocking the boat. "There is a conspiracy of silence in some [medical] marriages or a neurotic need to keep the peace at all costs" (Myers, 1988, p. 127). They would live in quiet desperation (Smith, Mary Evelyn, ed., 1987). Neither member of the couple knew any better than to accept the life they had together, no matter what the quality of their personal relationship.

Another theory suggests that a physician is so poor at intimate interpersonal relations (he's trained to be so detached) that his intimacy needs are met through his medical practice, so a more intimate marriage never is needed or missed (Gerber, 1983; Myers, 1988).

So he was too busy, too detached, and his wife was making life pretty comfortable and doing many supportive tasks at home to free him to succeed at work. She, on the other hand, had money, security, and prestige, either real or vicarious, and enjoyed a rich social and community life as his wife.

It was a fair trade. He had a quiet, stable place to return to after curing the ills of the world, and she had her bills paid for, along with some financial and social fringe benefits. They both were the pillars of a society that revered the power of science and medicine. Neither, especially him, had the time to even think about divorce as an option.

Then came the divorce revolution, bringing easier divorce, less stigma attached to it, less risk to reputation, and various feelings of "fulfilling oneself," "do your own thing," "life is too short," and "everyone deserves whatever life can give," including the best in personal relationships. Now the very thing that kept medical couples from divorcing—finances—was actually making it easier to go through the expensive and time-consuming details and procedures required for mediation, custody battles, and divorce settlements. Doctors would then become, as members of the privileged class, better able to afford the expense and luxury of divorce. More would file and more would have serial divorces. He still had no time to think about divorce, but the new girlfriend in the wings could more easily collude with him to leave his present home situation and begin again. She could show him that he really wasn't happy with his wife, and in today's world why should they settle for a long-term affair when they could be together and live happily ever after?

Oddly enough, after the divorce, often the abandoned wife would be grateful for the opportunity to discover life as someone other than a doctor's wife. Repeatedly I heard this general cry:

> As terrible and humiliating as that time was for me, and as abandoned as I felt by all of our friends and his colleagues, I wouldn't go back to the marriage I had for anything. It's true I wouldn't have ever left him, but since it's happened, I'm a new, alive, thinking, feeling woman, not just someone else's lady.

Those who felt blessed are more fortunate than those who went through a divorce and custody battles having the scars and hellish communications continue.

My divorce was eight years ago. For eight years we have been fighting over our two boys. Whenever Oliver gets it into his head, he pulls some horrendous trick to get at me with the kids. Here he has a new wife, 15 years my junior, they've had two kids of their own. He can afford whatever he wants and still he begrudges me my time with my sons. The divorce was his idea. I can't figure it out. It's as if he's still married to me — bossing me around and controlling our lives. Only now his young lady lives under his roof. So he bosses both of us I guess. I can't move away yet until my sons are in college, but I don't think I'll be free of him until I move and start over.

We've heard about problems with divorce, astronomical divorce settlements, the fact that men remarry much more quickly than women after a divorce, and that women and children are much worse off financially through increased divorce rates. Much has been written about the effects of divorce on the doctor (Myers, 1988; Glick and Bores, 1984; Gerber, 1983; Fine, 1981).

What about the doctor's wife? We have moved into an era in which more and more women are filing for divorce. It is no longer the stereotypical doctor husband leaving the wife for a younger woman.

The women married to doctors are saying that this can't be all there is. I want more than an absentee, autocratic, arrogant narcissist for a husband. Younger wives who want careers of their own are finding it almost impossible to tolerate the demands of being a physician's wife and having what they want and need to develop their own careers. Major conflicts over careers and children (to have or have not) are causing women to review their choices and not settle for seconds.

Middle-aged woman are risking less security for greater personal communication and connection with someone other than a stoic, distant physician. Now even middle- and older-aged women are starting divorce proceedings against their doctor husbands, often to the complete and utter shock of their husbands. Josephine, in her late forties, tells of her experience:

Ross couldn't believe it when he was served with divorce papers. I know it was like he was hit over the head with a water balloon. I still almost chuckle now about that. Here for four years I tried to get Ross to come with me to see my therapist. He would say, "That's good, dear. You take care of it." So I did—I left. When I finally gave up the big fears I had of no money, and worse yet, that no one else out there would ever love me, I could let go of a dull and really lifeless liaison. I can't even call what Ross and I had a marriage. My interactions with my women friends were always so much more invigorating and stimulating than my time with Ross. I thought I married a brilliant and interesting man, a man interested in his work and in the world around him. Medical school strips its students of interest in anything but healing and money. The more they heal the more money they get and the more powerful they feel. Well what about me? I became deadened, hopeless, and totally lost all pride and faith in myself. I was crying a lot and Ross was prescribing pills. All that you hear about doctors fixing their families with medicine instead of tender loving care is as true as I'm standing here talking. I didn't want pills, I wanted Ross. Well it took four years of therapy to realize in my heart of hearts that Ross was incapable of tender loving care. He used up all his "tender" when he was at the office, I guess. Anyway, I left and he was so shocked he got violent. I had to get a restraining order to keep him away from me and my daughter. He vandalized my house, left scary notes around, called our friends and threatened them not to talk to me. His family started calling me names and harassing my daughter. It was a nightmare. My daughter still has dreams about it and had to have counseling for a while. Talk about guilt—I'm the bad wife and the bad mother for acting on something that I really tried to work at for years. Why did we have to be punished? He stopped all of my charge cards and shut our joint bank accounts. I couldn't believe this shy, retiring man who was disinterested in me for years could turn on us that way. I'm not sure I would do it again if I had the chance.

If it wasn't that he connected with a female colleague of his right away, ten weeks after I filed and left, he would have killed us if he could. I lived in total terror those ten weeks. Here I had lived in isolation for years and now that I was saying I can't take it any more, I was going to be punished, brutally, or worse yet my daughter would be hurt.

Getting over the guilt of leaving a doctor is also difficult for a woman. He is the caretaker, the kindly, giving guardian of humanity, and how dare she leave him. What do her children think?

The following was reported by a 36-year-old woman married for 13 years:

> They were furious — how could I leave their daddy? He's so helpless. He can't take care of himself. But the worse part from their viewpoint is that if they stay with me (they are eight and eleven years old, boy and girl) they'll never have the things they had when we were a family. They're very materialistic at those ages. My daughter says — how will I face my friends in those clothes, or my son worries about not going to camp in the summer. I can't earn nearly what they were used to us having. So I feel guilty about that. Was I being selfish to leave? I don't know yet. Come ask me in a few years if I did the right thing.

Perhaps children as well as wives of physicians suffer a severe identity crisis in the case of divorce. They too may lose prestige if they live with their mothers.

For women, the decision to leave is riddled with conflict. To be assertive in that way, claiming their right to something more for themselves, is still quite punishable. The doctor-husband has the means and power to make it hellish for his wife. I'm in great admiration of those wives who choose, after trying so many other options, to repair the damaged marriage, but finally leave and start their lives anew. Knowing that the task of leaving, or worse yet divorcing a doctor can be an uphill battle, they are willing to risk it. Now the women leaving may be treated with great disdain. Courts, lawyers, and mediators may be looking at the wife as a deserter, undeserving of her children and undeserving of her fair share of financial remuneration. She is often punished dearly for choosing to leave.

"I left and gave up without much of a fight," says Ruth of her divorce after a 23-year marriage:

> I feel that Edward had the judge and the court in his hip pocket in our small town. How was I going to face a horrible trial and scandal that I and my children would have to live with the rest of our lives? I felt that if I wanted out I should go, quietly. My lawyers were devastated by my stance. I know now [three years later] that I was stupid—23 years, I deserved mega-bucks—but the court proceedings were so demeaning as it was. I couldn't stand the lack of privacy and the innuendos that I was a slut who slept around because of a professional friendship I developed with a colleague of mine; the message was loud and clear—"Who do you think you are, lady, trying to stand up for yourself. And married to a doctor too! How ungrateful can you be?!!"

Funny how now that women are sensing a greater freedom of choice there is such a strong pull to regression. Ruth gave up a great deal to leave a bad marriage. She gave up what was rightfully hers economically for her freedom. Not only was she not paid for her work as wife, mother, and director of house and family, but upon dissolution of the marriage she again was told that she was worthless and extremely replaceable. She continues:

> I went into the world with nothing. No money, a new job, low status—no one acknowledged me as Ed's wife, so I was no longer welcome in our circles. Those medical circles are so tight that even if you've been in them for 23 years, if you leave it's goodbye and good riddance forever. I was terrified. Ed still had money, a great profession, status, power. The women started calling him right away (still I'll never understand that!), and I was the heavy. I left the ranks. I said to all the others, "Your marriage isn't so sacred and safe as you thought. It's just as fragile as the rest of this life. Just because you're medical people, you're not safe from the world out-side." They shunned me. They couldn't wait to let me know who Ed was marrying. "A pretty young thing," they said. After my initial rage at this woman who would have all that I

worked my buns off for, I thought sanely: Good luck to you, Mrs. B. He's all yours in good health!

Now the stigma is on the ex-wife of the doctor. She stays single longer. She's scarred in ways that affect her deeply and lastingly. Women of divorce are at a disadvantage, especially if they have children. But women divorced from doctors feel as if they've been fired from an elite company and are blackballed by those around them. Places where they formerly shopped ignore them or humiliate them. Organizations for which they volunteered are less apprecia- tive of their efforts and often try to discourage their help altogether. Their social life may drop to zero, and even their church or syna- gogue may deny them the same treatment and respect they had as Mrs. Doctor. Carla Fine, in her book, *Married to Medicine*, clearly outlines the dilemma of the doctor's wife who divorces. The frus- tration and bitterness of ex-wives makes one wonder why the doctor is still considered such a good catch.

From the marriage counselor, psychiatrist, to judge and jury, the wives report feelings of being on the wrong, unfavored side. To protect herself, a realistic paranoia is honed and makes the woman suspicious, cautious, and eventually bitter and disillusioned.

My friends told me to take him for all he was worth when Lenny wanted to divorce me. I felt that to be independent and a true feminist meant to send him on his way and make it on my own. Little did I know that you're damned whatever you do.

The traditional medical husband-wife partnership is so en- trenched in the system that trying to adjust to a more egalitarian marriage has been excruciating. She wants and needs more options and a chance at a life, interests, and career for herself. He demands a wife to free him up for his career. In this time of role transition, and amidst the confusing definitions of the cooperation and interde- pendency of medicine/career/home/family, divorce rates rise. I sus- pect the doctor will keep looking for a woman who will fulfill the roles of a traditional doctor's wife, and there will be unsuspecting women out there who hope they will be fulfilled in the role.

For a doctor it's just as if he gets a new muffler for his car and it keeps on going as usual. For his wife a divorce means no muffler, no car, and perhaps losing her license to drive, and having to learn to drive all over again. And to top it off, she feels guilty.

Chapter 40

Wife Number 2 or 3 or 4: A Powerful Legacy

I can't believe I fell in love with another doctor. Is it an addiction or what? — Dot

In a warmly lit breakfast room with charming flowered chairs and matching tablecloth on the table, flowers in fall hues in the center, sit four women, including myself, all having tea and conversation. The house is simply decorated in tones of mauve and grey. The sun is streaming through the south-facing windows and there is a cuddly Scottish terrier nuzzling our ankles occasionally.

I am especially struck by an exciting array of artwork on the walls of the downstairs of the home. The watercolors are done by the woman of the house, and an assortment of macrame and other woven wall pieces, she tells me, are attributed to crafts people she admires in the area. The affinity for color is even obvious in the hostess's attire. She wears fall colors on her person the way her table's centerpiece carries itself — lightly, comfortably, and unassumingly. Even the soft music playing in the background, drifting into the kitchen from a central speaker system, adds to the careful, almost perfect setting for our tea and breakfast cakes.

With me are three women, all of whom have been married to the same man. The hostess is currently married to him and has graciously agreed to this somewhat unusual request of mine to interview them all at once. The husband is a neurosurgeon of excellent reputation, and from the looks of this home, is probably quite successful. He is in his mid-forties and is now supporting three families of assorted ages. We will hear more of that later.

The women appear quite relaxed and even excited about the idea of sharing their experiences with me for what may be a book. They are aware that it isn't often someone entertains ex-wives simultaneously, and I feel that they are as intrigued with the idea as I. It was easy to arrange this interview because all the women have remained in the same town even after divorcing Charles (MD), whom they all call Chuck. And I gather from the atmosphere of familiarity that these three women have a rather easy, accessible relationship with one another, also quite unusual from my perspective. It is rare for ex-wives to relate to each other with so little strain. I comment on that very observation. "It seems that you are so comfortable with each other. How has that happened?"

Sheila, the hostess, answers almost immediately:

> We have had to figure out some system of communication in order to deal with all of our mutual children. At first, since I'm the newest Mrs. Medicine [for lack of a better surname!], when we were dating I thought it was overwhelming to take on this job. Can I deal with seven children of all ages and two ex-wives? What am I getting into here?

The two others looked at each other and smiled in agreement quite knowingly.

Sheila is 34 years old. She's bright and cheerful, constantly chattering. In fact, she seems uncomfortable when there's a silence. She was married once before to a teacher and has one 11-year-old son from her first marriage. It's fun to listen to her talk; her speech sounds as if she was originally from the South.

> Yes, I'm from Louisiana, and I guess I still talk like a Southerner even though I've been away from there since college.

Sheila is a green-eyed redhead, quite stunning really, although I believe she has no idea how she looks to others.

> I thought it would be fairly easy to learn to deal with the assortment of children because I grew up with six brothers and two sisters, and we were not well-off. So I thought with Chuck's circumstances, money and all, as a doctor, we could manage just fine.

Sheila met Chuck working as a medical receptionist at a local hospital. When she had been divorced and on her own for four years, she felt:

> really ready to settle down again and find someone to help with my son. I never really liked doing everything on my own or living alone, actually. Chuck was just through his second divorce, from Carlene, when we started dating. I knew Carlene because she worked at the hospital too and we had been friendly before I started seeing Chuck. We were determined that my dating him was not going to interfere with our friendship.

Carlene jumps into the conversation.

> Yes, when I married Chuck, eight years ago, I had gone through a bitter divorce from my first husband. He left me for another woman whom I detested. So when Sheila started dating Chuck I thought, if this becomes serious I have to get along with Sheila and stay friends. I couldn't go through another sordid painful experience. My ex-husband and his new wife still make it hard for me to speak to my kids when they have them at their house.

Okay, I'm already starting to get confused by whose children are whose and from what marriage, but I forge ahead blindly. Carlene continues:

> After my divorce from Chuck I thought I'd never marry again, and look—I'm engaged to another doctor. I must be crazy! But working at the hospital, the only interesting men I meet are doctors. Or am I addicted?

Carlene is a smaller, darker version of Sheila. I am struck as I spend time with these women with how similar they are in looks and in mannerisms. Sure there are individual differences, but overall there are true likenesses—body type, degree of neatness, clothing style and general overall appearance, amount and type of jewelry. For instance, all three are wearing small gold bracelets and tiny pinky rings of pearl and gold. They all have mid-length hair, different colors but the same neat and tidy style.

Carlene shared the history of meeting Chuck while she was a surgical nurse on his operating floor at the hospital. Chuck had left his first wife, Fran, who was depressed after the death of their fourth child. Carlene worked with Chuck every day quite closely as an O.R. (operating room) nurse. Carlene continues:

> After my divorce, I was ready for someone to shower me with attention. Chuck doted on me then, called all the time whenever we weren't working together, and was quite romantic and flirtatious while we were in O.R. I moved in within two months after we began dating. I had two kids, and my first husband and his new wife were suing for custody. I was a wreck and needed Chuck to help me regain composure and self-confidence. Looking back, I think I also hoped that marriage to Chuck, a doctor, would help me to regain or keep custody of my two kids.

Carlene's first husband was in the auto business for himself. She had supported him as a nurse in the lean times and was aware of her financial capabilities. However, she felt emotionally depleted through her divorce and felt quite rejected when her place as mother and wife was taken over by another woman.

The third woman at the table, Frances, or Fran as she likes to be called, is the oldest and the most quiet. Her dark, deep-set eyes, I'm certain, are totally absorbing everything that is going on around her. I estimate her age at 48. Although trim and youthful for her years, her expression in her lower face tells me she has endured much of life's tribulations. She interjects:

> It's amazing to me how you two women [Carlene and Sheila, I assume] hoped for Chuck to be your savior. Don't get upset, Sheila, I wish you and Chuck all the best, but it seems clear to me that with our joint history you should be realistic in terms of what you can expect from marriage to him.

Sheila takes this remark in her stride. Presumably she's heard it from Fran before. Fran goes on:

This is almost funny. I married Chuck at 19, practically 20. I was an infant. I left my mother's house to move to Chuck's and mine. He had just started medical school, and I was going to college in the same town in the Midwest. I did the usual— dropped out of school to get work as a secretary to put him through residency, internship, the whole schmear. Then I had three kids and a job, and a husband who was out all this time. After he made chief resident at Chicago General he started behaving strangely: bossy, impatient, not satisfied with any-thing I did, or the kids for that matter. My oldest son and he argued all the time. And my baby got very sick. I wanted Chuck to make him well. We stopped being intimate and soon I became depressed and couldn't work any more. Fourteen years of marriage, hard work, putting up with a nonexistent husband and father, and he says he needs someone who is more up, more lively, someone he can move up the ladder with. He packed his bag in August and I moved back home with my three kids in September, devastated. The horror sto-ries of others who said: "Don't marry a doctor, especially a surgeon," turned out to be so right on! He'd turned into a tyrant, from a sweet, quiet, thoughtful boy to a bull-headed egomaniac!

The other women began trying to calm Fran. Sheila says:

She's still bitter, and I don't blame her, but Chuck was differ-ent. I think all that pressure and responsibility went to his head. He was scared. He's told me all about it.

Carlene chimes in,

Maybe so, but Fran left out the clincher. When her baby boy died, Chuck died a little too, and didn't know how to deal with her depression. I doubt if he's ever gotten over that loss.

Fran says:

Don't excuse him any more. I was a perfect doctor's wife. All the auxiliary meetings. I entertained the residents and the staff any time Chuck said I should. I looked good. The apartment looked good. I didn't complain about his hours or his coldness. What did it get me? Where was he when I needed comfort for my dying son? At the hospital taking care of other people's children! I'll never forgive him for that.

I tried to change the focus. My anxiety was rising, although Sheila and Carlene seemed strangely familiar with the outburst from Fran. Clumsily I asked how they all ended up living in the same town and if that presented problems. Carlene started:

Chuck wanted to leave Chicago. I guess it was too painful there for him. So we came out here to practice. He had visited a friend from medical school, and he and his wife seemed to like it, so we decided to try. Then Chuck and Fran, through a long time of dealing with their three kids, decided that Fran should come to live here so the kids could be near their father. She agreed.

Fran says:

Yeah, my kids pressured me and said if I didn't move out west they would come live with their dad anyway. So I saw the writing on the wall and did what I had to do. Actually, I love it here now and I'm happy they forced me. Although once Chuck and Carlene had two kids of their own, mine felt rejected somewhat. But that's the breaks, I guess.

More and more of Fran's bitterness shone through. My heart went out to her, a victim of very difficult circumstances.

"How do the new wives deal with the title of Mrs. Dr., and what happens when you're no longer his wife?" I asked.

They all piped in and started talking over one another.

Esther, you've been a doctor's wife long enough to know as long as you're in the club you're okay; when you leave you're shunned!

I said "I've never left, so tell me more." Sheila said:

> The auxiliary ignores you, the other wives treat you like you
> have the plague, people seem to look at you with pity, scorn,
> or as if you're not there. Shopkeepers no longer fuss over you.
>   As soon as everyone realized I was marrying Chuck they
> welcomed me with open arms. Here I was frightened to go
> from a mere clerical worker at the hospital to Chuck's wife.
> But most everyone gave me automatic status. I go to all auxil-
> iary meetings and volunteer a lot of support to their causes.
> Except for the occasional comments — "Carlene did it this way
> and Carlene was so great." But everyone else is more embar-
> rassed at that than I.

Carlene said:

> I had it easy in some ways. Soon after we married we moved
> away. So I didn't feel the pressure of living up to Fran's super
> job as doctor's wife. Except with the kids, and we still have
> our share of confusion and tension around the kids.

Our tea and cakes were getting cold. There was so much more to
find out. What does Fran do now? I know she never remarried and
has finally gotten a degree in art appreciation, which she was studying when she first met Chuck. She's a devoted mother and has been
in counseling for many years trying to work out her feelings about
the death of her fourth child and her divorce. Does she miss being a
doctor's wife?

> Only when I go into a store and people no longer act as if I'm
> a millionaire. I'm used to it now, though. At least I can buy
> cheap things now and no one raises eyebrows.

Carlene explained that her life will be same although her last
name will be different.

> Marry one doctor, and you marry them all. I'll still be alone a
> lot, be expected to be a perfect host, a perfect money manager,
> never get angry, wait a lot, keep quiet about interrupted sex
> [the others break into hysterics at this], and often lonely. But

it's all I know, and Bruce seems to be more talkative and understanding with me than Chuck was.

Sheila expressed her desire to do this again since I seemed to
have many more questions. Were they as cool as they appeared? As
resolute and resigned to their lives? What suggestions could these
women offer to others from their experience? What would they do
differently? What was it about the medical profession that resulted
in their experiences?

When I left at noon I had the increased sense of women's strength
and women's struggle. These three wives and women represented
today's world personified: women as victims of a male profession,
there to help, to provide nurturing, and to be cast aside!

The deference shown by the later wives to the earlier was shown
on occasion, even if it was mixed with an invisible thought, "It's
different with me. Chuck's different with me." I wondered if they
ever discussed and compared their sexual experiences with Chuck.
When queried Carlene said,

> Sure we talk about it because we all need to think we are better
> in bed than his last wife! Or we're such good lovers that Chuck
> has more fun with us than with his last wife! We've even com-
> pared his techniques and little idiosyncrasies, like the way he
> thinks it's so romantic to slobber in our left ear, only the left
> one, mind you. Right before he's unzipping his pants, he
> thinks he's such a stud!

All three women got giggly and shook their heads in agreement.
Such uninhibited communication—I was refreshed by their ease
and candor. What about this combination of deference, doubt, and a
smug, self-righteous attitude of the newer wives toward the earlier
ones? Fran said:

> It's always there. When we go to the baseball games or PTA
> meetings the new and old wives are face to face in an effort to
> keep things smooth and supportive for the kids. Thoughts like,
> "Oh, I see Carlene has a new diamond," or is driving a new
> car, or "How could she dress my daughter in those jeans?" or
> "Does Chuck look more relaxed with her?" Then she comes

to me and says, "I hope it's all right but I told the kids to call you about their school project and get your permission to help at school if you want to." Then I get suspicious about the consideration. It's always complicated. I was there first and the others know it, and I guess that gives me seniority.

Others corroborate this experience, the passing of the gavel from doctor's wife number one to number two and three and four has a ritualistic quality yet to be explored. Is it curious that knowing of the idiosyncrasies of this man and the negative impact on two women's personal lives, a third went into marriage with him with her eyes open? Does this attest to the powers of accommodation of all three of these wives? Or is it more a strong sense of both resignation and hope — the hope that their experience will be different, somehow better; or the resignation and knowledge that this is all there is when married to a doctor?

I felt a vague confusion. Why, when three interesting, vital people could share and communicate their experiences on this level — open, unreserved, uninhibited, and unashamed — why was it that they must live a life of such grossly distorted equality? A life in which they are the recipients of whim, moods, and demands of another, no matter how unpleasant or unreasonable? I was baffled about the draw of marriage to this physician, and what it was that made at least these three women put up with him! Was their self-esteem so low? Was their socialization so strong and complete? To be good women, this is a life that was to be admired, cherished, envied, and above all endured, no matter what the cost to her self!

I am inclined to think that these women (as all females) held shared unconscious beliefs from their early socialization process. That is, that when a marriage fails, it must truly be the woman's fault and/or responsibility — not the man's (especially if he is a physician). Hence, the current wife clings to the hope and magical belief that she will do better than the former wife. In a sad way, the distorted sense of poor self-esteem and magical, wishful thinking led each of these women into a situation that would hold few if any differences for any of them.

In observing the chart below notice how the patient (and the society of health care consumers) and the doctor (and the entire medical community) interact in a circular fashion to maintain the system, i.e., the patient demands and expects an all-honoring, readily available caregiver and the doctor sacrifices his health, well-being, and personal life to provide that care. Both the caregivers and the consumers of medical care make assumptions and harbor expectations of one another, sometimes false and often unwitting, at other times purposeful. The system is nurtured and perpetuated through the myths, needs, and beliefs of its participants.

COLLUSION OF SOCIETY
AND
MEDICAL ESTABLISHMENT

(Patients)	(Doctors)
Society Views Medicine	Institution of Medical Practitioners
Religion, worship, elevated status	Medical training, psychology of sacred calling
Demands and expectations	Home life disturbed, sacrifice of health and well-being
Dependent for health and life	Fear of failure, cannot save from death
Economics, health care megabucks	Overwork, obsession, treadmill to maintain success
Mysterious and exclusive club	Overcautious, paranoid, social separation
God-like, sacred dependence	Disdainful of patients' dependency, perfectionistic expectations, fear of failure
Love-Hate	Malpractice threat, peer review, reverence

Privileged, socioeconomic,
political

Curiosity, extreme preoccupation
(TV, media, books, etc.)

Aura, protect MDs, fears
MD's impotence

Sacrifices, addictions, personal breakdown, false
esteem

Reserved, private, fearful,
seduced by flattery of dependency and magi-
cal powers.

Isolated, threatened by truth
of frailty

Denial, play game of altruistic saving of lives, illusion of
avoiding death forever

Chapter 41

Caught Between Medicine and Society: Collusion Is in There Somewhere!

"If you are a nonmedical spouse of a doctor, you may prefer seeing a nonmedical therapist because you will not have to worry about dual doctor alignment, that is, that your physician spouse and the treating physician will collude in a two-against-one dynamic. This is a very realistic fear . . ." (Myers, 1988, p. 174)

Barbara Ehrenreich and Deirdre English studied the rise of the medical expert and his influence on women (*For Her Own Good*, 1978). In the last 150 years middle- and upper-class women have been the primary focus of medical advice, treatment, and cures. At various times these women were either confined to their beds for extended periods, operated on, set on with leeches, or medicated when the ovaries were considered the perpetrator of all sorts of problems with women. At that time poor women and those of minority groups (including blacks) were being ignored by the new male "regular physician." Their health was cared for by women healers, usually from their cultural group. Later, however (late 1800s, early twentieth century), the deprived women were used in experiments and training the students of the new formal medical profession. Hospital wards and clinics were filled with poor women who were to get care as a trade for being guinea pigs for men of medicine. At the same time the rich and middle-class women filled doctors' waiting rooms or were at home getting treatment by the newly renowned physicians.

Then Freud came along in Austria and proposed that it was not just the ovary, but the unconscious that drove women to their behaviors and illnesses. Women needed fixing. There was great money to be made, and if not through gynecology and surgery, then psychiatry would emerge as the savior. The mind was the new focus. Therapy, less painful than leeches and surgery, constituted a long and arduous process which women would require for years in order to be better. Their innate weakness and inferiority would benefit from the expert touch of the shrink.

How does the doctor's wife fit into this picture? She is certainly not counted among the indigent poor who were and still are the first to get new and experimental treatment in large city hospital wards. Rather, the doctor's wife is the perfect patient to receive the expert treatment of the doctor who formerly came to her home and now whom she sees in the most advanced, highly technological, most well-appointed office around. She is a member of the middle- to upper-class, usually not working outside the home, a perfect target for the male expert cult which has existed in different forms for over 100 years. As a woman in that economic class, the latter is true. As a woman married to a physician she already lives with the expert.

By virtue of her womanhood she is an imperfect, inferior being (so told by years [eons] of experts, be they religious, political, educational, and now scientific). Her husband belongs to the profession which is dedicated to helping, curing, and healing, and for the most part he does so in an authoritarian manner, mostly to women. The doctor's wife, though, is caught in a bind.

She ends up unwittingly colluding to maintain the medical-society-expert liaison. She is the right-hand person to her husband, given neither equal value nor equal rights in his world; nonetheless she stands by her man. She must believe his expertise or deny her loyalty to him. Several years ago I was walking on the beach with my husband and innocently asked whether he knew why the seals came so close to shore in a storm. I trusted implicitly and totally that he must know that answer since he's a doctor and a man, and never for a moment did he flinch or suggest that he had no answer for my question. Never for a moment did I expect him to say no, nor did I feel qualified or powerful enough to search out the answer myself. Then I realized how quickly both he and I played our roles—he the all-knowing expert on any subject, not necessarily related to his field of medicine, and I so willing to be the naive, ignorant, helpless woman—even at age 50! I caught myself just in time. I turned to him and said, "Jerry, did you realize what just happened?" He was totally innocent and oblivious to the transaction. I recounted my automatic response and told him how surprised and ashamed of myself I was. Am I still a dumb, helpless girl waiting for my hero to give me the answers to everything? At first I was upset at myself. Then I got angry at Jerry. "Why didn't you say you didn't know the answer?" I inquired. "Because I like to pretend I do," he said. "You must admit you almost bought it!" he continued. Still, he acted as if I were overreacting, and he changed the subject as quickly as possible. When will I learn?

So the myth of the expert with the power to think and to heal is in the hands of men and in the hands of our husbands, the doctors. I am again reminded of the spectacular works of women researchers who unlock the doors to the past and shake our long preserved views that men are the intelligent, creative, all-knowing, leaders, builders and law makers. Not so, according to Renee Eisler, Barbara Ehrenreich, Deidre English and Merlin Stone, Maria Gimbutas, plus numerous archaeologists, anthropologists, social scientists, and futurists who have collected unquestionable data to refute the so-called truth. We (humans) have lived with peace, equality, and harmony where women were viewed as valuable, even goddesses. In prehistory to as recently as 3,200 years ago in Crete, women raised crops, were architects, and craftspeople, held cities together, enriched life, and were instrumental in passing their history through millennia via paintings or the beginnings of written script. That women were healers as well as givers of life through birth and through harvesting crops and raising agriculture is a view more accepted in the halls of academia. It is hopeful to think that women were valued and valuable members of the species for thousands of years before they were systematically reduced to supporters of men, seen as inferior, and looked upon only as producers of babies and servants of "mankind."

The irony for a doctor's wife is that he and his profession embrace the caring, helping, and curing of our health, the nurturing values that women are known to possess, and the values that our society tends to denigrate at present. To be a helper, a caretaker, a role usually reserved for women and condemned as demeaning, is the script the doctor is supposed to play out in order to heal. Somehow this is a paradox, or ironic at least. How to fulfill both a macho, masculine-dominant, authoritarian role and still be a helper and caretaker of humanity is the question. What of his wife?

A recently appointed chairman of the local medical auxiliary was sitting in on medical association board of directors' meetings:

> I was so surprised to find out how opportunistic and materialist the medical association is. Their focus is on political power, getting laws passed that will ensure their position in society as the revered experts. But the most important part of the political antics of the board didn't focus on ways to heal, improve access to health for the impoverished or destitute. No, the focus, the obsession, was money, increasing fees, and ways to bring more people in to see the doctor. . . . I was so devastated by the meetings. The ideology blew me away. Here I am, a very active and proud auxiliary member, protecting doctors and their reputation at every turn. My children and I have always jumped in to stand up for medicine as a humane, idealistic way of life. Maybe I've been naive all these years [married 27 years], or stupid, but boy it's been an eye opener for me. Here I am in a position to see the medical society and how it works. Compared to the auxiliaries, we women are the humane and caring ones who cherish life! We offer our services free to children's groups, hospitals for underprivileged, make money by volunteering for the needy. What are our husbands, the doctors, doing! Looking for ways to dupe the public, finding ways the public will be more dependent on them for their health and well-being, which of course brings more dollars into their pockets.

What about our pockets – how do you justify your lifestyle?

Probably, at least the best way I can explain it now, is that while I was thinking that the medical profession was idealistic and focused on preserving life and making the quality of life better for all people, I was happy to be involved, to volunteer my services as a helper and supporter of what my husband was trained to do. I've enjoyed the financial rewards because I thought there was also so much altruism to balance it off. We all (or I should say men all) get reimbursed for their services, so I thought that hard work and ideals of altruism deserved good pay. Now I feel used, like we women do the real service-oriented work with compassion and hope; the men look for devious ways to create reasons for people to need their services. They get paid. We don't. Who wins? It's a mockery of service!

What can you think of doing to improve your dilemma?

I really don't know. If I confront my husband, he disagrees and immediately shuts me up. If I confront the medical board, I'll be expelled from sitting in and lose the one inroad we women of the auxiliary have finally achieved. So for now I sit and listen and am astonished and depressed. I think the ideology is wacky somewhere — can we be altruistic and mercenary at the same time? I feel so torn here.

We have had such a rich history of mixed messages, especially regarding those characteristics that make up the more female orientation — the intuitive, empathetic, life supporting, caring and feeling, sharing parts of ourselves. Men are discouraged from developing these traits and women are told these traits are unimportant. Women were at one time the guardians of health and well-being, and gradually that job was taken over by men, professional men. However, the traits conducive to healing were still not reinforced in the male healers, so a new type of relationship betwen patients and healers developed. In fact the more the technology became specialized and refined, the more distant from the patient did this male doctor become.

His wife began to develop her cool, detached attitude. She even repressed her fears and perhaps even her physical ailments. It became her job as the link between her husband and the society to project the image of professional detachment, a representative of the new scientific medical model.

Now it would be the nurses who could express the female traits of caretaking and nurturing, being empathetic and understanding to the sick. If the doctor's wife is a nurse, she is a helper on all fronts, but she must do the doctor's bidding at work, often soothing the sick before or after the doctor briefly graces the patient with a moment of his time. Then if that nurse goes home as a wife, she reverts back to the reserved, composed, less feeling, undervalued, or overlooked shadow of her husband. He dominates her life at work, her time, her activities, her thoughts, and at home, the same system undergoes a strange repetition.

She is told to be feeling and caring at work, but at home she is told to perform menial tasks first; feeling and caring is only useful in small doses. Eventualy she too forgets how to truly relate. Competition, jealousies, pettiness, and insecurities may override the sense of harmony that a family requires for health and survival. Just as in society, autocracy or androcracy* pervades the household. Female values are eschewed for male values. Beating out the next guy wins over sharing and preserving our relationships.

If this rampant, unpeaceful co-existence in the home (and in the hospital also) is to change, the ideologies must be clarified. Is overpowering, possessing, and dominating in order to win or be the best going to continue? What about the hierarchy of the big boss over the little people? The expert over the ignorant? The winners over the losers? Are we as doctors' wives comfortable to sit back and allow the continuation of such hypocrisy in the very field which espouses life enhancement and empathetic understanding?

If our households are not empathetic partnerships where we are valued equally as productive, creative, caring humans, how can we pretend to be achieving it outside?

Encouraging peace at home, not ignoring conflict or repressing feelings but maintaining open lines of sharing and interaction, and honesty without fear of humiliation or punishment, is what a healing, healthy family entails. In order to heal, and in order to be credible, the family of the physician, and in the larger sense, the family of humans, must encourage peace, deal with conflict, express real feelings, maintain open lines of sharing and interaction, and value honesty without fear of humiliation or punishment.

---

*Riane Eisler, in her 1987 book *The Chalice and the Blade*, introduced this term, explaining it was derived from the Greek root words *andros* (man), and *kratos* (ruled).

MARRIED TO MEDICINE

We are all married to medicine
whether we like it or not
what's the difference
　　between wife, patient, nurse or whore?

Medicine dictates our health
of mind, body and soul
a religion all its own
　　as long as we believe.

Sacred are the Gods of Medicine
Hippocrates king of them all
to worship with both joy and fear
　　hoping for life eternal.

We eat, drink and move as they say
gaining or losing on cue
most of the Gods say, "Do as I say
　　not as I do."

Women, children and the poor
seem to be prey to these gods
tested, sacrificed and scarred to provide
　　answers to their prayers.
At first it seemed innocent enough
a new way to care and cure our young
ways to give birth, feed and breed
　　then even death was prolonged.

What of the natural order of things
life, living, growing, ageing and death?
Medicine's Gods would have us believe
　　we can overcome nature and win.

Daily doses of health herbs, trips to the doctor
　　on time
Check-ups, x-rays, prevention and clinics
inoculations to our babies
　　whether we want them or not.

The sterile white walls and light blue shirts
of the Gods and ladies who wait
no one can touch or cry or feel
    the chemicals will heal on their own.

Is it a blessing, this healing by rote
this magic of test tubes, findings and scopes?
If the gods deem it necessary we all flock
    to the place of worship and wait.

We can't remember our lives before
the great word of Medicine came down
charts, scales, proportions, heights and weights
    fats, sugars, all according to them.

If he gives it to his child, so do we
if she says it works for days
we pack up our old remedies, our warmth and love
    and try her genuine round pills.

Elevator going up to the heights of curing all ills
never mind that only some are cared for
never mind that some are helpless just the same
    and only some can come down

The Gods don't justify their treatments
no matter what the price
praying, worshipping, believing, blindly following
    the word of the Medicine Gods.

The Gods don't justify their treatments
there is much to be learned yet, they say
this marriage means worshipping, believing
    blindly following until the
        reckoning day.

PART IV:
CONCLUSION

THE INVISIBLE DIPLOMA

As I walk into my house
Over the entrance to my special room
I see a framed picture
All glowing and glittery.

The words are clear to those who know
How long and hard I've worked
How many days and nights.

The names are those of women
Mothers, daughters, and aunts
Who went through the training before me.

The sorority we belong to
Entitles us to recognition
That a mere diploma would deny.

But even so I have this fantasy
That one day on my wall
Will say indelibly
    Woman, In recognition of your persistence
    your fortitude, your loyalty, dedication
    and accomplishments
    the board of directors of humankind
    bestows lifelong, honorary recognition and
      licensing

for your competence in your wifehood,
motherhood, and householderhood,
caretakerhood and personhood.
Respectfully, the Goddesses.

Chapter 42

Metaphorical Relationships:
Wife-Husband, Patient-Doctor

He has no bedside manner, but is he ever a good surgeon.
—patient to friend

Much of what is true about the relationship between wives and their physician husbands can also be applied to patients and the health care system.

Perhaps the most alarming similarity is the condescension with which the patient is often treated. An absolute essential to the livelihood of the medical doctor and the institution of medicine, the consumer is still viewed with wariness and contempt by the health care professional. Those of us who have been ignored by medical personnel, been kept waiting unreasonably long in sterile waiting rooms, who have been kept in the dark regarding diagnoses and treatments of frightening illnesses are living examples of society's marriage to physicians.

Can the doctor's wife be viewed as the symbol and barometer of society's view of the medical profession? I think so. Take her vow of secrecy and isolation, for example. She cannot penetrate his world. The language is obscure. People around him make it hard for her to access him. He remains aloof, mysterious, reserved. She thinks he contains knowledge and information that he alone can use and understand.

How does our society behave toward the medical practitioner? The medical schools teach separatism, elitism, special words only those allowed in can understand. Others are in awe, confused by the language and the surrounding mysteries. In school, he pledges confidentiality within the profession. His wife colludes by not asking

361

him about his work, patients' cases, or what his life is really like. She is also in collusion when she doesn't question her existence with him.

Again our society encourages mystery—there is little communication with medical schools, societies, and professional groups. How can we as lay people communicate and understand what is said, felt, discovered, questioned, and learned? The language and ethics preclude that possibility.

His wife feels that secretaries, nurses, technicians et al., block her way to him. He is inaccessible to her. They protect him from outside interferences. Our society encourages this inaccessibility by the insider-outsider stance. Only members allowed! What's the password? Medical lingo, or admission to the correct club only. She feels ignorant, lonely, and isolated, which only fosters the tremendous dependence inherent in the relationship.

So do we in society. We believe we are dependent on medicine for our survival. Medicine and its practitioners are canonized as a sacred religion. Our longevity, health, well-being, and our society's economic health may depend on the physician to the extent that the medical-economic-political complex is carefully intertwined.

What does this dependence do in the marriage? It fosters insecurity, anger, poor self-esteem, and rage in both parties. Unrealistic expectations which can't be met promote general unrest. We both love and hate that which we think we cannot survive without—like a child-parent relationship. We need food, love, affection, and protection for our survival. The physician in our society has been chosen or has chosen to be our symbolic father-god. He will protect us from hurts, pains, sickness, and maybe death. He is the ultimate expert over our well-being.

The demands on him are incredible; he stands for responsibility, invulnerability, irreplaceability, strength, omniscience. Time demands that the doctor sacrifice his personal, inner world. His wife experiences her permanent place as second, with various combinations of awesome appreciation, envy of him, insecurity, fear, doubt, anger, rage, resentment, and impotence.

Feminism has helped to point out some of the inequalities between the sexes related to medical marriage. It is symbolic to me that as women have become more assertive, questioning, open, less secretive, more confident, and increasing in knowledge and capacity to explore, so has the society as a whole begun specifically to question the health care system and physician vulnerability.

We could even say that the increase in malpractice suits against physicians coincides with the doctor's wife's assertive questioning. All at once she is expressing her concern, her curiosity, her need to be involved in his world. She wants to share in decisions, and share in the future of her relationship with him especially. Society too, by questioning his performance, reasons, ethics, and decisions, and even by taking a greater part in its own medical and health care needs, is sharing and becoming more connected to him.

He can be more human, less mysterious. His wife can benefit by being a valued and contributing family member. She need not stay at home idly or as a service volunteer, unappreciated and undervalued yet essential to our culture. By prioritizing her jobs and services, she can be involved in the mainstream of life. We too can become involved and connected. Our lifestyle changes — exercise, diet, relaxation, stress management — are all indicators that we are sharing in our health care. We can interact, converse, question him, be direct, disagree or, if necessary, choose another physician; the doctor's wife can do the same, and, if necessary, leave the marriage.

I believe that the myth of mystery, confidentiality, and inaccessibility in both the public and private lives of physicians has been a cycle which may be fostered by fear, intimidation, the bullying style or "macho mentality" learned in medical school, and perpetuated by economic greed, insecurity, and a basic fear of death. At home the myth is perpetuated by the wives' families and other doctors' wives. No one shares or talks about what is really going on! Alcohol, drug abuse, violence, incest, depression, suicide, and general anxieties all plague our society, but no one would believe that a physician, his wife, or child could suffer from them.

He worries about his quality of work. Can he be what society and family demand? He feels he has no choices. She's lonely, angry, impotent, dependent, not privy to his world. Her world is often the children, an arena where she can express the feeling, warmth, flexibility, vulnerability, and humanness that he can't display to his professional world or personal world without great anxiety and fear of professional unethical judgment. Perfectionism is something they both experience. He lives with risk taking; she fears risks. All this sounds like the overview of really traditional male-female roles and values.

That's what our society wants of him, really; to be omnipotent, cure all, develop miraculous paths to longevity. We (as patients) and his wife are willing to remain ignorant and powerless for the assurance that he can touch, medicate, and cure us, save us from pain and death. Underneath all of this implies that he is better, above, more powerful (through knowledge, position, and intimidation) than his patients, most often women, and especially his wife and children.

As wives we try competing with him with our determination to run as fast, ski as hard, win fights over money, control sex, and successfully parent the children. We want so desperately to be let in, to learn the secret. Of course, competition among other wives is also rampant. Like children we fight for approval and recognition, but most of all to show the medical and other communities that our husbands are truly the best providers, therefore the best doctors, and therefore perhaps he could be the very best parent figure!

What if the competition ceases? We become cooperative in marriage and health care in a society that stresses more communication, intimacy, shared responsibility, and less mystery, secrecy, confidentiality. Bring him down to Earth, be next to him, and all of us share in keeping ourselves healthy. Review our institutions. What's the greatest fear? Perhaps the doctor fears his obsolescence; necessary no more, he faces no money, no security, no prestige, no reverence. Other institutions are also heavily involved and committed to the institutions of health care and medicine as it has developed in the past 25 to 50 years; insurance companies, the legal profession, educational institutions, pharmaceutical companies, legislatures, and hospitals themselves all interconnect with medicine. All are married, if you will, to the traditional physician and medical model. So, would our economic system collapse if cooperation replaced competition in the world of medicine? Not being an economist, it would be presumptuous of me to make a judgment.

I can imagine, however, that the doctor's wife brings much more to the union and family as she becomes more involved in the marriage, more relaxed, more confident, less guilt ridden and ambivalent, has priorities and expectations which are more realistic, is involved in finding solutions, and is available to contribute to the economy of the family, not just the psyche, by being stronger as an individual. Change from secrecy to openness, competition to cooperation, denial to admission, passiveness to assertiveness, dependence to interdependence can only mean more knowledge, which would then lead to solutions. Greater equality frees them both from an unjust and oppressive system.

We can't fix the doctor's marriage, or the medical health system, so simplistically. But it's important to recognize problems and openly discuss them. Through inquiry, we can allow peers and non-peers to come in and provide input, ask questions, share in the exchange, and suggest the solutions. There will always be room for healers in our society. But we may be able to look at more efficient, less costly ways to care for ourselves and others if we shake our myths of medicine as God, the physician as his messenger, and the hospital as his miracle workroom. Magic and mystery breed great fear and anxiety. As a doctor's wife I feel it personally, and when my health depends on it, I feel it in the profession. I see how it can affect the practitioners and those related to them. The cost is high for us all.

Someone said to me during my research of doctors' wives that because I'm married to a physician, I get to sleep with a god. A colleague of mine also described the ambivalent feelings directed towards doctors' wives as one in which his patients are envious of her because she's sleeping with their symbolic father. It's time we let go of godly, fatherly images of the physician, and the symbolic incestuous liaison that leaves for his wife and those who are his patients. Medicine is not a religion unless we believe it is. Personally, I'd like to be freed up to enjoy the person I married as a man who works at a job and is also a warm, fun-loving human being. If I can't view him with humanity and imperfection, how then can I view myself?

We all seem to need permission to let go of preconceptions and outmoded myths. For me, I resent having to be seen only as the self-sacrificing dilettante who lives upon the hill with "him." And I would think that our society as a whole is getting tired of being overprotective, underinformed, powerless, pedestalizing. Maybe we are all married to medicine. Rather than divorce, I'm advocating awareness, recognition, and an ability to look for solutions. Perhaps as a society, instead of being in an unequal marriage we can become consulting colleagues. We can and must change our relationship, both yours and mine, into a partnership.

Chapter 43

Solutions:
Anger, A Case for Conflict Resolution

We need permission to disagree and negotiate our disagreements in an atmosphere of equality. — Karen

If we could just not be so afraid to disagree, we might find something to agree on. — Phyllis

A distinct thread runs throughout my interviews with women married to doctors, a rumbling of anger and protest which becomes a harsh, loud scream of rage and oppression when given expression. Along with the anger is the confusion about feeling it so strongly, and the question — what do we do with these feelings?

Even the silent, stoic women who chose the traditional role of wife to a prominent professional feel the sting of unspoken conflict. They may not express anger or rage openly, or may not be aware of feeling those emotions. However, they are aware that there are inconsistencies, and below all of this are the disturbing, uncomfortable, indescribable emotions of conflict. It's easily understood as the tightening in the pit of one's stomach or the cramping in one side of the neck when something is wrong but we cannot articulate the problem. These feelings occur between people, and most often are noticed between those closest in our lives.

What to do about the differences of opinion or the differences of feeling?

In our entire society it is thought important to maintain order, so conflict is kept under control by law and proper punishment for breaking those laws. We are taught to behave in ways that are socially acceptable, or "appropriate," as the psychologists say. In a society which has inequality among social classes and especially among genders, as does ours and those in most of our present world, the oppression required to keep the less favored and valued in their place is constant. Conflict and individual expression need to be kept at a minimum. In fact, to keep the oppressed down, conflict and the mere thought of it becomes terrifying. Soon it is terrifying to everyone. To raise one's voice is a sign taken to mean danger and violence, if it comes from a man, and yet a woman with raised voice is considered hysterical, crazy, wild, and out of control, to be tamed as an animal, burned at the stake, or systematically annihilated.

How does that translate in the family of a woman married to a doctor today? Probably as it does in the bigger world—his voice being the threat of nuclear war and hers representing the injustice and inequality in humanity, which is turned to rage and ignored as crazy and must be quieted, calmed, and sedated.

It seems obvious to me that by not teaching conflict resolution to young people, by not enabling our individual differences to be aired, accepted, and seen as acceptable, we are all maintaining the current of fear of loud voices in the world. In fact, voices won't be loud and frightening, and needn't be so if all voices can be heard equally with respect and caring. If the different timbres and qualities of the sounds and the meanings are not feared even if they are varied and don't blend with mine or yours, why not cherish the difference, listen carefully, and try to understand the sound and meaning even if ours feels more comfortable?

In other words, the physician's wife and her children must have an equal voice with the doctor in the household. If his voice is always feared, even if it's not raised and angry, her voice will fail to articulate. Not articulated, the fear she experiences, unexplained and misunderstood, can turn to rage, which at best perpetuates the cycle of oppression and violence, she being the one oppressed and violated, or her children.

Medicine is supposedly a helping profession of compassion, caring, and reaching out to the sick and pained. The paradox of a strong-armed doctor taking care of a weak, helpless, dependent patient is outmoded. But the fear of conflict underlies the patient's reserve. Should she or he raise a question in conflict with the doctor's judgment or medical call, the patient risks reprisals. If the doctor is angered by the patient, the doctor can and does deny the patient compassion, and could punitively (though less obviously) deny access to the most effective healing process. Is it not true that healing occurs in an atmosphere of safety, caring, trust, and understanding, and not in an atmosphere of force, domination, and fear?

If there is anger in a woman married to a doctor but she feels afraid and powerless to express her feelings, what can we expect of her growth and development? What can be expected within her relationship with her husband? He is dominating and she is oppressed.

Open exchange of information, desires, goals, and feelings is essential for humankind to survive. The fear of reprisals for expression must be reduced somehow. People will not speak freely and express themselves if they are afraid of humiliation or of emotional or physical punishments. It is essential that young people learn that to disagree or to be in conflict with another is acceptable and negotiable. If it's done in an atmosphere of equality, it is healthy!

We have heard hurt, angry, frustrated, disappointed voices of women throughout this book. Perhaps those feelings are favored more because this is an open forum for expression available to them. It is the only place where someone really listened and heard their viewpoint and shared much of it. It would have been easy and certainly acceptable to report only happy thoughts and feelings. In fact, humor, laughing, and joking were safe ways of experiencing their conflict. Or the women themselves could have just said everything was wonderful, life married to a doctor is pure joy and ecstasy all the time. But when given time to think and talk, and someone to listen and hear, they reached the usually reserved and secret voices inside, the sounds that aren't so pretty to hear, or for them, to feel. At times women felt ugly saying the angry words out loud and were even frightened knowing someone would be reading these words.

It is especially sad for me to think that angry thoughts or negative thoughts and feelings make us feel so ugly, repulsive even to ourselves. If we were taught that all parts of us are acceptable, changeable, viable, and if there were a safe environment to express these, they would not be ugly and repulsive or scary.

A woman who is married to a controlled and controlling person feels the underlying anger in his control. She is well aware, even unconsciously, that to cross him she will be hurt somehow. The concept of power, control, and aggression must be shattered and replaced by communication of equality, responsibility, and caring. Power and control breed fear and destruction. Sharing responsibility, caring, and equality of reason and respect breed conflict resolution and creative life enhancement.

Both the women and their husbands must be committed to a new understanding of conflict, an acceptance of its existence and awareness of the tools for expression and resolution. Not the tools of power and destruction like voices of night and fear, but tools of free expression, exchange of ideas, listening, hearing, negotiating and renegotiating. "True anger arises in legitimate protest over one's rights," Dr. Teresa Bernadez-Bonesatti says, and "the personal cause of dignity has been served" (*Journal of American Medical Women's Association*, 1978, p. 236). A worthy goal is the willingness to find solutions in which no one loses, no one is defeated, but rather both parties look for and find goal enhancements that please them. Both achieve humanitarian accomplishments.

Realistically, conflict is difficult to resolve if one person, group, country, or people holds more power over the other with whom they are in conflict. The healthy anger of people expressing a legitimate protest over their rights turns to rage in an unequal system where rights are in disequilibrium. Perhaps then the dominator power principle must be reworked and reevaluated, replaced by Eisler's partnership model in which feminine values of linking, sharing, creativity, individuality, and nurturing are encouraged (1987). Certainly I can think of no better placement for these values than in the marriage and family of women and men in the healing arts. The marriages of doctors and their wives need healing as well. Conflict must be allowed to exist, to be nurtured safely, and to be resolved. Anger can then be expressed safely, not as aggressive, dangerous rage with its implied retaliatory vengeance, but merely as an emotion to signal a conflict.

Kelly, a wonderfully expressive woman married 18 years who has been involved with her husband in the peace movement for the last ten years spoke:

At first in our marriage Wayne kept quiet even if he was seething underneath the cool exterior he was so good at. I love to express my feelings. I would rant and rave at the slightest upset or disturbance that struck my fancy. The kids [she has two] would easily push my buttons. I would react or yell or use my sarcastic tone of joking to express my feelings of the moment. The kids and I learned to banter back and forth, and we would usually eventually get to the core of our disagreement. With Wayne, though, there was difficulty reaching a core, or even disagreeing at all. If my voice raised, he'd raise his hand and point it in a quietly awesome way, and you know, bringing his finger to his mouth as if to say, "Quiet. Calm down." But somehow the look in his eye said, "Calm down or else!" I either started screaming louder or ended up in tears. "Let me talk," I'd say. "Let me finish my thought! Let me be upset for a minute. Please!"

Eventually though, with our involvement in the peace movement and many, many hours of courses in interpersonal communications and nonviolent conflict resolution, we have changed our reactions to our differences, our upsets, and our disagreements. We've tried everything but have come to the conclusion that holding in feelings doesn't serve anyone well. We're trying to help the kids deal with better ways to disagree and resolve conflicts and still be themselves and feel okay about who they are. Just respecting each other's personality differences and values and needs has been helpful. In fact most of the time a struggle continues only when we've stopped listening to each other or when we refuse to work on solving a problem to everyone's benefit.

Can you give me an example?

Let me think. Okay. Wayne comes home late, tired and irritable, and asks if I've remembered to make some calls about a meeting we'll be having at our home that night. I've been busy all day. My son is home from school with a sore throat. I'm also distracted and exhausted from my day. Formerly, because I'd have forgotten my responsibility and promise to call eight people and make sure they knew their jobs for the meeting, I would have felt guilty, attacked, incompetent, and blamed for being lazy and wrong. I'd have yelled that it was Wayne's job anyway, and he would have snapped back and either belittled or embarrassed me in some flippant way to quiet my reaction to his attack. Then he would have felt abused also. Soon we'd both be upset, frustrated, and enraged at each other and the situation. I'd be yelling. He'd be seething, sulking, or patronizing me. The most important aspect of this soon-to-be-over-reaction on both of our parts, plus the upset and confusion that the kids are feeling by watching us not deal well with our interaction, is that we are locked in a struggle of power — who's right, who's wrong. And we are trying to hurt and get back at each other. We have clearly ignored the issue at hand: the successful arrangement of a meeting at our home that night!

How did you handle it?

When he came home and asked about the calls, I'd have been totally flustered that I'd overlooked that job, in spite of our discussing it that very morning. I'd have explained my embarrassment, without fear of humiliation or reprisals, and we would have then had to sit down and figure out how the meeting could still happen. In fact, we both wanted the meeting to happen and to be successful. So in that case it was easy to each make some calls and get to our goal. If it was something that one of us really didn't want that night, the other options would be talked about until some resolution occurred. Talk, talk, talk. So far we have no better way of resolving conflicts, short of the threat of death and destruction to all!

Talking and listening, hearing what the feelings and goals are of the individuals in the discussion, and moving in different directions — totally new ones if necessary — can resolve conflict and dissipate anger. Ignoring a conflict increases tensions and feelings of confusion and fear. Anger, in fact, becomes a tool and not a weapon. We can use anger to signal a problem and the need for a settlement, or a negotiation, or a discussion, not as an excuse to attack and demolish. The goals are more humanistic, less militaristic, and more effective. Finally, knowing that creative options and nonviolent solutions are the way to resolution, we can be encouraged by possibilities we have yet to imagine.

Chapter 44

Where Are We Now?

It might be worse with someone else! — statement repeated by
Jerry numerous times.

Jerry and I may be a fortunate couple. We have weathered long
dry spells in our relationship and have emerged enriched. It is probably our humor and our particular temperaments that account for the
longevity of our marriage. It may also be sheer determination due to
an abiding discomfort with major changes in our lives.

I also credit Jerry's being a family physician with giving us a
different perspective of living in a medical marriage. He has never
been a workaholic by nature, which has kept him away from the
more demanding specialties and kept him in a group practice. Consequently, the politics of medicine as a way of life eluded us. We
have made time for leisure and fun, by ourselves and with our sons.
Had Jerry been more ambitious or driven by his profession, our
lives would be quite different.

Rather, I was the driven one. I felt compelled to continue my
education as my children grew, and that has kept me somewhat
separate and creative in my own right. I like to view myself as a
realist in search of truths about our humanness. I suspect this has
kept Jerry and me from taking ourselves too seriously.

Although the pitfalls have always been there, it has been possible
to sidestep them, or having fallen in, to pick ourselves up and move
on. As you are well aware by now, I have taken issue with a great
deal that is inherent or traditionally built into a medical marriage.
All these years, I guess I have seen myself as the watchdog for
fairness and equality within this system. Sometimes it has taken me
a long time, but whenever I am finally aware of personal injustices,
I try to confront the problem and find an equitable resolution.

Living in a house of men, it was important to me to present a feminine influence. Becoming a feminist and humanist and my work as a counselor helped raise the consciousness of my husband and sons. I am now convinced that change evolves only from knowledge and awareness of inequity. Once we could truly see the power struggles and the demands of life within medicine, we would begin to draw the picture of a marriage that makes us more fulfilled and contented as individuals.

We have been fortunate not to have been drawn into an impossible situation which puts medicine above all else. We have learned that materialism and the potential self-importance given to those with great incomes are difficult in a marriage where the earning power is very unequal among the partners.

We are still working at our marriage. Now our sensitive areas are out in the open and respected by us. I'd like to take credit for bringing Jerry into the '90s regarding the essential feminist values. No doubt my insistence on the importance of respect for women has helped him in his work as well as our marriage. Although he still tends to be paternal at times, he is trying, just as I continue to strive to be an adult who values herself and her capabilities as a feeling person. Today, Jerry appreciates counseling and emotions in ways that he would never have during our early years together. I credit myself for that.

I am well aware that there are wives of physicians who are exceptions to the experiences of those in this book. The wife of one of Jerry's former partners comes to mind. She is presently a dean of the School of Social Work in a large, northeastern university. She said she could not relate to the experiences reported here. When her children were young, her husband parented and took responsibility for the household while she completed her Ph.D. "As a matter of fact, I love housework. What's wrong with that?" reports her husband.

I look back on their relationship and admire their ability to take on the roles required of them at the moment. Each has always had mutual respect and pride for what the other was doing. Both of their children have had equal parenting from their mother and their father. They also have role models of accomplishment and self-reliance from both parents. In many ways, Marlene and Jeff (not their real names) were ahead of their time. Equality of opportunity to develop as individuals and fulfill personal potential was a priority for them. Medicine was never allowed to take on proportions that overshadowed them as individuals.

There are couples who thrive even when the male is a physician; not, however, without constant vigilance, awareness, open communication, respect, and love. We must not forget that medicine is a traditional institution, moving very slowly into the next century.

For each Marlene who feels she never had the problems outlined in this book, there are many who have and never articulated them. While the rest of us were thinking about how to improve our husband's chances for becoming head of the department of neurosurgery, Marlene was writing another textbook on social work. In fact, Jeff was probably worrying about Marlene's promotion to dean. As mothers and doctors' wives, we diligently insisted our children behaved perfectly in front of hospital personnel even though they may have broken an ankle from falling off a bicycle. Jeff, with gentleness and softness and concerned primarily for his children, got the hospital personnel to entertain his baby girl while his crying son was being treated for an allergic reaction and his wife was elsewhere, taking an exam. Both Jeff and Marlene were willing to make their own rules, in spite of the system.

It has taken Jerry and me longer to realize the requirements for success in a medical marriage. Only through our failures and regrouping have we become willing participants in the continuous search and process. I'd like to think there is a chance for more of us to look at the status quo and say, "It can be more equitable. It can be better for us all. Look at Marlene and Jeff."

Chapter 45

A Look at the Future

It is apparent that our present system of marriage and family life of women and their husbands the doctors is too often not an equitable, successful system for either party. The constant tensions created between the sexes and the inequalities and imbalance that have existed for years are proof the system isn't working, hence statistics on mental illness, alcohol and drug abuse, incest, household violence, sexual dissatisfaction, poor communication, loneliness, suicide, distressed children, and finally, serial divorces.

Taking a leaf from the book *The Chalice and the Blade* (Eisler, 1987), I would like to propose a look at the future.

To deny that technological advances in medicine have been a boon to our cultural well-being would be foolish. However, we must look at the disparate social and cultural stunting that occurs simultaneously with our high rate of technological progress. It is essential that medical care and discoveries and advances in medical science be available worldwide to all people. The humanitarian aspects of health care cannot continue to be shoved aside for commercialism. To provide for only those who can afford it leaves too great a gap in the human condition. All the discoveries of medical sciences must be encouraged to continue and to be utilized for the betterment of humanity at large. As this occurs through education available to all people, and by valuing the growth and development of all people, the face of the doctor as we know him today will change.

Medical research and health care will be developed, using a model of community and partnership and affiliation and sharing, rather than the present view of the sacred god, expert authoritarian, protector, knower, and healer to the ignorant, obedient ones who are oppressed by fear of punishment, power, and might. A view of equally accessible health care and human existence on the planet can then emerge. When everyone is healthier, well-nourished, free to become better educated, and has choices for her/his future development, a creative environment will be an alternative. Without fear of overpowering punishment or starvation or death by violence, and with shared resources for health, cultural, social, economic, environmental, physical, scientific, and technological advancement, prioritizing elimination of human suffering through caring compassion, and interpersonal understanding, we will survive on this planet.

To look at our marriages and nuclear families and admit to inequalities and imbalances initiates a surge toward freedom of the human spirit and the possibility of achieving our heretofore unimagined potential.

Feminists, futurists, humanists, and scientists are saying that now is the time for change and we have the choice, the power, and the ability to make those changes. They are sociocultural changes which will then affect our political-economic systems.

The doctor's wife of the future will have options to assume many roles. Her choice to be with a doctor will be based on a clear, free choice, not on an inequitable dependency. The household tasks will be shared equally, as will child rearing. She will, if she chooses, also have a meaningful career outside the home, creative and nurturing, rewarded and valued by society. The tasks formerly done just by women, those of taking care of men, children, and households, will be rewarded and valued, and will include taking care of women and men and children, interactively and humanely. There will be shared economics and ownership of properties. Children will bear the names of those who parented them, not just their fathers. Married people will carry the names of their own choosing, not just the male lineage.

Actualization of the self, humane values of community health, actualization of world health, and actualization of the planet environmentally and socially will be highly prized and rewarded. A vocabulary of formerly female values—sensitivity, creativity, intuition, caring, loving, sharing—will be incorporated into the world system of language, approved and cherished most highly. Formerly male values of violence, oppression, aggression, annihilation, armament, weapons, and killing will be withdrawn from the world language. Valuing life will be the only acceptable legacy passed from one generation to the next.

Education and knowledge will be encouraged as an effort of many, sharing and learning from one another, not withheld as sacred or limited by social class. The former concepts of stratification in society will be forgotten in favor of humanhood and interconnectedness of all peoples, as we learn to balance individuality, differentness, uniqueness with the bond of being human and sharing the Earth and its bounties. We will use technology to spread advances and to research for unthought-of possibilities for an enriched life together. Men, women, and children work and play together, not competing for limited resources but sharing equally and being valued equally for their humanness.

Individual physical health and mental health will be prized in all children and adults. And in so valuing and accomplishing these goals for all people, the environment will be cherished as essentially limited and interconnected with our human experience.

Women are a creative and essential part of this view of the future. By speaking out now, valuing ourselves and our connected world view, we can act to work toward the changes necessary. Our minds can change if we are motivated.

Again I would like to note the impressive research and broadening outlook of futurists like Riane Eisler and those acknowledged in her book *The Chalice and the Blade*. Their inspired world view and research can be an impetus for all of us interested in improving human relations, family life, community health, and world peace.

A TRIBUTE TO HER

I understand it better now
the women who stand by their men
supporting, staunchly
tolerating, bravely
carrying on, quietly.

You who don't see any separation
between yourselves and them
their work is for you
your work is for them
both with one goal—success.

A life of devotion, unselfish
as a parent dotes on her child
you dote on your partner in life
enabling his future and his present,
ever mindful of what ails him.

Ever watching for the downfalls
the worries, the troubles he encounters
True there's little time for you
but you truly may not want any
your goal is his success.

You have many feelings
which you never reveal
your interchange is practical and brief
if there is a problem
he tends to look for an answer.

You are somewhat less direct and stoic than he
but have adapted to his style
He's strong, cool, accomplished and
only angers when pushed too far
Next to him, you feel out of control and impulsive.

You bought him his first black bag
or microscope or instrument of healing

He was grateful then but may have gone on
to forget the origin of the gift
You sigh and then quickly recover from reverie.

Looking ever forward to a time, sometime,
your time when you will touch again
as children do in a special way
recalling only the existence of each other
you know him well and hope that he knows you.

There was never a moment's regret
Your job was to make his life complete
to provide solace and comfort
to sing him to sleep, to sing him to sleep
   I see now you have done well
      Your song is for two
         For him and for you —
            Sing on.

APPENDIXES

Appendix I:
How the Medical Wife is Symbolic
of the Health Care Consumer

Medical Wife	Society of Health Care Consumer
Reveres doctor	Doctor is superhuman, powerful (media obsession with medicine)
Poor self-esteem; he knows more	Patient has no power; doctor knows answers
No choices, powerless	Doctor alone can cure; limits health care options; public's anger and rage, illness within society
Caters, caretakes, supports	Deferent, high economic status, take care of him
Must keep him healthy; denies troubles, hers, his, family's	Don't explore and/or solve problems

Medical Wife	Society of Health Care Consumer
Poor communication	One-way communication: doctor to patient
Mysterious, excluded; his workers cover up; patronized	AMA keeps lay people from reviewing procedures, etc.; doctors are condescended to
Her economic survival needs met	Health and economic contribution to society
Economic advantages	Make him highest paid professional; megabucks into medical research
Waiting, accommodating, deferring	Waiting in office, defer to his judgment
Nonassertive, passive	Fear of reprisals, lay public not knowledgeable enough
Represses anger and rage	Powerless to self heal, more needy, patronized; medical personnel act arrogant, insensitive
Pedestalizes husband	God-like, religious, sacred profession; exclusive, above human
Keeps secrets or no referrals; fears economic demise	Fear institutional (medicine) economic collapse and personal incurable illness
Perfectionistic picture to outside world (self, home, and family life)	Illusion of God-Father strength and health care magic; system perfect
Poor level of intimacy; isolated and separated	We know doctors don't touch; distant, cool; improve health with chemicals and technology

Appendix II:
Solutions and Options

Change From	Opt For
Confidentiality and secrecy	Open communication; peer review; shared knowledge
Competition	Cooperation
Denial of problems	Admission; find solutions and treatments
Passive behaviors and communications	Assertiveness; share intimacies, more fun, more choices; equalize power and responsibilities
Dependence	Healthy independence and interrelatedness; less guilt, less anger, less depression and dissatisfaction
Overwork; God-like, magical expectations	Realistic and possible; no longer feeling important
Inflexible roles and expectations	Flexible roles; shared lives

Appendix III: Bibliography

Allard, J. "The Disease of Being a Doctor." *Medical Journal of Australia*. 1974. Vol. 2: 318–322.

Archterberg, J. *Imagery in Healing: Shaminism in Modern Medicine*. New York: Random House, 1985.

Barbach, Lonnie Garfield, PhD. *For Yourself: The Fulfillment of Female Sexuality*. New York: Signet, 1975.

Barrand, John. "Masochism, Masturbation and Matriarchy: The Doctor's Family." *Australian Family Physician*. June 1979, Vol. 8: 663–667.

Bass, Ellen and Laura Davis. *The Courage to Heal: A Guide for Women Survivors of Sexual Abuse*. New York: Harper and Row, 1988.

Bernadez-Bonesatti, Teresa. "Women and Anger: Conflicts with Aggression and Contemporary Women." *Journal of American Medical Women's Association*. 33 (1978) No. 5.

Bissel, LeClair, and Robert W. Jones. "The Alcoholic Physician: A Survey." *American Journal of Psychiatry*. 133 (1976): 1142–1146.

Bolen, Jean Shinoda, MD. *Goddesses in Every Woman*. New York: Harper and Row, 1985.

Bowman, M., and M. L. Gross. "Overview of Research on Women in Medicine: Issues for Public Policy Makers." *Public Health Report*. 101: 513–21 S/O 1986.

Branden, Nathaniel. *The Psychology of Romantic Love*. New York: Bantam Books, 1981.

Brewster, Joan M. "Prevalence of Alcohol and Other Drug Problems Among Physicians." *Journal of the American Medical Association*. April 11, 1986, Vol. 255, No. 14: 1913–1920.

Brook, M. F., J. D. Hailstone, and I. E. J. McLauchlan. "Psychiatric Illness in the Medical Profession." *British Journal of Psychiatry*. 1967. 113: 1013.

Chesler, Phyllis. *Women and Madness*. New York: Doubleday, 1972.

Clements, William M., and Randy Paine. "Family Physician's Family." *Journal of Family Practice*. 1981. Vol. 13(1): 105–152.

Coombs, Robert H., and J. Fawzy. "The Effects of Marital Status on Stress in Medical School." *American Journal of Psychiatry*. Nov. 1982. 139: 1490–1493.

Corea, Gena. *The Hidden Malpractice: How American Medicine Mistreats Women*. New York: Jove Publications, 1979.

Dalrymple-Champneys, Sir Weldon. "Wives of Some Famous Doctors." In *Proceedings of the Royal Society of Medicine*. November 1959. Vol. 52: 937–946.

de Beauvoir, Simone. *The Second Sex*. New York: Alfred A. Knopf, Inc., 1952.

Derdeyn, Andrew, P., MD. "The Physician's Work and Marriage." *International Journal of Psychiatry in Medicine*. 1978–79. Vol 9 (3 & 4): 297–306.

Dowling, Colette. *Cinderella Complex: Woman's Hidden Fear of Independence*. New York and London: Summit Books, 1981.

_____. *Perfect Women*. New York and London: Summit Books, 1988.

Duffy, John. *The Healers: The Rise of the Medical Establishment*. New York: McGraw Hill Book Company, 1976.

Ehrenreich, Barbara, and Deirdre English. *Complaints and Disorders, The Sexual Politics of Sickness*. New York: Feminist Press, 1974.

_____. *For Her Own Good*. New York and London: Doubleday, An Anchor Press Book, 1978.

Eichenbaum, Luise, and Susie Orbach. *Between Women: Love, Envy and Competition in Women's Friendships*. New York: Penguin, 1989.

_____. *Understanding Women: A Feminist Psychoanalytic Approach*. New York: Basic Books, 1983.

Eisler, Riane. *The Chalice and the Blade*. San Francisco: Harper and Row, Perennial Library, 1987.

Epstein, Cynthia Fuchs. *Women's Place: Options and Limits in*

Professional Careers. Berkeley: University of California Press, 1971.

Evans, James L. "Psychiatric Illness in the Physician's Wife." *American Journal of Psychiatry*. 1963. 122: 159–163.

Filene, Peter G. *Him/Her/Self: Sex Roles in America Today*. 2nd Edition. Baltimore/London: Johns Hopkins University Press, 1986.

Fine, Carla. *Married to Medicine*. New York: Athenia, 1981.

Fowlkes, Martha Richmond. *Behind Every Successful Man: Wives of Medical and Academe*. New York: Columbia University Press, 1980.

Franklin, Penelope, editor. *Private Pages, Diaries of American Women 1830s–1970s*.

Freeman, Lucy, and Herbert Strean. *Freud and Women*. New York: Continuum, 1987.

Freud, Sigmund. "Female Sexuality." In *Collected Papers*, Vol. 5. New York: Basic Books, 1959.

————. *On Narcissism: An Introduction*. In Standard Edition, Vol. 14. London: Hogarth Press, 1957.

Friday, Nancy. *My Mother My Self: The Daughter's Search for Identity*. New York: Delacorte Press, 1977.

Friedan, Betty. *The Feminine Mystique*. New York: Dell, 1963.

Gabbard, Glen O., MD, Roy W. Menninger, MD, and Lolafaye Coyne, PhD. "Sources of Conflict in the Medical Marriage." *American Journal of Psychiatry*. May 1987. 144:5: 567–572.

Garvey, Michael, MD, and Vincente Tucson, BMD. "Physician Marriages." *Journal of Clinical Psychology*. March 1979. 40(3): 129–131.

Gerber, Lane A. *Married to their Careers: Career and Family Dilemmas in Doctors' Lives*. New York and London: Tavistock Publications, 1983.

Getz, Kay. Director of Family Component Program of Florida Physicians Recovery Network. Telephone communication. September 1989.

Giele, Janet Zollinger. *Women and the Future: Changing Sex Roles in Modern America*. New York: Free Press, 1978.

Gilligan, Carol. *In a Different Voice: Psychological Theory and*

Women's Development. Cambridge, Massachusetts and London, England: Harvard University Press, 1982.

Glick, Ira D., MD, and Jonathan F. Borus, MD. "Marital and Family Therapy for Troubled Physicians and their Families: A Bridge Over Troubled Waters." *Journal of the American Medical Association*. April 13, 1984. Vol. 251, No. 14: 1855–1858.

Goldberg, Martin. "Conjoint Therapy of Male Physicians and their Wives." *Psychiatric Opinion*. 12 (1975): 19–23.

Goode, W. "Theory of Role Strain." *American Sociological Review*. 25 (1960): 283–299.

Gordon, Benjamin L., MD. *Between Two Worlds*. Bookman Associates, Inc., New York, 1952.

Gornich, Vivian, and B. K. Moran, editors. *Women in Sexist Society*. New York: Basic Books, 1971.

Greenspan, Miriam. *A New Approach to Women and Therapy*. New York: McGraw-Hill Book Co., 1983.

Hall, Alyson. "Medical Marriage: No Bed of Roses." *British Medical Journal*. January 16, 1988. Vol. 296: 152–153.

Hall, R. C., S. K. Stickney, and M. K. Popkin. "Physician Drug Abuser." *Journal of Mental Disorders*. Nov. 1978. Vol. 166, No. 11: 787–793.

Harding, O. G. "The Doctor, His Practice and His Wife." *Medical World News*. 1973 June: 88.

Harrison, Mrs. Julian. "Characteristics of Physicians and their Families: Casefinding Problems and Techniques." *Journal of Florida Medical Association*. May 1978. 65(5): 351–353.

Helfrich, Margaret. *The Social Role of the Executive's Wife*. Columbus, Ohio: Ohio State University Bureau of Business Research, 1965.

Hite, Shere. *The Hite Report on Male Sexuality*. New York: A. Knopf, 1981.

_____. *Women and Love*. New York: St. Martin's Press, 1987.

_____. *The Search for Self*. Vol. 2. Editor Paul H. Ornstein. New York: International University Press, 1970.

Holmstrom, Lynda Lytle. *The Two Career Family*. Cambridge, Massachusetts: Schenkman, 1973.

Howell, Elizabeth, and Marjorie Beyes, editors. *Women and Mental Health*. New York: Basic Books, 1981.

Johnson, R. P., and J. C. Connally. "Addicted Physicians: A Closer Look." *Journal of American Medical Association*. 245 (1981): 253–257.

Jones, Robert E. "A Study of 100 Physician Psychiatric Patients." *American Journal of Psychiatry*. 134 (1977): 1119–1123.

Jung, C. G. *Collected Works of C. G. Jung*. Edited by Sir Herbert Read, Michael Fordham and Gerald Adler; translated by R. F. C. Hall, Executive Editor, William McGuire, Bollingen Series 20, Princeton, N.J.: Princeton University Press.

————. "Archetypes of the Collective Unconscious." In *Collected Works of C. G. Jung*. Vol. 9, Part 1, 1968.

————. "Psychological Types." In *Collected Works of C. G. Jung*. Vol. 6, 1971.

Kessler, David R. "The Gay and Lesbian Physician: Unique Experiences, Opportunities and Needs." *The Physician*. J. P. Callan, editor. Norwalk, Connecticut: Appleton-Century-Crofts, 1983: 329–351.

Kohut, Heinz. *Analysis of the Self*. New York: International University Press, 1977.

Konner, Melvin, MD. *On Becoming a Doctor*. New York: Viking Press, 1987.

Krajeski, James P., MD. *Living with Medicine*, Mary Evelyn C. Smith, Editor. Washington, DC: American Psychiatric Association Auxiliary, 1987.

Krell, Robert, and James E. Miles. "Marital Therapy of Couples in which the Husband Is a Physician." *American Journal of Psychotherapy*. 1976. 30: 267–275.

LaCombe, Michael A. "Never Marry a Doctor." *Journal of the American Medical Association*. September 2, 1988. Vol. 260, No. 9, p. 1292.

Lerner, Harriet Goldhor, PhD. *The Dance of Anger*. New York: Harper and Row, 1986.

Lewis, Norman. *The New Roget's Thesaurus in Dictionary Form*. New York: G. P. Putnam & Sons, 1978.

Lorch, Barbara, and Lou Ellen Crawford. "Marriage to a Physician: The Stresses and Responsibilities." *Col. Med.* March 1983. 330(3): 84–86.

————. "The Physician's Wife: A Case for Caste." *Sociological*

Abstracts. Colorado Springs: University of Colorado. 1978. 18A, Supp. 82.

_____. "Physicians' Wives: An Examination of their Place in the Stratification System." *Social Sciences Journal*. January 1981. Vol. 18, No. 1: 69–80.

_____. "Role Expectations, Performance and Satisfaction: A Comparison of Physicians' and Lawyers' Wives." *International Journal of Sociology of the Family*. Spring 1983. Vol. 13: 117–128.

Luger, Rosalind Massaw. "The Doctor's Wife." *Physicians World*. 1974. 11(4): 21–27.

Maddison, David. "Stress on the Doctor and his Family." *Medical Journal of Australia*. 1974. 2: 315–318.

Martin, Del. *Battered Wives*. New York: Simon and Schuster, 1977.

Maslow, Abraham. *The Farther Reaches of Human Nature*. New York: Penguin Books, 1971.

_____. *Motivation and Personality*. New York: Harper, 1954.

_____. *Toward a Psychology of Being*. New York: Van Nostrand and Reinhold, 1968.

McClinton, James B. "The Doctor's Own Wife (His Fourth Investment)." *The Canadian Medical Association Journal*. November 1942: 472–476.

McPherson, Myra. *The Power Lovers: An Intimate Look at Politicians and their Marriages*. New York: G. P. Putnam and Sons, 1975.

Medical Economics:

"Why Not Consider the Doctor's Wife?" by an Alabama Doctor's Wife. February 1924: 14–15.

"Friend, Help-Mate, Wife," by a Tennessee Doctor's Wife. July 1924: 21, 44.

"Are You Your Husband's Partner . . . Mrs. Doctor's Wife?" by Mrs. Charles F. Heider. February 1925: 17–18.

"If I Were A Doctor's Wife—!" by May Andes. September 1926: 20, 44–46.

"Phinancial Philosophy of a Physician's Wife," by Dolores B. Bingaman. September 1927: 23–24.

"Some Fibs I Tell for My Husband's Sake," by a Physician's Wife. April 1928: 29–31.

"That Isn't the Half of Being a Doctor's Wife!" A few replies to "Some Fibs I Tell for My Husband's Sake" in April *Medical Economics*. July 1928: 29–32.

"Just What Can We Do About the Future?" by a Physician's Wife. October 1928: 47, 57–63.

"Daddy Has a Patient," by a Physician's Wife. January 1929: 12, 71–79.

"Is There A Doctor in the House?" by a Physician's Wife. March 1929: 27, 59–61.

"How To Be A Doctor's Wife," by Lois Marlowe (pseudonym). October 1953: 161–179.

"How To Be A Doctor's Wife," by Lois Marlowe (pseudonym). November 1953: 203–215.

Mendelsohn, Robert S. *Male Practice: How Doctors Manipulate Women*. Chicago: Contemporary Books, 1982.

Miles, James E., Robert Krell, and Tsung-Yi Lin. "The Doctor's Wife: Mental Illness and Marital Patterns." *International Journal of Psychiatry in Medicine*. 1972. Vol. 6(4): 481–487.

Miller, Jean Baker. *Toward a New Psychology of Women*. Boston: Beacon Press, 1976.

Mogul, Kathleen M. "Overview: The Sex of the Therapist." *American Journal of Psychiatry*. January 1982. 139: 1–11.

Morris, William, editor. *The American Heritage Dictionary of the English Language*. Boston; New York: American Heritage Publishing Co., Inc. and Houghton Mifflin Co., 1970.

Myers, Michael F. *Doctors' Marriages: A Look at their Problems and Solutions*. New York and London: Plenum Medical Book Co., 1988.

———. "Treating Troubled Marriages." *American Family Physician*. 29 (January 1984): 221–226.

Myrdal, Alva, and Viola Klein. *Women's Two Roles*. London: Routledge and Kagan Paul, 1968.

Oakley, Ann. *Women's Work: The Housewife Past and Present*. New York: Random House, 1974.

Ochs, Carol. *Behind the Sex of God: Toward a New Conscious-*

ness – *Transcending Matriarchy and Patriarchy*. Boston: Beacon Press, 1977.

Pahl, R. E., and J. M. Pahl. *Managers and their Wives: A Study of Career and Family Relationships in the Middle Class*. London: Allen Lane, The Penguin Press, 1971.

Paul, Jordan, PhD, and Margaret Paul, PhD. *Do I Have to Give up Me to Be Loved by You?* Minneapolis: CompCare Publishers, 1983.

Pearson, M. M. "Psychiatric Treatment of 250 Physicians." *Psychiatric Annals*. 12 (1982): 194–206.

Peters, Ann. "Real Life for the Doctor's Wife." *Today's Health*. June 1964: 24–57.

Phelps, Stanler, MSW, and Nancy Austin, MBA. *The New Assertive Woman*. California: Impact Publishers, 1988.

Prather, L. "Stress and Strain of a Medical Marriage from a Wife's Point of View." *Journal of Florida Medical Association*. Feb. 1977. Vol. 64, No. 2: 103–104.

Robbins, Jhan and June Robbins. "Never Marry a Doctor." *McCalls*. Sept. 1969. 69: 126–127.

Rogers, Natalie. *Emerging Woman: A Decade of Midlife Transitions*. California: Personal Press, 1980.

Rome, Howard P. "The Doctor's Wife." *Psychosomatics*. 1976. 17: 14–20.

Rose, Daniel K., and Irving Rosow. "Marital Stability Among Physicians." *California Medicine*. March 1972. 116: 95–99.

Rothstein, William G. *American Physicians in the Nineteenth Century: From Sects to Science*. Baltimore: The Johns Hopkins University Press, 1972.

Roy, Alec. "Suicide in Doctors." *Psychiatric Clinics of North America*. June 1985. Vol. 8, No. 2: 377–387.

Rubin, Lillian. B. *Women of a Certain Age: The Midlife Search for Self*. New York: Harper and Row, 1979.

Safinofsky, S. "Suicide in Doctors and Wives of Doctors." *Canadian Family Physician*. 1980. 26: 839–844.

Sagan, Eli. *Freud, Women and Morality: The Psychology of Good*. New York: Basic Books, 1988.

Sager, Clifford J. *Marriage Contracts and Couples Therapy*. New York: Brunner/Mazel, 1976.

Sanford, Linda Tschirhart, and Mary Ellen Donovan. *Women and Self Esteem*. New York: Penguin Books, Viking Penguin, Inc., 1984.

Scarf, Maggie. *Unfinished Business*. New York: Doubleday and Co., 1980.

Scarlett, E. P. "Doctor out of Zebulun: The Doctor's Wife." *Archives of Internal Medicine*. March 1965. Vol. 115: 351–357.

Schoicket, Sally, PhD. "The Physician's Marriage." *Journal of the Medical Society of New Jersey*. Feb. 1978. 75 (2): 149–152.

Scheiber, Steven C., and Brian B. Doyle, Editors. *The Impaired Physician*. New York: Plenum Press, 1983.

Scolaro-Moser, Rosemary. Telephone communication. September 1989.

Shahar, Shulamith. *The Fourth Estate, A History of Women in the Middle Ages*.

Sheehy, Gail. *Passages: Predictable Crises in Adult Life*. New York: E. P. Dutton, 1974.

Shortt, S. E. D. "Psychiatric Illness in Physicians." *Canadian Medical Association Journal*. 121 (1979): 283–288.

Simon, Kate, Editor. *Bronx Primitive, Portraits in a Childhood*. New York: Harper and Row, 1983.

Skipper, James K. and Werner A. Gliebe. "Forgotten Persons: Physicians' Wives and their Influence on Medical Career Decisions." *Journal of Medical Education*. Sept. 1977. Vol. 52: 764–766.

Smith, Manuel J., PhD. *When I Say No, I Feel Guilty*. Toronto: Bantam, 1975.

Smith, Mary Evelyn C., Editor. *Living with Medicine*. Washington, DC: American Psychiatric Association Auxiliary, 1987.

Sontag, Susan. *Illness as Metaphor*. New York: Farrar, Straus and Giroux, 1978.

Spada, James. *Grace: The Secret Lives of a Princess*. Garden City, New York: Doubleday, 1987.

Stone, Merlin. *When God Was a Woman*. San Diego, New York, London: A Harvest/HBJ Book, Harcourt Brace Janovich, 1976.

Stone, Michael. "New York Hospital On the Spot." *New York*. June 22, 1987, Vol. 20, p. 40.

Symonds, Alexandria. "Violence Against Women: The Myth of

Masochism." *American Journal of Psychotherapy*. 1979. 33, No. 2, pp. 161–173.

Vaillant, G. E., J. Brighton, and G. McArthur. "Physicians Use of Mood Altering Drugs: A Twenty Year Follow-up Report." *New England Journal of Medicine*. 1970. 282:365.

Vaillant, G. E., N. C. Sobawale, and C. McArthur. "Some Psychological Vulnerabilities of Physicians." *New England Journal of Medicine*. 1972. 287: 372–375.

Viorst, Judith. *Necessary Losses*. New York: Fawcett Gold Medal Ballantine Books, 1986.

Vincent, M. O. "Doctor and Mrs.: Their Mental Health." *Canadian Psychiatric Association Journal*. 1969. 14: 509–515.

_____. "The Doctor's Marriage and Family." *Nova Scotia Medical Bulletin*. Dec. 1971. 50(6): 143–146.

Wallis, Claudia. "A Hospital Stands Accused, But Mystery Still Surrounds Andy Warhol's Death." *Time*. April 27, 1987, Vol. 129, p. 64.

Wallot, H., and J. Lambert. "Characteristics of Physician Addicts." *American Journal of Drug and Alcohol Abuse*. 10(1) (1984): 53-62.

Webster, Thomas G. "Problems of Drug Addiction and Alcoholism Among Physicians." *Impaired Physician*. Eds. Stephen C. Scheiber and Brian B. Doyle. New York: Plenum Press, 1983, pp. 27–38.

Webster's Dictionary of English Usage. Springfield, Massachusetts: Miriam Webster, Inc., 1989.

Wehr, Demaris S. *Jung and Feminism: Liberating the Archetypes*. Massachusetts: Beacon Press, 1987.

West, Gilly. "Poor Little Rich Girl of American Medicine." *Social Problems*, Vol. 31, No. 3, February 1984, pp. 285–295.

Witkin-Lanoil, Georgia. *Female Stress Syndrome: How to Recognize and Live with It*. New York: New Market, 1984.

Wilson, W. P., MD, and D. B. Larson, MD. "The Physician and Spouse: Happiness, Marriage and Family Life." *North Carolina Medical Journal*. March 1981. Vol. 42, No. 3: 176–180.

_____. "The Physician and Spouse: Problems and Some Comments on Solutions." *North Carolina Medical Journal*. April 1981. Vol. 42, No. 4, 274–277.

Index

395